Iron Deficiency Anemia

Iron Deficiency Anemia

Edited by Macey Sharp

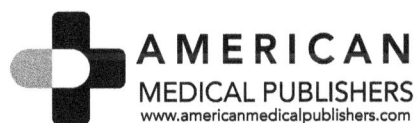

AMERICAN
MEDICAL PUBLISHERS
www.americanmedicalpublishers.com

American Medical Publishers,
41 Flatbush Avenue,
1st Floor, New York,
NY 11217, USA

Visit us on the World Wide Web at:
www.americanmedicalpublishers.com

ISBN: 978-1-63927-183-2

Cataloging-in-Publication Data

Iron deficiency anemia / edited by Macey Sharp.
     p. cm.
Includes bibliographical references and index.
ISBN 978-1-63927-183-2
1. Iron deficiency anemia. 2. Iron deficiency diseases. 3. Iron deficiency anemia--Diagnosis.
4. Iron deficiency anemia--Treatment. I. Sharp, Macey.
RC641.7.I7 I76 2022
616.152--dc23

Table of Contents

Permissions

List of Contributors

Index

Preface

The decrease in the number of red blood cells or the amount of hemoglobin in the blood is known as anemia. The anemia that is caused by lack of iron is referred to as iron deficiency anemia. It shows almost vague symptoms such as fatigue and short breaths, when it occurs slowly. However, if it comes quickly it often shows severe symptoms including confusion and increased thirst. Blood loss, poor absorption of iron from food or insufficient dietary intake, are some of the major causes of iron-deficiency anemia. Symptoms may include chest pain, restless leg syndrome, palpitations, irritability, poor appetite, etc. It can be prevented by taking iron supplements or by eating a proper diet containing adequate amounts of iron such as nuts, meat and spinach. This book provides comprehensive insights into the field of iron deficiency anemia. It presents researches and studies performed by experts across the globe. It will serve as a reference to a broad spectrum of readers.

This book is the end result of constructive efforts and intensive research done by experts in this field. The aim of this book is to enlighten the readers with recent information in this area of research. The information provided in this profound book would serve as a valuable reference to students and researchers in this field.

At the end, I would like to thank all the authors for devoting their precious time and providing their valuable contribution to this book. I would also like to express my gratitude to my fellow colleagues who encouraged me throughout the process.

Editor

Direct Comparison of the Safety and Efficacy of Ferric Carboxymaltose versus Iron Dextran in Patients with Iron Deficiency Anemia

Iftikhar Hussain,[1] Jessica Bhoyroo,[1] Angelia Butcher,[2]
Todd A. Koch,[2] Andy He,[2] and David B. Bregman[2,3]

[1] Vital Prospects Clinical Research Institute, PC, Tulsa, OK 74136, USA
[2] Luitpold Pharmaceuticals, Inc., Norristown, PA 19403, USA
[3] Department of Pathology, Albert Einstein College of Medicine, Bronx, NY 10461, USA

Correspondence should be addressed to Iftikhar Hussain; iftikhar.hussain@aaicenter.net

Academic Editor: Aurelio Maggio

Several intravenous iron complexes are available for the treatment of iron deficiency anemia (IDA). Iron dextran (DEX) is associated with an elevated risk of potentially serious anaphylactic reactions, whereas others must be administered in several small infusions to avoid labile iron reactions. Ferric carboxymaltose (FCM) is a nondextran intravenous iron which can be administered in high single doses. A randomized, open label, and multicenter comparison of FCM to DEX in adults with IDA and baseline hemoglobin of ≤ 11.0 g/dL was conducted. A total of 160 patients were in the safety population (FCM $n = 82$; DEX $n = 78$). Adverse events, including immune system disorders (0% in FCM versus 10.3% in DEX, $P = 0.003$) and skin disorders (7.3% in FCM versus 24.4% in DEX, $P = 0.004$), were less frequently observed in the FCM group. A greater portion of patients in the FCM group experienced a transient, asymptomatic decrease in phosphate compared to patients in the DEX group (8.5% in FCM versus 0% in DEX, $P = 0.014$). In the FCM arm, the change in hemoglobin from baseline to the highest observed level was 2.8 g/dL, whereas the DEX arm displayed a change of 2.4 g/dL ($P = 0.20$). Treatment of IDA with FCM resulted in fewer hypersensitivity-related reactions than DEX.

1. Introduction

Iron deficiency is one of the most common deficiencies in the world and can lead to anemia [1–3]. Patients with reduced absorption of dietary iron (e.g., patients with inflammatory bowel disease, gastrointestinal surgery, or who have had gastric bypass) or patients with increased utilization or loss of iron from the body (e.g., pregnancy/childbirth, heavy uterine bleeding, lactation, hemodialysis, or surgery) are particularly at risk [1, 4–6]. IDA may adversely affect cognitive function, physical activity, immune response, inflammatory conditions, and pregnancy outcomes [7]. Different kinds of therapies from oral iron to blood transfusion are currently used to treat IDA. The aim of the treatment is to return both hemoglobin and iron stores to normal levels. Oral iron therapy is the treatment of choice for the majority of patients

with IDA because of its effectiveness, safety, and low cost. Even though many patients can tolerate oral iron without difficulty, up to 40% may have side effects attributable to oral iron replacement therapy [8]. The incidence of side effects increase with the dose and adversely affects compliance. Also, oral iron is often not capable of replenishing severe iron deficits [9]. As a treatment of last resort, blood transfusions are used, but they may lead to the transmission of known and unknown pathogens, immunological impact, and transfusion reactions.

Intravenous (IV) administration of iron is preferred in patients who are unable to absorb sufficient iron from the gastrointestinal tract or those who do not tolerate oral iron, in patients in whom blood transfusions need to be avoided for medical or religious reasons, and in patients with chronic iron loss exceeding the rate of replacement possible with oral treatment. First generation intravenous iron formulations, namely, iron dextran (DEX), have been used as an alternative to oral iron in the treatment of IDA of multiple etiologies although it is known to cause severe immunological responses, including fatal anaphylactic reactions [3, 4, 10]. Second generation, nondextran IV irons, such as iron sucrose and sodium ferric gluconate, do not contain dextran, or modified dextran, but they have significant dosage and administration rate limitations. They are characterized by a risk of adverse reactions called labile iron reactions at higher doses which may include hypotension, cramping, diarrhea, or chest pain [11]. Feraheme (ferumoxytol) is a recently approved IV iron administered as two injections of 510 mg [2]. Although Feraheme was designed with a modified dextran shell to reduce immunogenic potential, anaphylaxis in individuals with previous hypersensitivity to iron dextran has been reported [12]. Ferric carboxymaltose (FCM), a novel IV iron, is a stable Type I polynuclear iron (III) hydroxide carbohydrate complex [1] that has been approved in Europe for the treatment of iron deficiency since 2007. After IV administration, FCM is mainly found in the reticuloendothelial system of the liver, the spleen, and bone marrow [1, 13]. The iron slowly dissociates from the complex and can be efficiently used in the bone marrow for hemoglobin synthesis. FCM offers significant advantages compared to earlier generation IV iron preparations. Due to its structure, FCM is more stable than sodium ferric gluconate and iron sucrose. It is therefore possible to administer much higher single doses over shorter periods of time than sodium ferric gluconate or iron sucrose, resulting in the need for fewer administrations to replete iron stores [1, 4, 5, 13–15]. In addition, it is not a dextran or modified dextran so the risk of hypersensitivity reactions is reduced. In multiple studies, FCM has been shown to be an effective option in the treatment of IDA, and it also improves the quality of life of patients [1, 4, 5].

The aim of this study was to conduct a head-to-head comparison of the safety of an investigational IV iron regimen (FCM) versus IV iron dextran in the treatment of IDA when oral iron was not tolerated or the response was poor.

2. Materials and Methods

This was a Phase 3b, 7-week, multicenter, open label, randomized (1:1) study that evaluated the safety and efficacy of FCM versus DEX. It took place between July 2008 and July 2009 and involved 27 sites within the United States. The protocol was approved by the Institutional Review Board for each site, and the trial was performed in accordance with the Declaration of Helsinki. Informed content was acquired from each patient prior to inclusion of the study. A flowchart of the study is depicted in Figure 1. Clinical trials registration information: ClinicalTrials.gov number, NCT00704028.

The study treatment involved a single maximum dose (15 mg/kg body weight up to 750 mg) administered weekly until the total iron requirement (calculated by the Ganzoni formula) [16] or a maximum of 2,250 mg was reached. Patients were 18 years old and older with IDA and had

a history of intolerance to oral iron or an unsatisfactory response to oral iron. The screening visit hemoglobin had to be ≤11.0 g/dL, and the screening ferritin level had to be ≤100 ng/mL or ≤300 ng/mL when transferrin saturation (TSAT) was ≤30%.

Patients were excluded if they had a history of a hypersensitivity reaction to any component of FCM or DEX, required dialysis for treatment of CKD, had anemia not due to iron deficiency, were previously treated with IV iron, had red blood cell transfusion(s) or antibiotics during the 10 days prior to screening, were treated with erythropoiesis stimulating agents in a regimen exceeding product labeled dosing during the 30 days prior to screening (or during the study), were receiving treatment with radiotherapy and/or chemotherapy, or required a surgical procedure that necessitated general anesthesia. Additional exclusion criteria included infection other than viral upper respiratory tract infection, aspartate aminotransferase (AST) or alanine aminotransferase (ALT) >1.5 times the upper limit of normal, active hepatitis, human immunodeficiency virus positive, being treated for asthma, recent alcohol abuse, history of hemochromatosis or other iron storage disorders, systolic blood pressure ≥180 or <80 mmHg or diastolic blood pressure ≥100 or <40 mmHg at screening or Day 0, significant cardiovascular disease, breastfeeding, and sexually active females not willing to use an acceptable form of contraception.

After confirmation of eligibility, study site personnel randomly allocated participants using an integrated voice response system. Treatment assignments to study drugs were randomly generated in blocks of 4. Patients were stratified by baseline hemoglobin (≤8, 8.1–9.5, ≥9.6), baseline cardiovascular risk (Category 1–4), and use of immunosuppressive therapy. Cardiovascular risk was defined by using variables from the Framingham model [17]. Risk score was defined as Category 1 if there was no known risk factor, Category 2 if the subject had one of the following: age > 75, current smoker, hypertension or on antihypertensive medications, hyperlipidemia or use of a lipid lowering medicine, use of low dose aspirin, Category 3 if they had one of the following: diabetes or ≥2 of the risk factors used to define Category 2, and Category 4 if they had prior history of cardiovascular disease.

Patients who were randomized to FCM (Luitpold Pharmaceuticals, Inc.) received their study drug on Days 0, 7, and 14. Both of the doses of these two study drugs were calculated by the Ganzoni formula. The IV iron dose was calculated by the following algorithm: weight in kg × (15-current hemoglobin g/dL) × 2.4 + 500 = total iron requirement in milligrams (mg). The maximum total was not to exceed 2,250 mg. If the subject was postpartum, the prepregnancy weight was used. If TSAT >20% and ferritin >50 ng/mL, 500 mg was subtracted. Patients received up to 750 mg of iron as undiluted FCM (15 mg/kg up to a maximum of 750 mg) at 100 mg per minute via IV push injection weekly until the calculated iron deficit dose had been administered.

Patients who were randomized to DEX received their study drug between Days 0 and 42. On Day 0, a test dose of 25 mg of DEX was administered slowly over 5 minutes, and the subject was observed for 15 minutes to 1 hour, and

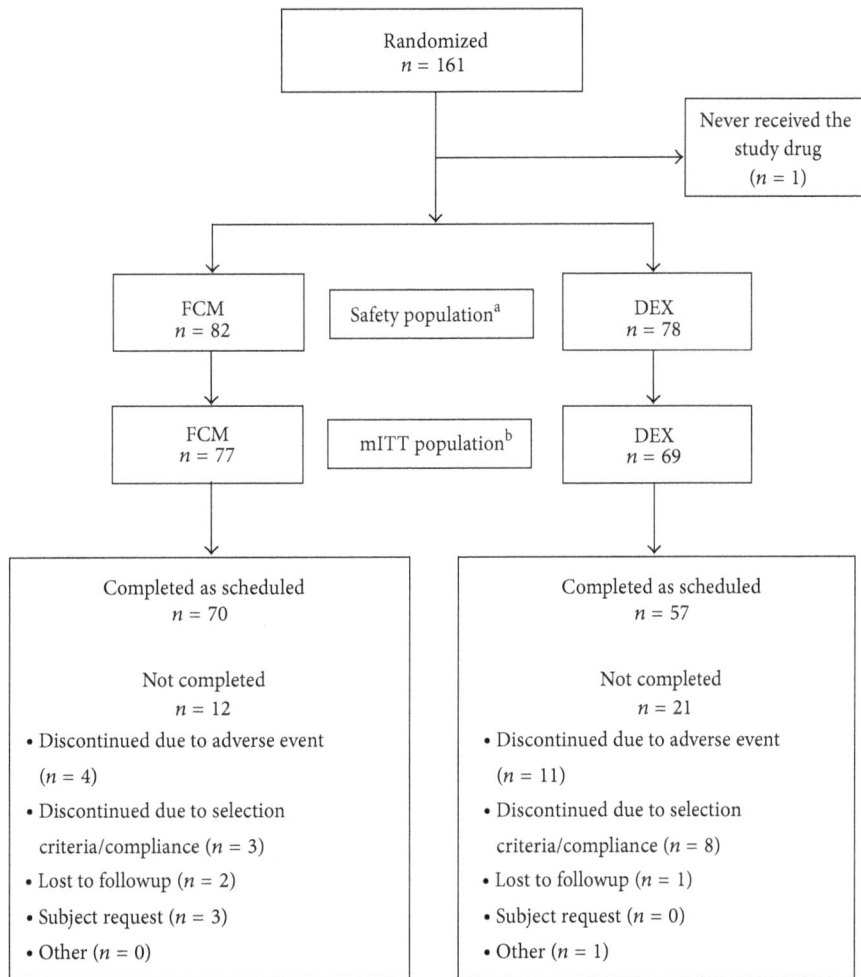

FIGURE 1: Flowchart of the study. [a]All subjects treated with FCM or DEX were included in the safety population. [b]mITT: all subjects in the safety population with 2 baseline hemoglobin values (with <1 g/dL difference between the 2 values) and at least 1 postbaseline hemoglobin value on or before Day 49 or intervention date, whichever came first.

if no reaction occurred, the remainder of the Day 0 dose was given. The total DEX dose was determined by calculating the total iron requirement and dividing this total amount into one or more single dose(s). They received DEX at doses and infusion times as determined by the investigator until the calculated iron deficit dose was administered (to a maximum cumulative dose of 2,250 mg). Investigators were allowed to administer either Dexferrum (American Regent, Inc.) or INFeD (Watson Pharma, Inc.). The dose and rate of administration of the DEX was up to the discretion of the investigator as this would mimic practice in the clinical setting.

The primary endpoint was the incidence of treatment-emergent serious adverse events (AEs) from Day 0 to Day 42, or 28 days after the last dose of study drug. Secondary endpoints included incidence of treatment-emergent AEs, incidence of treatment-emergent abnormal clinical laboratory values, and incidence of potentially clinically significant vital sign values. Assessments for safety were performed on Days 0, 7, 14, 28, and 42. Measurements of safety included AEs, physical examination, vital signs, and clinical laboratory

evaluations. Adverse events were collected from the time of the initial treatment of FCM or DEX on Day 0 to the end of the study (Day 42), or 28 days after the last dose of study drug, whichever was longer. Electrocardiogram (ECG) assessments were performed at screening, Days 0 and 42. A follow-up phone call to collect AEs may have been required for patients that discontinued early.

Adverse events were classified using the Medical Dictionary for Regulatory Activities Terminology. For the purpose of this study, allergic reactions (hypersensitivity) were classified by grade according to the National Cancer Institute (NCI) Common Terminology Criteria for Adverse Events (CTCAE), Version 3.0 [18]. The investigator classified the severity of all AEs as Grades 1 to 5 by CTCAE criteria if they existed or as Grade 1 if considered mild, Grade 2 if moderate, Grade 3 if severe, Grade 4 if life-threatening, and Grade 5 if the AE resulted in death. An AE was classified as serious if it met any one of the following: death, life-threatening, hospitalization, disability, congenital anomaly/birth defect, or important medical events. In addition, the investigator documented his/her opinion of the relationship of the event

TABLE 1: Baseline demographics and characteristics.

Demographic characteristic	FCM ($N = 82$)	DEX ($N = 78$)	P value
Age (years)			
Mean (SD)	46.2 (14.64)	48.2 (17.10)	
Minimum, maximum	20, 86	18, 84	
≤65	72 (87.8%)	63 (80.8%)	$P = 0.422$
66–75	5 (6.1%)	9 (11.5%)	
76–85	5 (6.1%)	6 (7.7%)	
Gender			
Female	73 (89.0%)	69 (88.5%)	$P = 1.00$
Male	9 (11.0%)	9 (11.5%)	
Race			
African American	27 (32.9%)	21 (26.9%)	
Asian	4 (4.9%)	3 (3.8%)	
Caucasian	41 (50.0%)	42 (53.8%)	$P = 0.639$
Hispanic	7 (8.5%)	11 (14.1%)	
Other	3 (3.7%)	1 (1.3%)	
Iron intolerance			
No	37 (45.1%)	33 (42.3%)	$P = 0.752$
Yes	45 (54.9%)	45 (57.7%)	
Weight (kg)			
Mean (SD)	79.89 (22.960)	82.18 (20.681)	$P = 0.509$
Height (cm)			
Mean (SD)	163.65 (7.965)	163.80 (8.245)	$P = 0.903$
Drug allergy			
No	44 (53.7%)	45 (57.7%)	$P = 0.636$
Yes	38 (46.3%)	33 (42.3%)	
Baseline hemoglobin (g/dL)			
Mean (SD)	9.63 (1.190)	9.49 (1.260)	$P = 0.472$
Hemoglobin category			
≤8.0 g/dL	9 (11.0%)	9 (11.5%)	
8.1–9.5 g/dL	23 (28.0%)	20 (25.6%)	$P = 0.857$
≥9.6 g/dL	50 (61.0%)	49 (62.8%)	
Use of immunosuppressive therapy			
No	79 (96.3%)	77 (98.7%)	$P = 0.621$
Yes	3 (3.7%)	1 (1.3%)	
Cardiovascular risk			
1	41 (50.0%)	40 (51.3%)	
2	19 (23.2%)	19 (24.4%)	$P = 0.809$
3	12 (14.6%)	10 (12.8%)	
4	10 (12.2%)	9 (11.5%)	
Baseline TSAT (%)			
Mean (SD)	10.05 (10.010)	10.95 (11.257)	$P = 0.596$
<20	72 (87.8%)	63 (80.8%)	
Baseline ferritin (ng/mL)			
Mean (SD)	12.89 (21.848)	23.12 (44.828)	$P = 0.067$
<100	80 (97.6%)	71 (91.0%)	
Past response to iron therapy			
Poor/no	17 (20.7%)	18 (23.1%)	$P = 0.849$
Poor/yes	65 (79.3%)	60 (76.9%)	

TABLE 1: Continued.

Demographic characteristic	FCM ($N = 82$)	DEX ($N = 78$)	P value
Etiology of IDA			
Heavy uterine bleeding	32 (39.0%)	27 (34.6%)	
Chronic kidney disease	4 (4.9%)	2 (2.6%)	
IBD/Gastrointestinal related	31 (37.8%)	30 (38.5%)	$P = 0.659$
Other	4 (4.9%)	9 (11.5%)	
Postpartum	2 (2.4%)	1 (1.3%)	
Unknown	9 (11.0%)	9 (11.5%)	

IBD: inflammatory bowel disease; IDA: iron deficiency anemia; SD: standard deviation.

TABLE 2: Treatment-emergent adverse events experienced by ≥5% of patients in either FCM or DEX group.

MedDRA SOC[a] Preferred term	FCM ($N = 82$) n (%)	DEX ($N = 78$) n (%)	P value[b]
At Least 1 treatment-emergent adverse event	60 (73.2%)	59 (75.6%)	0.856
Gastrointestinal disorders	24 (29.3%)	14 (17.9%)	0.099
Diarrhea	5 (6.1%)	3 (3.8%)	0.720
Nausea	12 (14.6%)	8 (10.3%)	0.477
Vomiting	5 (6.1%)	4 (5.1%)	1.000
Immune system disorders	0	8 (10.3%)	0.003[†]
Hypersensitivity	0	7 (9.0%)	0.006[†]
Metabolism and nutrition disorders	8 (9.8%)	4 (5.1%)	0.371
Hypophosphatemia	7 (8.5%)	0	0.014[*]
Nervous system disorders	16 (19.5%)	17 (21.8%)	0.845
Dizziness	6 (7.3%)	4 (5.1%)	0.747
Headache	6 (7.3%)	10 (12.8%)	0.297
Skin and subcutaneous tissue disorders	6 (7.3%)	19 (24.4%)	0.004[†]
Pruritus	2 (2.4%)	6 (7.7%)	0.160
Rash	2 (2.4%)	5 (6.4%)	0.268
Urticaria	0	7 (9.0%)	0.006[†]

MedDRA: medical dictionary for regulatory activities; SOC: system organ class.
[a]Each subject is counted only once per SOC when multiple preferred terms are reported for the SOC.
[b]From Fisher's exact test.
[*]Statistically significant at the $P = 0.05$ level.
[†]Statistically significant at the $P = 0.01$ level.

to the study drug either as none, unlikely, possible, or probably. Adverse events that followed the treatment with study drug were classified as treatment-emergent AE.

In order to assess the development of clinically significant signs and symptoms, the patients were evaluated prior to drug administration. Sitting heart rate and blood pressure were assessed before, immediately after, and 30 minutes after administration. Patients were monitored for serious acute reactions as hypersensitivity or labile iron reactions to IV iron products which have rarely been reported.

Efficacy measures included change in hemoglobin, ferritin, and TSAT from baseline to the highest value observed for all patients in the Modified Intent-to-Treat (mITT) population. Hematology and iron indices were measured at screening, baseline, Days 0, 7, 14, 28, and 42.

2.1. Statistical Analysis. No formal sample size calculation was performed for this trial, the primary objective of which was to assess the safety of FCM. However, the statistical precision of the endpoints (as measured by confidence interval width) was adequate with the planned sample size. Approximately 100 patients (up to 200) were expected to be randomized. Enrollment was ceased when 160 patients were randomized because subsequent to discussions with the FDA, two other efficacy and safety trials were initiated that fulfilled the same programmatic goals as this trial (ClinicalTrials.gov nos. NCT00981045 and NCT00982007). These trials did not compare FCM to iron dextran.

All patients were included in the safety population, which was defined as patients who received a dose of randomized FCM or DEX. All safety analyses were performed using

TABLE 3: Subjects who experienced serious adverse events.

Subject	Age/sex	Event	Severity	Causality
		FCM		
1	63/M	Syncope	Grade 4	None
		Asthenia	Grade 4	None
2	54/F	Abdominal pain	Grade 2	None
3	76/M	Crohn's disease	Grade 3	Unlikely
		Death	Grade 5	Unlikely
4	83/F	Syncope	Grade 3	None
5	53/M	Colon cancer recurrent	Grade 4	None
		DEX		
1	32/F	Hypersensitivity	Grade 4	Probable
		Atrial fibrillation	Grade 2	Probable
2	56/F	Vascular pseudoaneurysm	Grade 3	None
3	64/F	Anaphylactic reaction	Grade 4	Probable

TABLE 4: Patients who experienced adverse events that led to premature discontinuation from the study.

Subject	Age/sex	Event	Severity	Causality
		FCM		
1	28/F	Injection site reaction	Grade 2	Probable
2	56/M	Systemic inflammatory response syndrome	Grade 3	Probable
3	76/M	Death	Grade 5	Unlikely
4	53/M	Colon cancer recurrent	Grade 4	None
		DEX		
1	81/M	Dyspnea	Grade 4	Probable
2	19/F	Abdominal pain	Grade 1	Probable
3	29/F	Hypersensitivity	Grade 2	Probable
4	21/F	Hypersensitivity	Grade 2	Probable
5	57/F	Hypersensitivity	Grade 2	Probable
6	45/M	Hypersensitivity	Grade 3	Probable
7	37/F	Peripheral edema	Grade 3	Probable
8	32/F	Hypersensitivity	Grade 4	Probable
9	18/F	Dyspnea	Grade 1	Probable
10	64/F	Anaphylactic reaction	Grade 4	Probable
11	20/F	Hypersensitivity	Grade 3	Probable

the safety population. The mITT population was defined as patients from the safety population who had two baseline hemoglobin values and at least 1 postbaseline hemoglobin value on or before the Day 42 visit (no later than Day 49) or date of first intervention, whichever was earlier.

All statistical tests were two tailed and performed with a 0.05 Type I error. Data comparisons were performed using the one-way analysis of variance (ANOVA) and Fisher's exact test. The use of mean standard deviations (SD) was preferred as the use of the standard error mean. Some results were reported in percentages, and some data are mean +/− (SD). P values < 0.05 were considered statistically significant.

3. Results

A total of 160 patients were randomized to the FCM or DEX group. No statistically significant differences were observed between the FCM and DEX groups in the safety population for any of the demographic characteristics (Table 1). Most of the patients were females with a primary etiology of heavy uterine bleeding, inflammatory bowel disease, or other gastrointestinal pathologies. The majority of patients had a cardiovascular risk of 1 or 2 and had a poor response to iron therapy. Similar baseline values of mean hemoglobin and TSAT were observed between both FCM and DEX groups. A higher mean ferritin value at baseline was observed for patients in the DEX group compared to the FCM group; however, this difference did not reach statistical significance ($P = 0.067$) and was not of a magnitude considered to be clinically significant. In the safety population for subjects receiving FCM, the mean (±SD) total dose received during the study was 1450.9 (±372.02) mg and 1342.5 (±603.06) mg for patients receiving DEX. Of the patients that received FCM, 58.5% received 1-2 IV push injections and patients that received DEX, 57.7% received 1-2 infusions. In the DEX group, 32.1% of the patients received one infusion. Of the patients who were randomized to receive DEX, 73 patients received Dexferrum and 5 patients received INFeD. The mean single dose in the FCM group was 628.6 mg and in the DEX group was 649.5 mg.

The most commonly (≥10.0%) experienced treatment-emergent AEs in the DEX group were headache and nausea; the only treatment-emergent AE experienced by ≥10.0% of patients in the FCM group was nausea (Table 2). The majority of the treatment-emergent AEs experienced during the study were classified by the investigators as severity Grades 1 or 2. Compared to the FCM group, a statistically significantly greater proportion ($P < 0.01$) of patients in the DEX group experienced AEs associated with immune system disorders (i.e., hypersensitivity) or skin and subcutaneous tissue disorders (i.e., urticaria). Adverse events related to the immune system were classified by the investigators as severity of Grades 2, 3, or 4 and AEs related to skin and subcutaneous tissue disorders classified as severity of Grades 1 or 2.

In regard of serious AEs, 5 patients (6.1%) in the FCM group and 3 patients (3.8%) in the DEX group experienced at least 1 serious adverse event. Of the 5 subjects that experienced a serious AE in the FCM group, the causality was none in 4 subjects and unlikely in one subject. On the other hand, the causality of serious AEs in the DEX group were probable in 2 patients and none in 1 patient. A summary of subjects who experienced serious AEs is listed in Table 3.

One death occurred in the FCM group during the study which the investigator considered to be unrelated to study drug. The patient was a 76-year-old man with a history of coronary artery disease, myocardial infarction, hypertension, and Crohn's disease with small bowel resection who received

TABLE 5: Changes in laboratory values.

Chemistry parameter (units)	N	FCM Baseline mean (SD)	FCM Change to final value (SD)	N	DEX Baseline mean (SD)	DEX Change to final value (SD)	P value[a]
ALT (SGPT) (U/L)	82	16.0 (7.09)	5.6 (9.80)	76	17.2 (12.72)	2.1 (12.77)	0.052
AST (SGOT) (U/L)	82	20.0 (7.94)	3.1 (11.41)	76	21.0 (10.04)	−0.4 (10.93)	0.051
Albumin (g/dL)	82	3.83 (0.499)	0.14 (0.313)	76	3.77 (0.446)	0.13 (0.373)	0.930
Alkaline phosphatase (U/L)	82	76.2 (36.29)	11.3 (24.40)	76	81.7 (34.46)	3.6 (16.88)	0.023
C-reactive protein (mg/dL)	82	0.7356 (1.38596)	−0.1090 (1.19793)	76	0.6104 (1.02749)	0.1315 (0.52244)	0.109
Calcium (mg/dL)	82	9.44 (0.543)	0.06 (0.412)	76	9.49 (0.469)	0.15 (0.542)	0.233
Creatinine (mg/L)	82	0.88 (0.738)	−0.04 (0.324)	76	0.80 (0.203)	−0.02 (0.095)	0.531
GGT (U/L)	82	23.1 (24.21)	8.3 (25.50)	76	24.4 (26.24)	6.5 (13.20)	0.573
LDH (U/L)	82	168.0 (39.75)	−1.9 (29.17)	76	171.4 (34.45)	−3.8 (25.35)	0.661
Magnesium (mg/dL)	82	2.06 (0.198)	0.00 (0.187)	76	2.08 (0.218)	−0.04 (0.180)	0.227
Phosphorus (mg/dL)	82	3.71 (0.712)	−0.78 (0.770)	76	3.62 (0.502)	0.22 (0.580)	≤0.001
Bicarbonate (mEq/L)	82	21.37 (3.073)	−0.19 (4.064)	76	21.35 (3.282)	−0.02 (2.845)	0.770
Chloride (mEq/L)	82	104.8 (4.31)	0.2 (3.63)	76	105.4 (3.57)	−0.4 (3.35)	0.281
Glucose (mg/dL)	82	115.7 (60.83)	−6.7 (43.09)	76	111.4 (55.87)	−6.6 (35.87)	0.976
Potassium (mEq/L)	82	4.20 (0.473)	−0.03 (0.412)	76	4.27 (0.408)	−0.05 (0.495)	0.789
Sodium (mEq/L)	82	141.5 (3.71)	−0.1 (3.85)	76	141.3 (3.34)	0.8 (3.68)	0.141
Total bilirubin (mg/dL)	82	0.33 (0.143)	0.03 (0.142)	76	0.34 (0.222)	0.01 (0.125)	0.486
Urea nitrogen (mg/dL)	82	16.5 (20.88)	−0.8 (12.48)	76	14.6 (6.03)	0.1 (4.20)	0.546

[a]P value for difference between change for FCM versus DEX using a 1-way ANOVA.

a single dose of 750 mg of FCM. The cause of death, which occurred 28 days after the dose of FCM, was stated to be "possible myocardial infarction."

The majority of the AEs in patients who were prematurely discontinued were considered possibly or probably related to study drug. Six patients (7.3%) in the FCM group and 11 patients (14.1%) in the DEX group were discontinued from the study drug due to the occurrence of drug related AEs. Four patients (4.9%) in the FCM group and 11 (14.1%) patients in the DEX group were discontinued from the study due to occurrence of AEs (Table 4). The majority of the AEs leading to discontinuation from study for patients in the DEX group were due to hypersensitivity reactions. For the FCM group, causality ranged from none to probable, and the AEs varied.

One of the notable differences in clinical chemistry values reported between the groups was for the proportion of patients with significant phosphorus values below 2.0 mg/dL. Compared to the DEX group, a statistically significantly greater proportion of subjects in the FCM group experienced a transient decrease in serum phosphate (8.5% versus 0%, $P < 0.05$). A statistically significantly greater mean decrease from baseline to final value ($P \leq 0.001$) was observed in the FCM group (Table 5). Figure 2 illustrates the phosphorus change from Day 0 to Day 42. The mean value reached its nadir (2.05 mg/dL) at Day 14 and was within the normal range (2.5–4.5 mg/dL) by Day 42.

Statistically significantly greater mean increases from baseline to final value were observed in the FCM group compared to the DEX group for alkaline phosphatase ($P =$

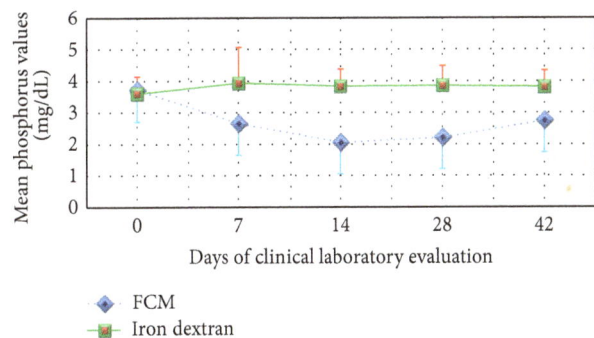

FIGURE 2: Mean phosphorus values for FCM and DEX patients.

0.023). Mean ALT and AST increased form baseline to final value ($P = 0.052$ and $P = 0.051$, resp.) in the FCM group but remained within their respective normal ranges. Thus, these increases were not considered clinically significant (Table 5).

Regarding measures of efficacy, there were no statistically significant differences in mean hemoglobin increase between FCM and DEX. The change in hemoglobin from baseline to the highest value was 2.8 g/dL in the FCM arm and 2.4 g/dL in the DEX arm ($P = 0.200$). Within each group, there were statistically significant increases in hemoglobin for both FCM and DEX from baseline to the highest value observed ($P = 0.001$). Change in hemoglobin is displayed in Figure 3. Mean changes in ferritin from baseline to the highest value observed was higher in the FCM group than in the DEX group (543.2 ng/mL versus 319.7, $P = 0.001$, resp.). In regards

TABLE 6: Changes in hemoglobin, ferritin, and TSAT values.

	FCM ($N = 77$)	DEX ($N = 69$)
Hemoglobin (g/dL)		
Baseline		
Mean (SD)	9.6 (1.18)	9.4 (1.31)
Median	9.9	9.8
Highest value		
Mean (SD)	12.4 (1.26)	11.9 (1.47)
Median	12.5	11.8
Change to highest value		
Mean (SD)	2.8 (1.44)	2.4 (1.71)
Median	2.7	2.7
P value (within group)[a]	0.001[†]	0.001
P value (versus FCM)[b]		0.200
Ferritin (ng/mL)		
Baseline		
Mean (SD)	11.6 (19.29)	21.2 (44.62)
Median	6.2	5.9
Highest value		
Mean (SD)	554.7 (287.84)	340.8 (245.46)
Median	503.5	278.8
Change to highest value		
Mean (SD)	543.2 (280.06)	319.7 (239.96)
Median	491.9	268.9
P value (within group)[a]	0.001[†]	0.001[†]
P value (versus FCM)[b]		0.001[†]
TSAT (%)		
Baseline		
Mean (SD)	10.2 (10.27)	9.6 (8.89)
Median	7.0	5.5
Highest value		
Mean (SD)	39.8 (15.45)	47.7 (20.73)
Median	39.0	48.0
Change to highest value		
Mean (SD)	29.6 (18.02)	38.1 (22.06)
Median	28.0	39.5
P value (within group)[a]	0.001[†]	0.001[†]
P value (versus FCM)[b]		0.012[*]

SD: standard deviation.
[a] P value from the paired t-test for the within group change from baseline.
[b] P value from 1-way ANOVA.
[*] Statistically significant at $P = 0.05$.
[†] Statistically significant at $P = 0.001$.

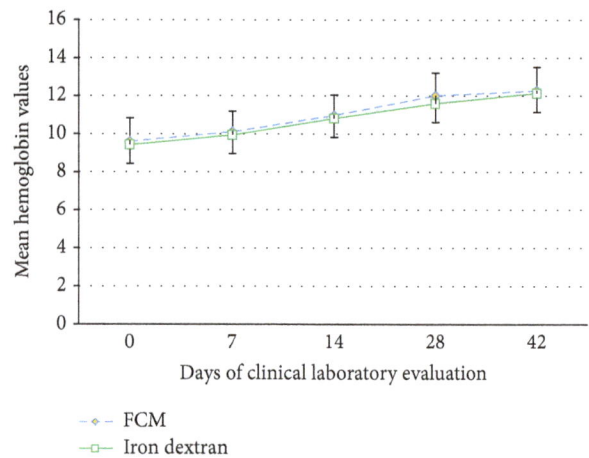

FIGURE 3: Mean hemoglobin values for FCM and DEX patients.

bleeding, inflammatory bowel disease, or other gastrointestinal pathologies. This trial confirmed the safety profile of FCM in comparison to another frequently administered IV iron, iron dextran.

Although the trial had a sample size of only 160 patients, several adverse events related to immune system disorders and skin disorders were observed more frequently in the DEX group than the FCM group. Two subjects in the DEX group reported serious AEs that were considered to be study-drug related as opposed to none in the FCM group. Moreover, about twice as many subjects in the DEX group were prematurely discontinued from study drug due to the occurrence of an AE (11 versus 4). The majority of AEs resulting in premature discontinuation from study drug were considered possibly or probably related to study drug. Many in the DEX group were related to allergy/immune response.

Many studies have shown that FCM has a relatively modest incidence of adverse effects [4, 4, 19]. The most commonly observed AEs were nausea, headache, abdominal pain, diarrhea, and rash [1, 13]. Serious AEs observed were considered to be unrelated to the administration of FCM [5, 13]. Iron dextran is currently the only IV iron approved in the US for use in ID patients (i.e., other than chronic kidney disease). It can lead to potentially dangerous clinical scenarios because of the possibility of inducing a severe immunological response. The risk of anaphylaxis/anaphylactoid reactions caused by DEX has been reported previously [10, 20]. The iron dextran utilized in this trial was mainly high-molecular weight iron dextran (Dexferrum). The difference between the high molecular weight and low molecular weight iron dextran formulations is due to the size of the iron cores, not the dextran shell, the suspected component responsible for iron dextran-related anaphylactic reactions [21]. The amounts of carbohydrate shell are approximately equal in the two iron dextrans [22, 23]. Studies have found that high molecular weight iron dextran compared with low molecular weight iron dextran had higher frequencies of anaphylactic-type reactions [24, 25], while another study found similar or higher frequencies with low molecular weight iron dextran [26]. The current study indicates a favorable safety profile

to mean change in TSAT, a greater difference from baseline to highest value was observed in the DEX group than the FCM group (38.1% versus 29.6%, $P = 0.012$, resp.). A detailed summary is shown in Table 6.

4. Discussion

The primary objective of this trial was to compare the safety of FCM to DEX in patients with IDA. Most of the patients were females whose principal cause of anemia was heavy uterine

for FCM as compared to that of high molecular weight iron dextran due to the small number of subjects that received low molecular weight iron dextran.

Compared to the DEX group, the proportion of patients experiencing a transient decrease in serum phosphate was higher in the FCM group. The mean value of phosphorus decreased from Day 0 to Day 14 in patients in the FCM group but increased after Day 14 to Day 42. The mean value at Day 42 (2.75 mg/dL) is within the normal range for the central laboratory used in this trial (2.2–5.1 mg/dL). None of the patients with reduced phosphorus levels were clinically symptomatic or received any medications to treat these changes in phosphorus level. A transient decrease in serum phosphate has also been reported in other trials of FCM [4, 5, 27, 28]. A possible mechanism is that FCM transiently increases the levels of intact fibroblast growth factor 23, which is a hormone that inhibits renal reabsorption of phosphate [29].

FCM was equivalently effective as DEX in the treatment of IDA. Both treatments improved hemoglobin by an average of approximately 2.5 g/dL over the study period, returning hemoglobin from starting value of about 9.5 g/dL to about 12 g/dL in around 4 weeks after first dose. Intravenous administration of FCM with doses of up to 750 mg delivered at a rate of 100 mg per minute also significantly increased ferritin level. As compared to iron dextran, FCM had a greater effect with respect to the restoration of iron stores (as indicated by an increase in ferritin).

Our results, consistent with the results of previous clinical trials, [1, 3, 4, 13, 30, 31] demonstrate that FCM is safe and well tolerated. In the current study, consistent with previous trials [4, 5, 13, 15, 30–32], FCM increased hemoglobin levels, replenished iron stores, and had a low incidence of AEs. In this study there was also a lower rate of allergic reactions in the FCM group with respect to the DEX group. Moreover, large doses of FCM (up to 750 mg) could be administered via rapid IV push injection (at 100 mg per minute) in this trial. Thus, FCM is a safe, effective, and convenient option for the treatment of IDA of any etiology [1, 5, 32].

Acknowledgments

The funding of this study was supported by Luitpold Pharmaceuticals, Inc. The authers would like to thank David Morris, Ph.D. for the statistical analysis.

References

[1] K. A. Lyseng-Williamson and G. M. Keating, "Ferric carboxymaltose: a review of its use in iron-deficiency anaemia," *Drugs*, vol. 69, no. 6, pp. 739–756, 2009.

[2] S. F. Clark, "Iron deficiency anemia: diagnosis and management," *Current Opinion in Gastroenterology*, vol. 25, no. 2, pp. 122–128, 2009.

[3] Anonyme, "Ferric carboxymaltose: a breakthrough treatment for iron deficiency anaemia," *European Journal of Hospital Pharmacy Practice*, vol. 15, pp. 62–65, 2009.

[4] D. B. Van Wyck, M. G. Martens, M. H. Seid, J. B. Baker, and A. Mangione, "Intravenous ferric carboxymaltose compared with oral iron in the treatment of postpartum anemia: a randomized controlled trial," *Obstetrics and Gynecology*, vol. 110, no. 2 I, pp. 267–278, 2007.

[5] L. T. Goodnough, D. B. Van Wyck, A. Mangione, J. Morrison, P. E. Hadley, and J. A. Jehle, "Large-dose intravenous ferric carboxymaltose injection for iron deficiency anemia in heavy uterine bleeding: a randomized, controlled trial," *Transfusion*, vol. 49, no. 12, pp. 2719–2728, 2009.

[6] C. Gasche, M. C. E. Lomer, I. Cavill, and G. Weiss, "Iron, anaemia, and inflammatory bowel diseases," *Gut*, vol. 53, no. 8, pp. 1190–1197, 2004.

[7] S. F. Clark, "Iron deficiency anemia," *Nutrition in Clinical Practice*, vol. 23, no. 2, pp. 128–141, 2008.

[8] B. G. Danielson, P. Geisser, and W. Schneider, *Iron Therapy with Special Emphasis on Intravenous Administration*, Vifor (International) Inc., 1996.

[9] S. B. Silverstein, J. A. Gilreath, and G. M. Rodgers, "Intravenous iron therapy: a summary of treatment options and review of guidelines," *Journal of Pharmacy Practice*, vol. 21, no. 6, pp. 431–443, 2008.

[10] S. Fishbane, V.-D. Ungureanu, J. K. Maesaka, C. J. Kaupke, V. Lim, and J. Wish, "The safety of intravenous iron dextran in hemodialysis patients," *American Journal of Kidney Diseases*, vol. 28, no. 4, pp. 529–534, 1996.

[11] D. B. Van Wyck, J. Anderson, and K. Johnson, "Labile iron in parenteral iron formulations: a quantitative and comparative study," *Nephrology Dialysis Transplantation*, vol. 19, no. 3, pp. 561–565, 2004.

[12] S. Santosh, P. Podaralla, and B. Miller, "Anaphylaxis with elevated serum tryptase after administration of intravenous ferumoxytol," *NDT Plus*, vol. 3, no. 4, pp. 341–342, 2010.

[13] S. Kulnigg, S. Stoinov, V. Simanenkov et al., "A novel intravenous iron formulation for treatment of anemia in inflammatory bowel disease: the ferric carboxymaltose (FERINJECT) randomized controlled trial," *American Journal of Gastroenterology*, vol. 103, no. 5, pp. 1182–1192, 2008.

[14] M. Auerbach and H. Ballard, "Clinical use of intravenous iron: administration, efficacy, and safety," *Hematology/the Education Program of the American Society of Hematology*, vol. 2010, pp. 338–347, 2010.

[15] S. Tagboto, L. Cropper, J. Turner, and K. Pugh-Clarke, "The efficacy of a single dose of intravenous ferric carboxymaltose (Ferinject) on anaemia in a pre-dialysis population of chronic kidney disease patients," *Journal of Renal Care*, vol. 35, no. 1, pp. 18–22, 2009.

[16] A. M. Ganzoni, "Total infusion of ferri-carbohydrate complexes," *Blut*, vol. 25, pp. 349–351, 1972.

[17] P. W. F. Wilson, R. B. D'Agostino, D. Levy, A. M. Belanger, H. Silbershatz, and W. B. Kannel, "Prediction of coronary heart disease using risk factor categories," *Circulation*, vol. 97, no. 18, pp. 1837–1847, 1998.

[18] Cancer Therapy Evaluation Program, "Common Terminology Criteria for Adverse Events, Version 3.0," DCTD, NCI, NIH, DHHS March 2003, http://ctep.cancer.gov/.

[19] P. Geisser and J. Banké-Bochita, "Pharmacokinetics, safety and tolerability of intravenous ferric carboxymaltose: a dose-escalation study in volunteers with mild iron-deficiency anaemia," *Arzneimittel-Forschung*, vol. 60, no. 6 a, pp. 362–372, 2010.

[20] G. Bailey, R. L. Strub, R. C. Klein, and J. Salvaggio, "Dextran-induced anaphylaxis," *Journal of the American Medical Association*, vol. 200, no. 10, pp. 889–891, 1967.

[21] S. Fishbane, "Safety in iron management," *American Journal of Kidney Diseases*, vol. 41, no. 6, pp. S18–S26, 2003.

[22] B. G. Danielson, "Structure, chemistry, and pharmacokinetics of intravenous iron agents," *Journal of the American Society of Nephrology*, vol. 15, no. 2, pp. S93–S98, 2004.

[23] R. Lawrence and M. Helenek, "Development and comparison of iron dextran products," *PDA Journal of Pharmaceutical Science and Technology*, vol. 52, no. 5, pp. 190–197, 1998.

[24] R. Fletes, J. M. Lazarus, J. Gage, and G. M. Chertow, "Suspected iron dextran-related adverse drug events in hemodialysis patients," *American Journal of Kidney Diseases*, vol. 37, no. 4, pp. 743–749, 2001.

[25] J. T. McCarthy, C. E. Regnier, C. L. Loebertmann, and E. J. Bergstralh, "Adverse events in chronic hemodialysis patients receiving intravenous iron dextran—a comparison of two products," *American Journal of Nephrology*, vol. 20, no. 6, pp. 455–462, 2000.

[26] B. A. J. Walters and D. B. Van Wyck, "Benchmarking iron dextran sensitivity: reactions requiring resuscitative medication in incident and prevalent patients," *Nephrology Dialysis Transplantation*, vol. 20, no. 7, pp. 1438–1442, 2005.

[27] C. F. Barish, T. Koch, A. Butcher, D. Morris, and D. B. Bregman, "Safety and efficacy of intravenous ferric carboxymaltose (750 mg) in the treatment of iron deficiency Anemia: two randomized, controlled trials," *Anemia*, vol. 2012, Article ID 172104, 12 pages, 2012.

[28] C. Charytan, M. V. Bernardo, T. Koch, A. Butcher, D. Morris, and D. B. Bregman, "Intravenous ferric carboxymaltose versus standard medical care in the treatment of iron deficiency anemia in patients with chronic kidney disease: a randomized, active-controlled, multi-center study," *Nephrology Dialysis Transplantation*, vol. 28, pp. 953–964, 2013.

[29] M. Wolf, T. A. Koch, and D. B. Bregman, "Effects of iron deficiency anemia and its treatment on fibroblast growth factor 23 and phosphate homeostasis in women," *Journal of Bone and Mineral Research*, vol. 28, no. 8, pp. 1793–1803, 2013.

[30] M. H. Seid, R. J. Derman, J. B. Baker, W. Banach, C. Goldberg, and R. Rogers, "Ferric carboxymaltose injection in the treatment of postpartum iron deficiency anemia: a randomized controlled clinical trial," *American Journal of Obstetrics and Gynecology*, vol. 199, no. 4, pp. 435.e1–435.e7, 2008.

[31] C. Breymann, F. Gliga, C. Bejenariu, and N. Strizhova, "Comparative efficacy and safety of intravenous ferric carboxymaltose in the treatment of postpartum iron deficiency anemia," *International Journal of Gynecology and Obstetrics*, vol. 101, no. 1, pp. 67–73, 2008.

[32] S. D. Anker, J. C. Colet, G. Filippatos et al., "Ferric carboxymaltose in patients with heart failure and iron deficiency," *The New England Journal of Medicine*, vol. 361, no. 25, pp. 2436–2448, 2009.

Iron-Fortified Drinking Water Studies for the Prevention of Children's Anemia in Developing Countries

Jose E. Dutra-de-Oliveira,[1] J. Sergio Marchini,[1] Joel Lamounier,[2] and Carlos A. N. Almeida[3]

[1]*Department of Internal Medicine, Ribeirão Preto School of Medicine, University of São Paulo, Av Bandeirantes 3900, 14049-900 Ribeirao Preto, SP, Brazil*
[2]*Department of Pediatrics, Medical School Belo Horizonte, Av Professor Alfredo Balena 190, 30130-100 Belo Horizonte, MG, Brazil*
[3]*Department of Pediatrics, Ribeirão Preto School of Medicine, University of São Paulo, Av Costábile Romano 2201, 14096-900 Ribeirao Preto, SP, Brazil*

Correspondence should be addressed to Jose E. Dutra-de-Oliveira, jeddoliv@fmrp.usp.br

Academic Editor: Fernando Ferreira Costa

Anemia and iron deficiency should receive special attention considering their high prevalence and serious consequences. For prevention, globally it is recommended to increase dietary iron intake, iron fortification of industrialized foods, and medical iron supplementation. Food fortification for the prevention of iron deficiency in developing countries should consider carriers locally available and consumed daily, requiring limited infrastructure and technology. Drinking water is the iron carrier we have been working for years for the prevention of iron deficiency and anemia in small children in Brazil. It was shown that studies with iron-fortified drinking water were proved to be effective on children's anemia prevention. Water is found everywhere, consumed daily by everyone may be easily fortified with simple technology, is low priced and was effective on the prevention of children's anemia. Fortification of drinking water with iron was locally implemented with the direct participation of the government and community. Government authorities, health personnel and population were part of the project and responsible for its community implementation. The mayor/municipality permitted and supported the proposal to supply it to children at their day-care centers. To keep the children drinking water iron fortified supply an officially authorized legislation was also approved.

1. Introduction

Iron deficiency and iron anemia are prevalent worldwide, affecting a large proportion of global population. It has been estimated the worldwide incidence of anemia to be 47% in children under five, 30% in no pregnant women of childbearing age, and 42% in pregnant women [1]. It has been identified as the most prevalent micronutrient deficiency in the world [2]. It is mostly present in developing world and is said to affect over 2 billion people. Infants, preschool children, and pregnant women are the main groups at risk for iron deficiency and iron anemia. Its prevention includes food with high-iron bioavailability and a nutritious daily diet. Alternative solutions involve selective plant breeding or genetic engineering that will increase iron content or reduce absorption inhibitors in dietary staples, iron enrichment of industrialized foods, and iron supplementation with pharmacological medicine products.

Food fortification has been regarded as the safest and most effective means to supplement diets with low-iron content. Industrialization required for preparation of iron food fortification has often been a problem requiring technology not available in less developed countries. Frequently, poor regions do not have the necessary infrastructure or even adequate local for processing food fortification. Or even in these poor and less developed countries or regions they do not produce or use international agencies food recommended to be fortified. Several foods have been used as nutrient carriers, with their own particularities. Important considerations are that international food-based suggestions for food fortification require changes in local diet habits and even food importation. Fortification of foods should include locally available and consumed foods. Another serious problem for prevention of iron deficiency through food fortification in developing and less developed countries as wheat flour, for example, is to have it available everywhere and consumed daily in amounts that could be sufficient to supply their daily need of iron. Small children can only eat small amounts of bread and infants have problems to eat solid foods. In Brazil where iron-fortified wheat flour was made mandatory by law, preliminary results have shown that under five children anemia did not get better [3]. Reality has shown that in spite of all available knowledge, new technologies, supplementation, and fortification programs, the problem of iron deficiency and iron anemia is kept as one of the greatest public health nutrition problems in less and developing world.

At the Micronutrient Forum held at Turkey in 2007 [4] several papers reported again the magnitude and severity of the world anemia problem. It was shown that the problem is far from being solved, especially in less developed countries and poor areas of the world. On the other hand it is also to be said that several studies on iron food fortification for the prevention of anemia keep going in several parts of the world. In Mexico [5], fortification of rice with iron using Ultra Rice technology was shown to be an efficacious strategy for preventing iron deficiency. In Guatemala [6] fortification of sugar with FeNaEDTA improved the iron status of the semirural population. In Vietnam [7] the use of NaFeEDTA fortified salt was shown effective to control iron deficiency in child bearing women. There are also a large number of other experimental studies using a variety of carriers, as iron-fortified soy sauce in Indonesia, fish sauce in Cambodia, and brown bread in South Africa. Mandatory flour fortification with iron and folic acid and of maize is going on in some countries, such as Pakistan, where the prevalence of anemia is quite high [8].

It has to be clear that a fortified food for anemia prevention in developing countries to be effective should use carriers locally available and legally implemented at the community. Certainly one such alternative is our proposed utilization of drinking water as an iron carrier. Water by itself is an essential liquid nutrient and to it could be dissolved other nutrients as iron and other minerals and vitamins. WHO held a meeting on water on health and published a report on the subject [9]. Water is available and used daily everywhere by everyone from infants at birth to old age, which does not happen with various other nutrient food carriers. An important characteristic of water as a carrier is that it is liquid, proper to be given to infants, children, and sick people. The bioavailability of nutrients carried in water increases with their solubility. Fortification of drinking water with iron is a simple process, and solutions may be prepared locally starting with a concentrate water iron sulfate solution at a drug medicine store or similar set-up, local always available even in small towns. A concentrated iron solution is bottled in 1 L pot and sent to the day-care centers where a diluted solution is offered to the children. At the day-care a calculated amount of the concentrated iron solution

is diluted to large drinking water bottles of 20 litters. We have worked with a final concentration of 10 to 20 mg/L of iron from ferrous sulfate, which by the usual daily children water intake was shown to be sufficient for the control of the children's anemia. This ferrous sulfate iron-fortified water shows a light yellowish color and has a small metallic taste. Starting the utilization with low amount of iron, the children get used to the fortified water with no problems.

Quite a few iron salts were tested by us and some of them like the NaFeEDTA did not change the color of the water, does not change its taste, and is biologically active. This salt is a little more expensive than ferrous sulfate. Our studies have also worked with different ways through which iron-fortified water could be supplied to the population in a large community. One of them was adding iron to the city water distribution system. This is the way through which fluoride has been carried out in several places in the world to prevent tooth decay; we thought to use it for the prevention of anemia at community level. Different iron salts as pills and tablets to be used at homes were also tested to supply extra iron to all members of a family, including one with a sparkling formulation with iron plus ascorbic acid. The fact is that water iron fortification solutions may be prepared locally and used for cooking and drinking water, supplying iron to all members of families or institutions. Drinking water iron fortified could also be used to increase the daily iron intake of pregnant and lactating women. An additional and important advantage of liquid iron water solutions over other kinds of solid food iron carriers as we appointed is that a liquid can be easily given to small infants and children, the largest iron deficient and anemia age groups. Recent data from Brazil has shown that 72.5% of infants 6 to 12 months of age were found to be iron deficient and anemic in a surrey in the Northwestern of Brazil [10].

Data on our previous experimental, animal, children, and community on the use of drinking water as an iron carrier and strategies for its implementation at community levels in Brazil will be presented and commented (Table 1).

2. Iron from Complex Salts and Its Bioavailability in Rats [11]

The objective of these laboratory experiments was to show the effect of adding different iron salts to drinking water and checking their effects on color, turbidity, and taste, through physical and chemical tests. Ferric ammonium citrate, ferric chloride, ferric gluconate, ferric hydroxide, ferric sulfate, and ferric nitrate, diluted in water, were tested. Iron citrate, chloride, gluconate, and ferrous sulfate produced small color changes at 1 mg/L and 5 mg/L concentrations, when measured initially and after seven days. Tests with iron sodium EDTA added to the water solution showed practically no color change and no metallic taste; the solution remained clear and transparent. The presence of chloride in iron-fortified water increased color and turbidity, though it had no effect on NaFeEDTA solution. Along with the physic-ochemical tests, acceptance trials of these different water-fortified solutions were run continuously with over 500

TABLE 1: Clinical work carried out in preschool children with iron fortified drink water in Brazil.

Reference	Age group (years)	Number of Participants	Place	Fortification compounds	Indicator of ID g/dL		Duration
					Before	After	
Dutra-de-Oliveira et al. [12]	2–6	31	Daycare Center of Ribeirão Preto Brazil	Ferrous sulfate (20 mg Fe/L)	Hb: 10.6 ± 1.1 FT: 13.7 ± 8.9	Hb: 13.0 ± 1.1 FT: 25.6 ± 10.5	8 months
Dutra-de-Oliveira et al. [13]	Families Adults + Children 1–6	88	Homes of Ribeirão Preto Brazil	Ferrous sulfate 10 mg/L + L-ascorbic acid 100 mg/L	Children: Hb: 10.9 ± 1.1 FT: 27.6 ± 21.6 Adults: Hb: 12.9 ± 1.7 FT: 74.8 ± 41.3	Children: Hb: 11.7 ± 1.1 FT: 33.8 ± 22.1 Adults: Hb: 13.7 ± 1.7 FT: 106.2 ± 93.9	4 months
Lamounier et al. [14]	Children 1/2–6	321	Daycare Center Belo Horizonte Brazil	Ferrous sulfate 10 mg/L + L-ascorbic acid 100 mg/L	Hb: 11.8 ± 1.3	Hb: 12.9 ± 1.4	5 months
Almeida et al. [15]	1–6	74	Daycare Center of Monte Alto Brazil	Ferrous sulfate (10 mg Fe/L)	Hb: 11.3 ± 1.3	Hb: 11.5 ± 1.3	6 months

children. Different from what many expected, our children rapidly adapted to the low metallic taste of ferrous sulfate.

It was also found that iron-fortified water turbidity decreases with the addition of ascorbic acid or citric acid to the solution. Water solutions of Fe gluconate, citrate, and sulfate had less color and turbidity than those of poli-maltosed $OHFe^3$ and Fe^3 nitrate. An anemic weanling rat test was carried out where a group of rats did not get iron in their drinking water and the other group receive water with ferrous sulfate, NaFeEDTA, iron-glycine chelate, and complex ferric orthophosphate. The control animals became anemic after 35 days, 9.1 g/dL of Hb, and the ones receiving ferrous sulfate, NaFeEdta, and Fe glycine chelate 13.0–13.9 g of Hb. The animals drinking iron Fe orthophosphate had 10.6 g Hb/dL. Weight gain, hemoglobin, hematocrit, transferring saturation, iron hemoglobin, and relative iron biological value were checked in all animals. NaFeEDTA and iron aminochelate produced similar results as ferrous sulfate. Orthophosphate iron had lower biological value.

3. Drinking Water as an Iron Carrier to Control Anemia in Preschool Children in a Day-Care Center [16]

In this study, we look at the effect of Fe-fortified drinking water offered to 31 preschool children under 5, during eight months. The children attended a day-care institution in the city of Ribeirão Preto, starting early in the morning and leaving around 5 pm in the afternoon. They received three meals a day and had free access to iron-fortified water. Iron sulfate solution was added to the drinking water, at a concentration of 20 mg of elemental iron per liter. Clinical and anthropometric data were obtained for each child. Blood was collected and hemoglobin and serum ferritin measured before, four and eight months after the

intervention began. Anemia decreased significantly after the introduction of iron-fortified drinking water (ferrous sulfate only). The number of Fe-deficient children decreased drastically after they started drinking the Fe-enriched water. Mean hemoglobin values increased from 10.6 to 13.7 g/dL and serum ferritin from 13.7 to 25.6 mcg/L, after eight months. There were no problems related to the ferrous sulfate addition or the acceptance of drinking the Fe-enriched water. It was concluded that the iron-enriched water is a practical alternative to supply iron and prevent anemia.

4. Iron Fortification of Domestic Drinking Water to Prevent Anemia among Low Socioeconomic Families in Brazil [17]

The objective of this study was to evaluate through blood parameters (hemoglobin and ferritin levels) the effect of an iron-fortified drinking water used in the preparation of family meals. Participants were families of small children with anemia who were previously seen at our University Hospital in the City of Ribeirão Preto. They had borderline blood anemia iron parameters. Twenty-one families of low socioeconomic status including 88 subjects participated in the project and were divided into two groups. Twelve families, 22 fathers and/or mothers, and 22 children less than 6 years old with hemoglobin levels ≤11 g/dL participate in the study. Daily intakes of selected nutrients were measured. A solution of water iron + ascorbic acid (AA) in small bottles was given to a group of 12 families mothers to be added to their cooking pots (concentration 10 mg of Fe and 60 mg AA/L). Nine other families (18 fathers and mothers and 26 similar children) were supplied with the same type of water, but without added iron or ascorbic acid, during four months. Blood samples were collected at the beginning and at the end of the trial to measure Hb and ferritin levels at the end in both children and adults. The group receiving the iron + ascorbic acid-fortified water increased their Hb and ferritin blood values and the control maintained concentrations similar to initial levels. It was concluded from this study that iron + ascorbic acid fortification can be add at home for their home food cooking and is effective to increase blood hemoglobin and ferritin in adults and children. It can be a simple and effective way to supply iron to low socioeconomic families where the iron intake may be found to be low.

5. Effect of Fortification of Drinking Water with Iron Plus Ascorbic Acid or with Ascorbic Acid Alone on Hemoglobin Values and Anthropometric Indicators in Preschool Children in Day-Care Centers in Monte Alto, Southeast Brazil [15]

Ascorbic acid is known to increase iron absorption. We ran a trial to look at the effect of ascorbic acid on iron utilization. This study was conducted with 150 children in six day-care centers of the village of Monte Alto. Their diet included approximately 10 mg of iron, mainly from vegetable sources and low levels of vitamin C (28% of daily requirements for the age group). Half of the children received iron plus 100 mg of AA in the water and the other half received only the 100 mg AA, with no added iron, during a six-month period. The prevalence of anemia (Hb $\leq$ 11 mg/dL) was 45% for the iron plus AA group and 31% for the AA group, at the beginning of the experiment, dropping to 31.7 and 17.1%, respectively, at the end of the study. This led us to the conclusion that the day-care diet already supplied some iron because there was found an anemia decrease in the children receiving only the day-care diet and that ascorbic acid alone increases its availability. We had also previously shown that fortification of orange juice with iron (8 mg a day) offered to preschool children during four months also increased significantly their iron status measured by hemoglobin levels [18].

6. Implementation of Iron Fortification Programs at Community Level

An important aspect of our studies, along with the demonstration that iron carried out by drinking water could control iron deficiency anemia in infants and small children, was planned in a way that the program should implanted locally as part of the local government children assistance program. The community-applied research studies on the use of drinking water as an iron carrier were always previously approved by the University Research Committee and the County Community Authorities where they were to be carried. The project always started with our close contact with the municipality mayor and public health authorities, linked to county children assistance programs. There were explained to them details of the project that would start with a clinical nutrition check-up of all children attending their day-care centers. We would check locally their blood

for anemia and all children would receive a fortified drinking water during 6 to 8 months, when a new clinical and blood test would be repeated. It was explained that we would supervise, train, and work with local people who already work at the center, like teachers, care takers, and helpers for them to know what to do in relation to the anemia project. The local healthy community personnel, physicians, nurses, dietitians, helpers, children, mothers, and educators were involved. Several meetings were carried out to explain the project, to look for the presence of anemia in the children, and to tell them on the importance of iron on health, growth, learning, and development of the children. The results were always shown to the mothers, day-care helpers, and local health authorities. The mayor was to have the compromise to support the research project and at the end of it to send to the city council a law project that would require mandatory addition and availability of iron water fortification to all children at the municipality day-care centers. A booklet on anemia printed with topics on food, nutrition, and anemia was distributed at the community.

7. Conclusions

This review has shown the following.

(i) Anemia is a hidden deficiency, present and out of control problem in Brazil as it is in several other parts of the world. It is affecting millions of persons, particularly infants, young children, future generations, and women.

(ii) World food fortification programs are going for more than 20–30 years concentrating efforts on the prevention of iron deficiency. Results are far from what it would be expected or desirable. This is an unacceptable situation.

(iii) A recent 2010 anemia prevalence data in a poor area of the Northeast Brazil, a children survey 6 to 60 months showed 45% occurrence of anemia. The highest incidence 75.2% was on the 60- to 12-month age-group [10].

(iv) Strategies on iron food fortification to control childhood anemia in Brazil have been recently reviewed. Iron food fortification for the control of childhood anemia in Brazil includes mandatory fortification of milled wheat and corn flour, fortification of milk, iron fortification of biscuits and bread rolls, and iron fortification of potable drinking water [3].

(v) Our Group at the Medical School of Ribeirao Preto, University of Sao Paulo have been working since 1994 with iron fortification of drinking water for small children [16]. It has all the perspectives to be a better worldwide carrier than other more traditional wheat flour, corn flour, soya, and so forth.

(vi) Iron fortification of drinking water has been shown to be efficient for the prevention of children's iron deficiency and anemia and easily implemented at community level. Water is consumed everywhere by everyone; infants drink water, can be iron fortified locally, and is quite cheap. Public level and mandatory legal law approach showed iron fortification drinking water to be feasible for local public implementation.

Acknowledgments

Medical School of Ribeirão Preto, University of São Paulo, Brazil, São Paulo Research Foundation—FAPESP, Brazil, SIBAN Foundation, Ribeirão Preto, São Paulo, Brazil, and FAEPA Teaching, Research and Assistance Foundation Clinical Hospital Medical School of Ribeirão Preto, Brazil, supported these studies.

References

[1] E. McLean, I. Egli, B. de Benoist, and D. Wojdyla, "Worldwide prevalence of anemia in preschool aged children, pregnant women and non-pregnant women of reproductive age," in *Nutritional Anemia*, K. Kraemer and M. B. Zimmermann, Eds., pp. 1–12, Sight and Life Press, Basel, Switzerland, 2007.

[2] R. J. Stoltzfus, L. Mullany, and R. E. Black, "Iron deficiency anemia," in *Comparative Quantification of Health Risks: The Global Burden of Disease Due to 25 Selected Major Risk Factors*, M. Ezzati, A. D. Lopez, and A. Rodgers, Eds., pp. 163–209, World Health Organization, Geneva, Switzerland, 2004.

[3] J. A. Lamounier, F. D. Capanema, D. S. Rocha, J. E. Dutra-de-Oliveira, M. C. Silva, and C. A. N. Almeida, "Iron fortification strategies for the control of childhood anemia in Brazil," *Journal of Tropical Pediatrics*, vol. 56, no. 6, pp. 448–451, 2010.

[4] J. E. Dutra-de-Oliveira and J. S. Marchini, "Drinking water iron fortification for the prevention of anemia at community level," in *Proceedings of the Micronutrient Forum: Consequences and Control of Micronutrient Deficiencies: Science, Policy, and Programs—Defining Issues*, Istanbul, Turkey, April 2007, abstract no. pp111-w52.

[5] C. Hotz, M. Porcayo, G. Onofre et al., "Efficacy of iron-fortified Ultra Rice in improving the iron status of women in Mexico," *Food and Nutrition Bulletin*, vol. 29, no. 2, pp. 140–149, 2008.

[6] F. E. Viteri, E. Alvarez, R. Batres et al., "Fortification of sugar with iron sodium ethylenediaminotetraacetate (FeNaEDTA) improves iron status in semirural Guatemalan populations," *American Journal of Clinical Nutrition*, vol. 61, no. 5, pp. 1153–1163, 1995.

[7] P. V. Thuy, J. Berger, Y. Nakanishi, N. C. Khan, S. Lynch, and P. Dixon, "The use of NaFeEDTA-fortified fish sauce is an effective tool for controlling iron deficiency in women of childbearing age in rural Vietnam," *Journal of Nutrition*, vol. 135, no. 11, pp. 2596–2601, 2005.

[8] N. Baig-Ansari, S. H. Badruddin, R. Karmaliani et al., "Anemia prevalence and risk factors in pregnant women in an urban area of Pakistan," *Food and Nutrition Bulletin*, vol. 29, no. 2, pp. 132–139, 2008.

[9] World Health Organization, "Nutrients in drinking water: water, sanitation and health protection and the human environment," 2005, http://www.who.int/water_sanitation_health/dwq/nutrientsindw.pdf.

[10] R. C. S. Vieira, H. S. Ferreira, A. C. S. Costa, F. A. Moura, T. M. M. T. Florencio, and Z. M. C. Torres, "The prevalence of and risk factors for anemia in preschool children in the State of

Alagoas, in Brazil," *The Brazilian Journal of Mother and Child Health*, vol. 10, no. 1, pp. 107–116, 2010.

[11] J. E. Dutra-de-Oliveira, M. L. Freitas, J. F. Ferreira, A. L. Gonçalves, and J. S. Marchini, "Iron from complex salts and its bioavailability to rats," *International Journal for Vitamin and Nutrition Research*, vol. 65, no. 4, pp. 272–275, 1995.

[12] J. E. Dutra-de-Oliveira, J. B. Ferreira, V. P. Vasconcellos, and J. S. Marchini, "Drinking water as an iron carrier to control anemia in preschool children in a day-care center," *Journal of the American College of Nutrition*, vol. 13, no. 2, pp. 198–202, 1994.

[13] J. E. Dutra-de-Oliveira, M. M. Amaral Scheid, I. D. Desai, and S. Marchini, "Iron fortification of domestic drinking water to prevent anemia among low socioeconomic families in Brazil," *International Journal of Food Sciences and Nutrition*, vol. 47, no. 3, pp. 213–219, 1996.

[14] J. A. Lamounier, F. D. Capanema, D. S. Rocha, J. E. Dutra-de-Oliveira, C. A. N. De Almeida, and R. C. Norton, "Effect of drinking water fortification with iron and vitamin C in nutritional status and reducing anemia among children in day care centers of Belo Horizonte City Brazil," in *Proceedings of the Micronutrient Forum: Consequences and Control of Micronutrient Deficiencies: Science, Policy and Programs—Defining Issues*, Istanbul, Turkey, April 2007, abstract no. pp. 73-t20.

[15] C. A. N. Almeida, J. E. Dutra-de-Oliveira, G. C. Crott et al., "Effect of fortification of drinking water with iron plus ascorbic acid or with ascorbic acid alone on hemoglobin values and anthropometric indicators in preschool children in day-care centers in Southeast Brazil," *Food and Nutrition Bulletin*, vol. 26, no. 3, pp. 259–265, 2005.

[16] J. E. Dutra-de-Oliveira, J. B. Ferreira, V. P. Vasconcellos, and J. S. Marchini, "Drinking water as an iron carrier to control anemia in preschool children in a day-care center," *Journal of the American College of Nutrition*, vol. 13, no. 2, pp. 198–202, 1994.

[17] J. E. Dutra-de-Oliveira, J. S. Marchini, and I. Desai, "Fortification of drinking water with iron: a new strategy for combating iron deficiency in Brazil," *The American Journal of Clinical Nutrition*, vol. 63, no. 4, pp. 612–614, 1996.

[18] C. A. N. Almeida, G. C. Crott, R. G. Ricco, L. A. Del Ciampo, J. E. Dutra-de-Oliveira, and A. Cantolini, "Control of iron-deficiency anaemia in Brazilian preschool children using iron-fortified orange juice," *Nutrition Research*, vol. 23, no. 1, pp. 27–33, 2003.

3

Study of Hematological Parameters in Children Suffering from Iron Deficiency Anaemia in Chattagram Maa-o-Shishu General Hospital, Chittagong, Bangladesh

Abu Syed Mohammed Mujib,[1] **Abu Sayeed Mohammad Mahmud,**[1] **Milton Halder,**[1] **and Chowdhury Mohammad Monirul Hasan**[2]

[1] *Industrial Microbiology Research Division, Bangladesh Council of Scientific and Industrial Research, Chittagong 4220, Bangladesh*
[2] *Department of Biochemistry and Molecular Biology, University of Chittagong, Chittagong 4331, Bangladesh*

Correspondence should be addressed to Abu Sayeed Mohammad Mahmud; sayedrism@gmail.com

Academic Editor: Aurelio Maggio

A total of 150 (30.61%) anemic patients out of 490 patients diagnosed to have iron deficiency anemia (IDA) have been selected for the first time in Bangladesh. For detailed study, blood samples from 150 anemic patients along with 25 controls were analyzed. Analysis of variance showed significant P value between mean platelet volume (MPV) in females (8.08 μm^3) and males (7.59 μm^3) ($P < 0.05$) in iron deficiency anemia patients. Besides, the value of white blood cells (WBC) in males (10946.08/cmm) was significantly higher than in females (9470.833/cmm) ($P < 0.05$). The significant correlation was observed among hemoglobin levels with hematocrits, hemoglobin with RBC, RBC with hematocrits, and MCV with MCH as well as MCH with MCHC. However, the negative correlation was observed between the hematological variables neutrophils and lymphocytes ($r = -0.989$). The common complaints we have found in the survey were weight loss 73.33%, attention problem 68%, dyspepsia 65%, decrease of appetite 72%, weakness 68%, diarrhea 65%, and headache 55% among IDA patients. ANOVA showed significant statistical difference in all the hematological and biochemical parameters. Analysis of variance test between anemias with only one of three biochemical parameters decreased and control showed that this group does not have iron deficiency.

1. Introduction

As the name implies, iron deficiency anemia is due to insufficient iron. Without enough iron, human body cannot produce enough hemoglobin; as a result, iron deficiency anemia causes tired and short breath. Worldwide, the most important cause of iron deficiency anemia is parasitic infection caused by hookworms, whipworms, and roundworms, in which intestinal bleeding caused by the worms may lead to undetected blood loss in the stool. These are especially important problems in growing children [1]. Malaria infections that destroy red blood cells (although the iron is recycled) and chronic blood loss caused by hookworms (where the iron is lost) contribute to anemia during pregnancy in most developing countries [2]. The principal cause of iron deficiency anemia in the developed countries is blood lost during menses in premenopausal women, which is not compensated by intake from food and supplements. Iron deficiency anaemia still remains the most common cause of anaemia not only in Bangladesh but also all over the world. According to the World Health Report, there are 1,788,600 people in this world suffering from iron deficiency anaemia. And iron deficiency anaemia is the foremost prevalent disease causing morbidity in the world [3]. Many surveys had been conducted in Bangladesh to know the prevalence of iron deficiency. A study of 114 healthy, socioeconomically privileged girls demonstrated that 24% of this group had no storage iron of and 42% of girls had suboptimal iron stores [4].

In a study of 85 men and 54 women in Finland, only traces of marrow iron were found in 4 to 7% of men, in 70% of women of 15 to 49 years of age, and in 23% of women of 50 years of age or older [5]. In a survey of 1105 Canadians, iron stores, judged by serum ferritin values, were greatly reduced in about 25% of children, 30% of pregnant women, and 3% of men [6]. In a study conducted by Looker AC. [7], it was found that 9% of toddlers aged up to 2 years, 9% to 11% of adolescent girls, and women of child bearing age were found to be iron deficient. Of these, iron deficiency anaemia was found in 3% and 2% to 5%, respectively. Also 7% of men over 50 years of age and 1% of young men and teenage boys had iron deficiency [8]. In Pakistan, anaemia was present in 47% of children and 30% of the adult females [9]. Iron deficiency is particularly common in infants and pregnant women. The iron deficiency in women occurs most often during the reproductive years, whereas in men the incidence is relatively high in adolescent and low during young adulthood; it increases thereafter with advancing age. In infancy, the occurrence of iron deficiency is equal in both sexes. It is usually detected between the ages of 6 and 20 months; the peak incidence is at a younger age in infants born prematurely than in those born at term.

2. Methods

2.1. Study Design. A cross-sectional study was conducted from November 2010 to June 2011. The subjects were selected depending on the availability in the hospital ward. The hospital has facilities for iron deficiency anaemia diagnoses, treatment, and monitoring.

2.2. Study Subjects. A total of 150 subjects were included in this study. There was no specific predilection for race, religion, and socioeconomic status. The study subjects comprised the following two groups:

group 1:

(a) IDA male: 102 (subjects),
(b) IDA female: 48 (subjects);

group 2:

(a) control male: 17,
(b) control female: 8.

2.3. Ethical Consideration. Informed parental consent was taken before enrolling the children into the study. The procedure was fully explained to the parents and they were informed that if they wish they will be able to withdraw them from the study and it would not in any way hamper the treatment. Permission was also taken from the hospital authority, departmental head of the haematology laboratory, and biochemistry lab in order to undertake the study.

2.4. Inclusion Criteria and Exclusion Criteria

2.4.1. Inclusion Criteria. Inclusion criteria are as follows:

(1) all cases of suspected iron deficiency anaemia belonging the age group of 18 yrs,
(2) all the patients having haemoglobin less than 11 gm/dL.

2.4.2. Exclusion Criteria. Exclusion criteria are as follows:

(1) patients previously transfused with blood within 120 days,
(2) patients already on iron therapy.

2.5. Control and Development of Questionnaire

2.5.1. Control. 25 patients having haemoglobin within normal range were taken as control.

2.5.2. Development of Questionnaire. A questionnaire was developed to obtain relevant information of demographic and socioeconomic data. The questionnaire also included anthropometric data, birth date, immunization history, past medical history, and clinical information. The questionnaire was coded and pretested before finalization. The questionnaire was both closed and open ended.

2.6. Blood Samples. Blood samples were collected by venepuncture using either the antecubital vein or the dorsal vein and dispensed into dipotassium EDTA anticoagulant bottles. Thereafter, informed consents were obtained from their parents/guardians and teachers. All haematological parameters were carried out by automatic methods. Adequate quality control measures were taken on each test procedure to ensure the reliability of the results. Haematological and biochemical investigations were done in haematology laboratory and biochemistry laboratory, respectively.

2.7. Serum Sample. Collect whole blood in a covered test tube. If commercially available tubes are to be used and should use the red toped tubes. These are available from Becton Dickinson (BD). BD's trade name for the blood handling tubes is Vacutainer. After collection of the whole blood, allow the blood to clot by leaving it undisturbed at room temperature. This usually takes 15–30 minutes. Remove the clot by centrifuging at 1,000–2,000 ×g for 10 minutes in a refrigerated centrifuge.

2.8. Biochemical Examination

2.8.1. Serum Iron Estimation. Serum iron estimation was done with the help of the automated Dimension IRON method by Dade Behring Dimension Biochemistry Analyser.

2.8.2. Total Iron Binding Capacity. TIBC estimation was done with the help of kit manufactured by Randox Laboratories LTD, UK.

2.8.3. Serum Ferritin Assay. Serum ferritin assay was done with the help of ferritin serozyme kit manufactured by Biochem Immunosystems, Italy.

2.9. Hematological Examination

2.9.1. Automated Blood Count (Complete Blood Count). A complete blood count (CBC), also known as full blood count

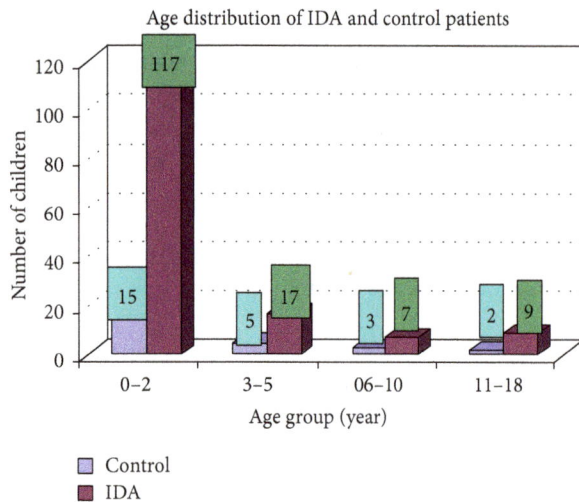

FIGURE 1: Showing age distribution of control and iron deficiency anaemia.

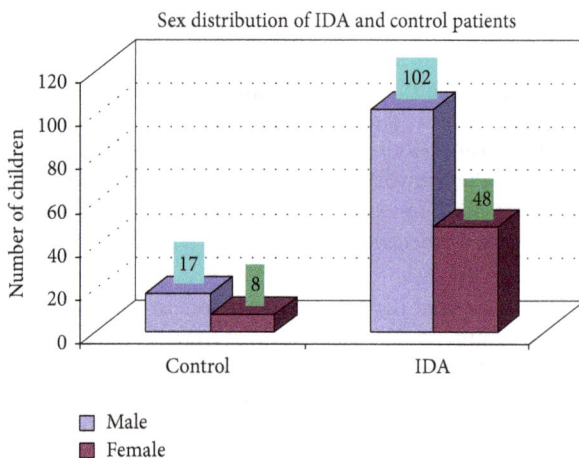

FIGURE 2: Showing sex distribution of IDA and control patients.

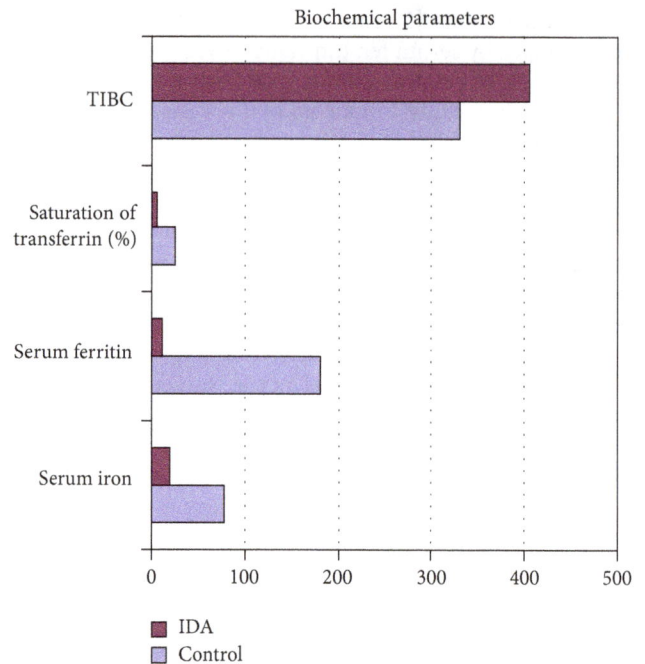

FIGURE 3: Showing biochemical parameters in control and IDA.

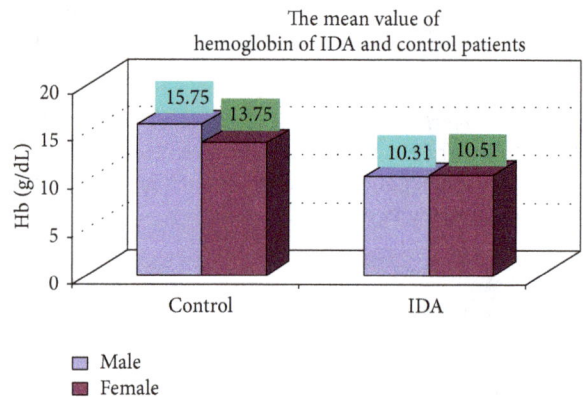

FIGURE 4: Showing the mean value of hemoglobin of control and iron deficiency anaemia.

(FBC), was analyzed by the ABX PENTRA 60 which is a fully automated (Microprocessor controlled) haematology analyser used for the in vitro diagnostic testing of whole blood specimens. The ABX PENTRA 60 is able to operate either in CBC mode (12 parameters) or in CBC + 5DIFF mode (26 parameters). A scientist or lab technician performs the requested testing and provides the requested medical professional with the results of the CBC. The blood is well mixed (though not shaken) and placed on a rack in the analyzer. This instrument has many different components to analyze different elements in the blood. The cell counting component counts the numbers and types of different cells within the blood. The results are printed out or sent to a computer for review.

2.9.2. HCT Measurement. The height of the impulse generated by the passage of a cell through the microaperture is directly proportional to the volume of the analyzed RBC.

The haematocrit is measured as a function of the numeric integration of the MCV.

2.10. MPV Measurement. The MPV (mean platelet volume) is directly derived from the analysis of the platelet distribution curve.

2.11. Erythrocyte Sedimentation Rate (ESR) Measurement. We have followed Westergren method, collecting 2 mL of venous blood into a tube containing 0.5 mL of sodium citrate. It should be stored no longer than 2 hours at room temperature or 6 hours at 4°C. The blood is drawn into a Westergren-Katz tube to the 200 mm mark. The tube is placed in a rack in a strictly vertical position for 1 hour at room temperature, at which time the distance from the lowest point of

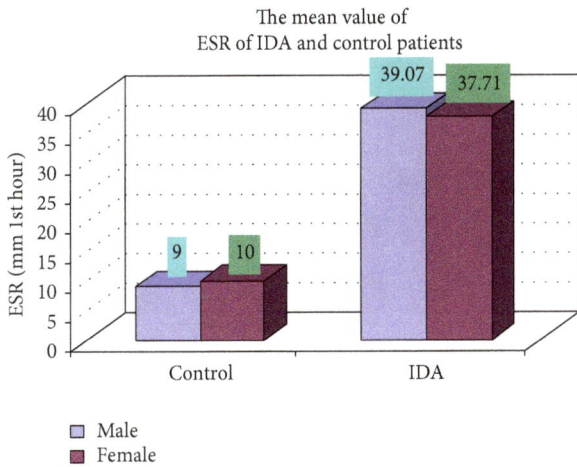

FIGURE 5: Showing the mean value of ESR of control and iron deficiency anaemia.

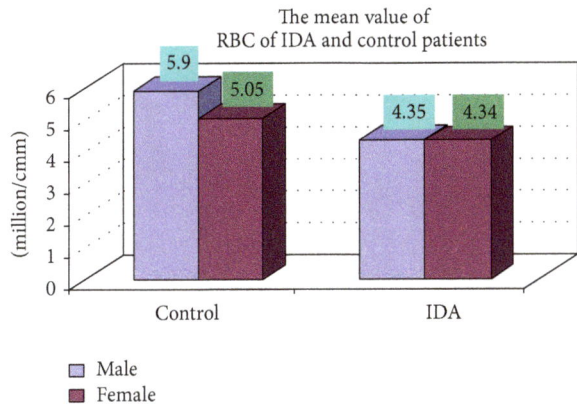

FIGURE 7: Showing PCV/hematocrit of control and iron deficiency anaemia.

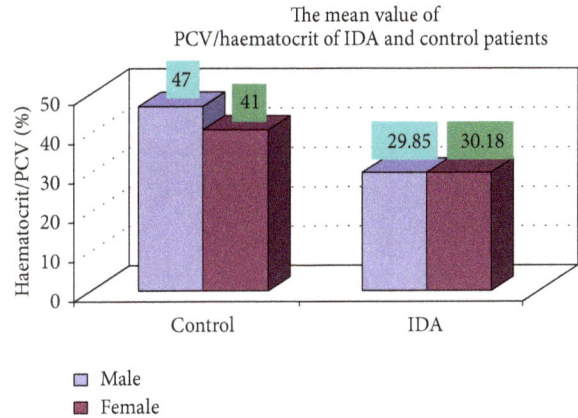

FIGURE 6: Showing the mean value RBC of control and iron deficiency anaemia.

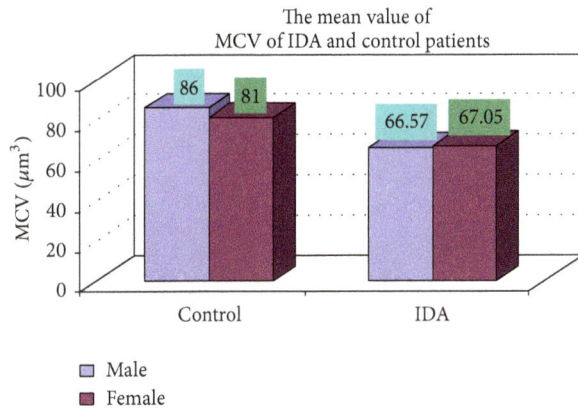

FIGURE 8: Showing the mean value MCV of control and iron deficiency anaemia.

TABLE 1: Mean biochemical parameters of IDA and control.

Biochemical parameters	Control	IDA
Serum iron (g/dL)	78.25	20.85
Serum ferritin (ng/mL)	180.33	9.94
% saturation of transferrin	25.51	5.73
TIBC (g/dL)	329.42	404.47

the surface meniscus to the upper limit of the red cell sediment is measured. The distance of fall of erythrocytes, expressed as millimeters in 1 hour, is the ESR.

3. Results

The diagnosis of iron deficiency anaemia was made only if all the three biochemical parameters like serum iron, serum ferritin, and percentage saturation of transferrin were below normal for the sex. By these criteria 150 (30.61%) out of 490 patients were diagnosed to have iron deficiency anaemia.

3.1. Age Distribution of IDA. Out of 150 patients of IDA, 117 patients were in the age group of 0–2 years, 17 in the age group of 3–5 years, 7 in the age group of 6–10 years, and 9 in the age group of 11–18 years. The age distribution of iron deficiency anaemia and controls is shown in Figure 1.

3.2. Sex Distribution of IDA. Of 150 patients with IDA patients, 102 were male and 48 were female and M : F ratio

is 2.1 : 1. Of 25 controls, 17 were male and 8 were female and M : F ratio is 2.12 : 1 (Figure 2).

3.3. Biochemical Parameters. The mean value of serum iron in IDA was 20.85 g/dL, which is markedly less than that in control. The mean total iron binding capacity was greater in IDA (404.47 g/dL) than in control (Table 1). The mean percentage saturation of transferrin in IDA was found to be 5.73% that is markedly less than control. The mean serum ferritin in IDA was 9.94 ng/mL, which is less than control (Figure 3).

3.4. Complete Blood Count. The blood samples were collected from suspected anemic patient and control group,

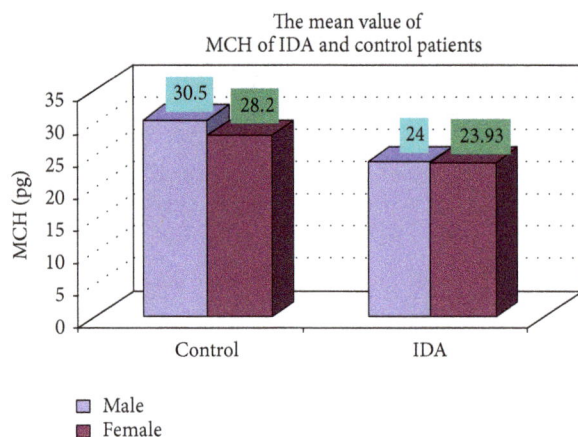

FIGURE 9: Showing mean value MCH of control and iron deficiency anaemia.

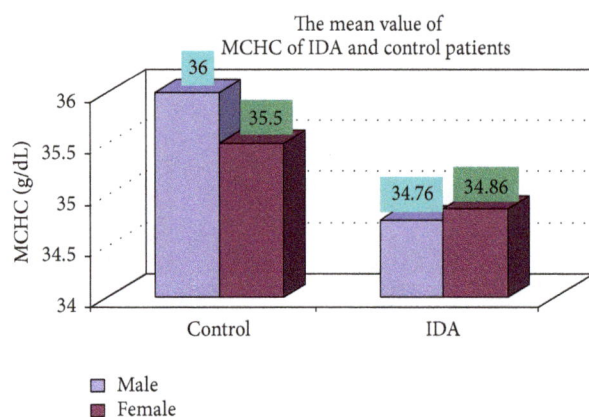

FIGURE 11: Showing the mean value RDW of control and iron deficiency anemia.

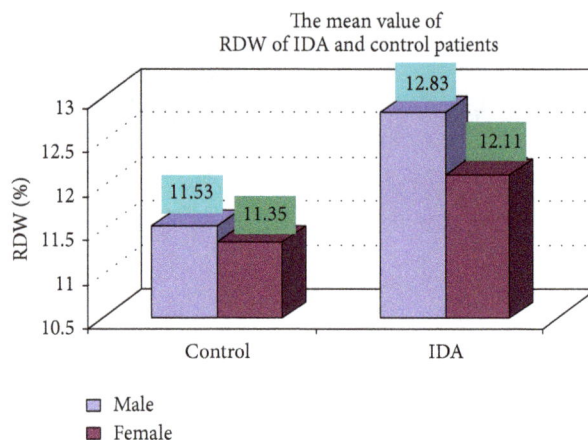

FIGURE 10: Showing the mean value MCHC of control and iron deficiency anemia.

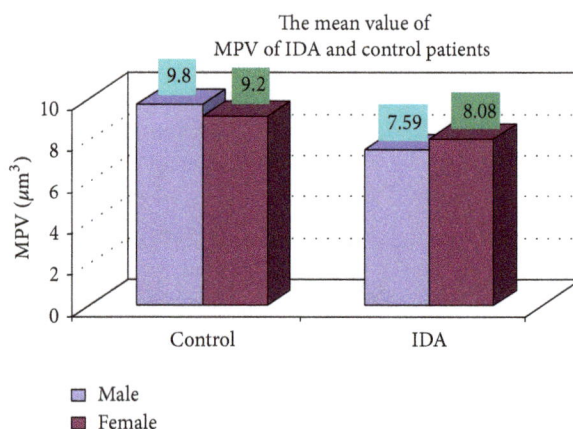

FIGURE 12: Showing the mean value of MPV of control and iron deficiency anaemia.

then complete blood count was conducted for the following hematological values like hemoglobin (Hgb), erythrocyte sedimentation rate (ESR), red blood cell (RBC), hematocrit (HCT), packed cell volume (MCV), mean corpuscular hemoglobin (MCH), mean corpuscular hemoglobin concentration (MCHC), red cell distribution width (RDW), mean platelet volume (MPV), platelet, white blood cell (WBC), neutrophil, lymphocyte, eosinophil, and monocytes. The results are represented graphically (Figures 4, 5, 6, 7, 8, 9, 10, 11, 12, 13, 14, 15, 16, 17, and 18).

3.5. Comparison of Hematological Parameters in Anemic Males and Females. We conducted complete blood count for various hematological values like hemoglobin (Hgb), erythrocyte sedimentation rate (ESR), red blood cell (RBC), hematocrit (HCT), packed cell volume (MCV), mean corpuscular hemoglobin (MCH), mean corpuscular hemoglobin concentration (MCHC), red cell distribution width (RDW), mean platelet volume (MPV), platelet, white blood cell (WBC), neutrophil, lymphocyte, eosinophil, and monocytes. The following (Table 2) is the comparative study of hematological values for IDA in males and females. Statistical

analysis was carried out using Statistical Package for Social Sciences (SPSS) version 11.5, and an independent-sample t-test (P < 0.05) and one-way ANOVA test were used for comparison of hematological parameters. Results were considered to be statistically significant when the two-sided P value was less than 0.05 or (P < 0.05). ANOVA (analysis of variance) showed significant P value between mean platelet volume (MPV) in females (8.08 μm^3) and males (7.59 μm^3) (P < 0.05) in iron deficiency anemia patients (Tables 2, 3, 4, and 5). On the other hand, the value of white blood cells (WBC) in males (10946.08/cmm) was significantly higher than in females (9470.833/cmm), (P < 0.05).

The positive correlation among hematologic and biochemical variables was between hemoglobin and hematocrit (r = 0.851), hemoglobin and RBC (r = 0.659), RBC and hematocrit (r = 0.736), MCV and MCH (r = 0.806), and MCH and MCHC (r = 0.620), but not with other parameters.

The best negative correlation among hematologic variables was between neutrophils and lymphocytes (r = −0.989) but not with other parameters.

TABLE 2: Showing comparative hematological values for iron deficiency anemic males and females.

Parameters	Male mean ± SD	Female mean ± SD	P value
Hb (g/dL)	10.31 ± 1.46	10.51 ± 1.07	0.339
ESR (mm 1st hour)	39.07 ± 27.40	37.71 ± 25.68	0.768
RBC (million/cmm)	4.35 ± 0.59	4.34 ± 0.52	0.918
PCV/haematocrit	29.85 ± 3.75	30.18 ± 3.23	0.589
MCV (fl)	66.57 ± 5.32	67.05 ± 4.86	0.584
MCH (pg)	24.00 ± 2.93	23.93 ± 2.59	0.87
MCHC (g/dL)	34.76 ± 1.43	34.86 ± 0.98	0.626
RDW (%)	12.83 ± 2.08	13.11 ± 2.28	0.485
MPV (μm^3)	7.59 ± 0.85	8.08 ± 0.82	0.001
Platelet (×1000/cmm)	340.49 ± 82.57	332.29 ± 80.99	0.567
WBC (/cmm)	10946.08 ± 3786.32	9470.833 ± 2969.49	0.011
Neutrophil (%)	49.32 ± 16.27	49.43 ± 17.50	0.97
Lymphocytes (%)	45.66 ± 15.98	45.85 ± 17.21	0.947
Eosinophil (%)	2.95 ± 2.95	2.48 ± 1.60	0.208
Monocytes (%)	2.13 ± 1.05	2.25 ± 1.05	0.052

TABLE 3: Showing comparative hematological values between control and iron deficiency anemia (IDA) males and females.

Parameters	Control Male Number (mean)	Control Female Number (mean)	IDA Male Number (mean)	IDA Female Number (mean)
Hb (g/dL)	17 (15.75)	8 (13.75)	102 (10.31)	48 (10.51)
ESR (mm 1st hour)	17 (9)	8 (10)	102 (39.07)	48 (37.71)
RBC (million/cmm)	17 (5.9)	8 (5.05)	102 (4.35)	48 (4.34)
PCV/haematocrit	17 (47)	8 (41)	102 (29.85)	48 (30.18)
MCV (μm^3)	17 (86)	8 (81)	102 (66.57)	48 (67.05)
MCH (pg)	17 (30.5)	8 (28.2)	102 (24.00)	48 (23.93)
MCHC (g/dL)	17 (con)	8 (28.2)	102 (34.76)	48 (34.86)
RDW (%)	17 (11.53)	8 (11.35)	102 (12.83)	48 (13.11)
MPV (μm^3)	17 (9.8)	8 (9.2)	102 (7.59)	48 (8.08)
Platelet (×1000/cmm)	17 (325.25)	8 (315.00)	102 (340.49)	48 (332.29)
WBC (/cmm)	17 (12500.3)	8 (12300.2)	102 (10946.08)	48 (9470.833)
Neutrophil (%)	17 (48.3)	8 (47.2)	102 (49.32)	48 (49.43)
Lymphocytes (%)	17 (29.22)	8 (28.2)	102 (45.66)	48 (45.85)
Eosinophil (%)	17 (2.4)	8 (2.2)	102 (2.95)	48 (2.48)
Monocytes (%)	17 (3)	8 (3.2)	102 (2.13)	48 (2.25)

TABLE 4: Showing correlation among hematologic and biochemical variables in iron deficiency anemia patients.

	Hb	ESR (west)	RBC	PCV/Hct	MCV	MCH	MCHC	RDW	MPV
Hb	1	−0.281**	0.659**	0.851**	0.441**	0.329**	0.159	−0.302**	−0.020
ESR (west)		1	−0.252**	−0.241**	0.016	0.008	−0.064	0.032	−0.138
RBC			1	0.736**	0.070	−0.118	−0.183*	0.040	−0.090
PCV/hct.				1	0.448**	0.289**	0.125	−0.289**	−0.121
MCV					1	0.806**	0.410**	−0.492**	−0.085
MCH						1	0.620**	−0.399**	−0.017
MCHC							1	−0.366**	0.084
RDW								1	0.004
MPV									1

**Correlation is significant at the 0.01 level (2-tailed). *Correlation is significant at the 0.05 level (2-tailed).

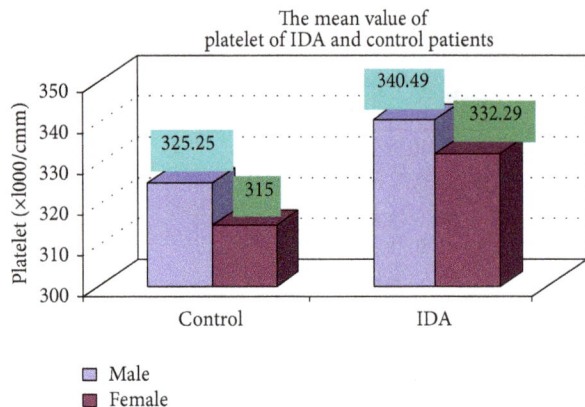

FIGURE 13: Showing mean value platelets of control and iron deficiency anemia.

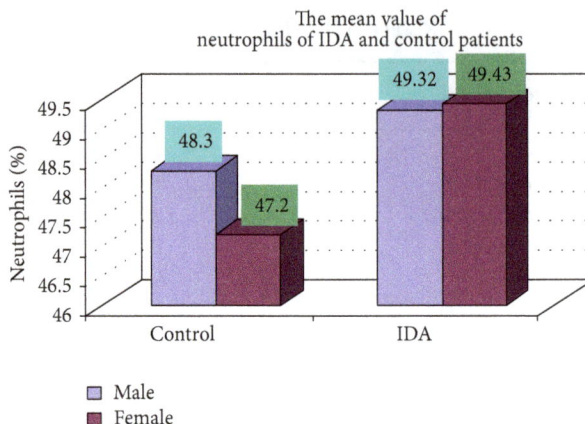

FIGURE 14: Showing mean value WBC of control and iron deficiency anaemia.

TABLE 5: Showing correlation among hematologic variables in Iron deficiency anemia patients.

	Neutrophils	Lymphocytes	Eosinophils	Monocytes
Neutrophils	1	−0.989**	−0.141	−0.035
Lymphocytes		1	0.035	−0.024
Eosinophils			1	−0.047
Monocytes				1

**Correlation is significant at the 0.01 level (2-tailed).

3.6. Clinical Features of IDA. Regarding the clinical presentation the most common complaints were weight loss 73.33%, attention problem 68%, dyspepsia 65%, decrease appetite 72%, weakness 68%, diarrhea 65%, and headache 55% (Table 6). Pale skin color and premature baby were the least common clinical presentation. The results regarding clinical complaints of iron deficiency have been shown graphically (Figures 19, 20, 21, 22, 23, and 24).

4. Discussion

In our study out of 150 IDA patients (102 males and 48 females) 78% were in age group between 0 and 2 years, 11.3% in age group between 3 and 5 years, 4.7% in age group

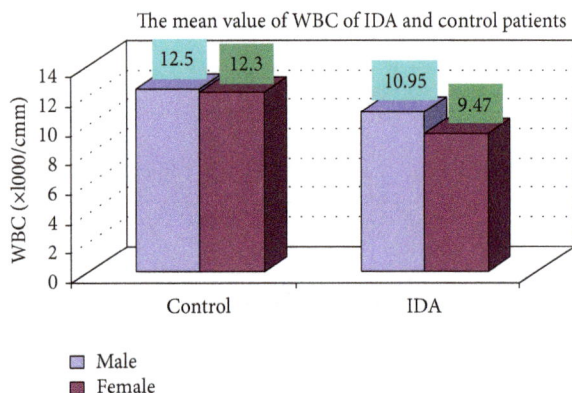

FIGURE 15: Showing mean value of neutrophils of control and iron deficiency anemia.

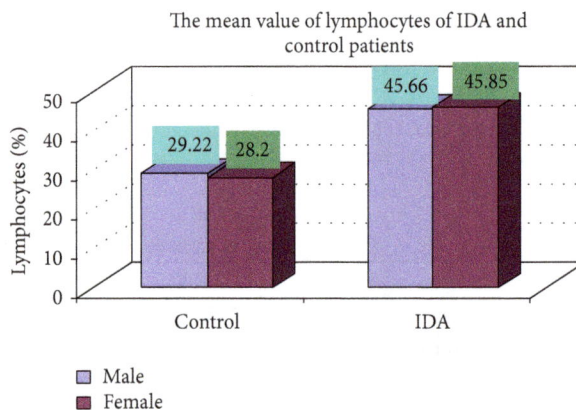

FIGURE 16: Showing means value of lymphocytes of control and iron deficiency anemia.

TABLE 6: Showing the frequency of clinical features of IDA and control patients.

Clinical features	Control Number (%)	IDA Number (%)
Weight loss	8 (32%)	110 (73.33%)
Attention problem	4 (16%)	102 (68%)
Pale skin colour	3 (12%)	51 (34%)
Dyspepsia	5 (20%)	97 (65%)
Diarrhoea	6 (24%)	98 (65%)
Premature baby	2 (8%)	52 (35%)
Weakness	4 (16%)	102 (68%)
Decrease appetite	5 (20%)	108 (72%)
Headache	7 (28%)	83 (55%)

between 6 and 10 years, and 6% in age group between 11 and 18 years. It should be noted that iron supplements and increased iron stores have recently been linked to maternal complications [10]. In contrast, our study showed that IDA is most commonly prevalent in the 0–2-year age group which includes 78% (male and female) and the sex ratio is

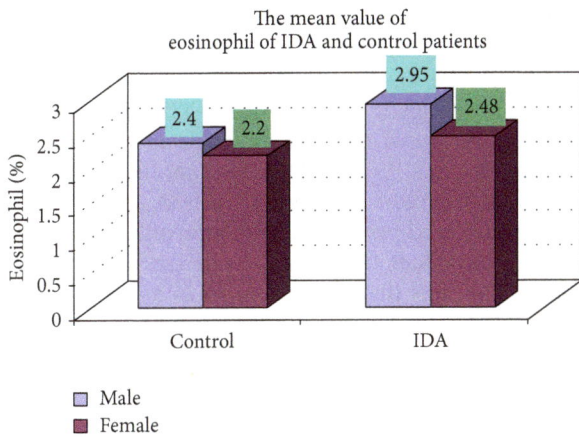

FIGURE 17: Showing mean value of eosinophil of control and iron deficiency anaemia.

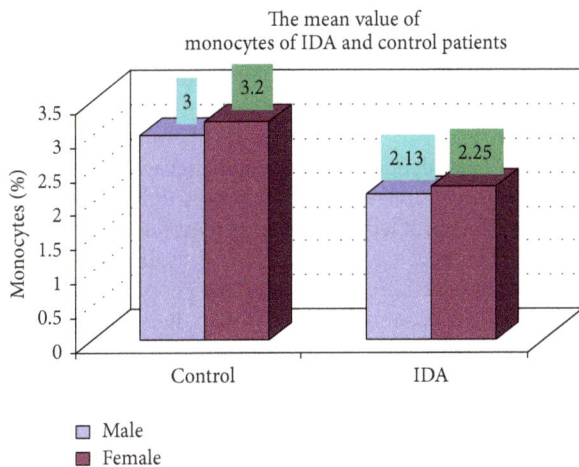

FIGURE 18: Showing the mean value of monocytes of control and iron deficiency anaemia.

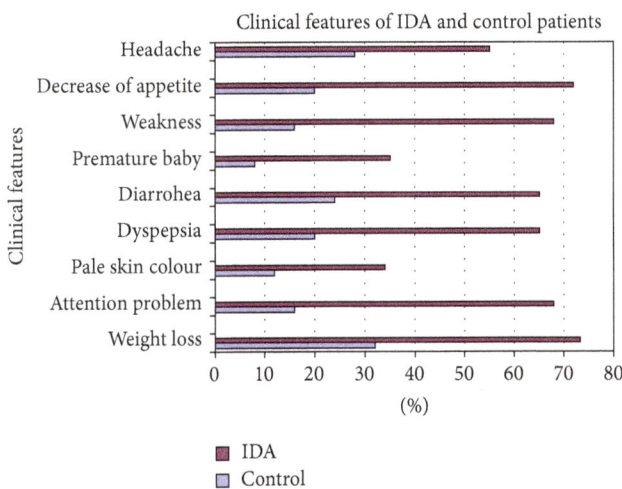

FIGURE 19: Showing clinical features of IDA and control patients.

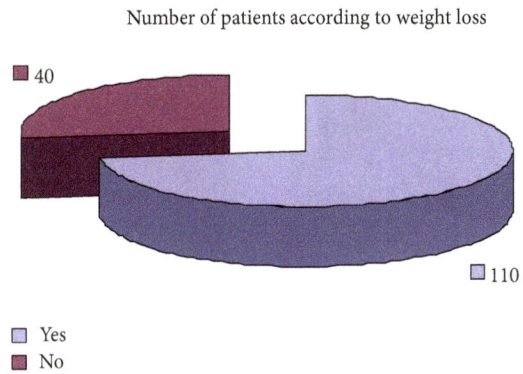

FIGURE 20: Showing the distribution of patients according to complaints of weight loss.

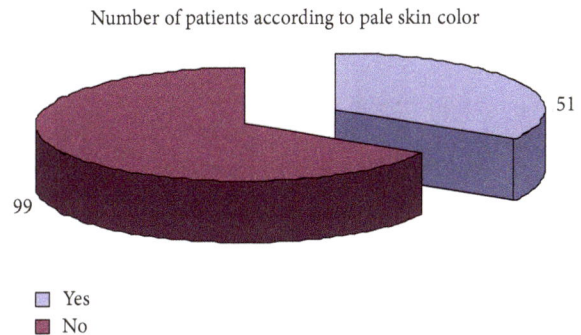

FIGURE 21: Showing the distribution of patients according to complaints of pale skin colour.

also 2.12 : 1. These observations were taken from patients of medical OPD and ward. Moreover, hookworm infestation is more common in our context. Various researches have shown that hookworm is second most prevalent parasitosis in Nepal, incidence of which varies from 11% to 100% [11–13]. This could be the probable factor for the difference in the observations as stated before. Lower class (54%), middle class (31%), and upper class (15%) were mostly affected. These observations show that economically deprived and ignorant people are mostly affected. In clinical manifestations, weight loss, decrease of appetite, diarrhea, attention problems, and weakness were the most common complaints of the patients with IDA. Also, it is equally common among the anaemic individuals who were not iron deficient. Moreover, premature baby, pale skin color, dyspepsia, and headache were other complaints almost equally common among IDA and controls. These are symptoms of anaemia but not specifically concerned with IDA. These observations are in accordance with the previous reports of Elwood [12]. In our observation, the average MCV in IDA was 66.81 fl. Similarly the mean value of MCH was 23.97 pg, mean value of MCHC was 34.81%, and mean hemoglobin was 10.41 gm/dL in IDA. These observations are similar to the report by Bainton [14] and Finch C. A., which showed mean MCV to be 74 fl, mean MCH to be 20 pg, mean MCHC to be 28%, and mean hemoglobin to be 7.6 gm/dL in patients with IDA [15].

Number of patients according to dyspepsia

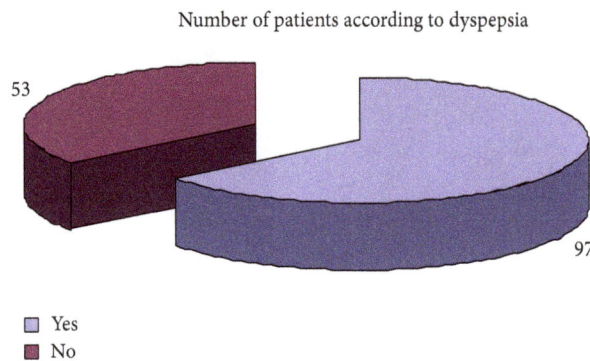

FIGURE 22: Showing the distribution of patients in accordance with complaints of dyspepsia.

Number of patients according to decrease of appetite

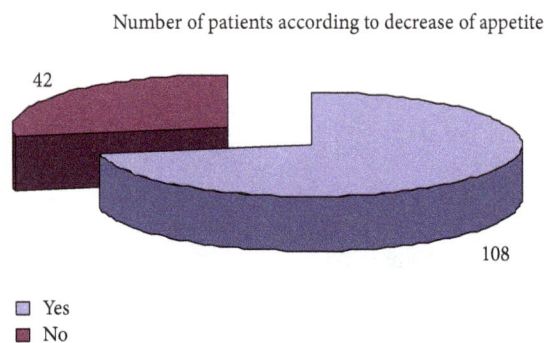

FIGURE 23: Showing the distribution of patients in accordance with complaints of decrease in appetite.

Number of patients according to headache

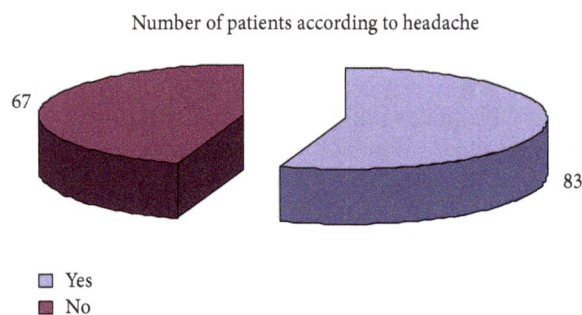

FIGURE 24: Showing the distribution of patients in accordance with complaints of headache.

In the present study, the mean value of serum iron in IDA was 20.85 g/dL, which was significantly lower than control group (78.25 g/dL). In a study conducted in geriatric patients the mean was found to be 22.7 g/dL [16] which is almost similar to our result. The principal limitation of the serum iron determination is variability in the values [17], which may be due to both technical and physiologic factors [18] such as contamination of glassware and reagents with iron although the use of disposable, plastic equipment has reduced such contamination considerably. Among the biochemical tests, total iron binding capacity (TIBC) was increased in 42% out of the IDA patients (102 male and 48 female). The mean value of TIBC in IDA was 404.47 μg/dL, which

was significantly higher than control group (329.42 μg/dL). A study done in children IDA patients the mean TIBC was found to be 413.6 μg/dL, which is also closer to our observation. Though increased value of TIBC indicates iron deficiency, the normal or even lower value may occur in iron deficiency anaemia [19]. So, TIBC was not included among the three biochemical parameters. Instead, in the present study, we have used percentage saturation of transferrin, the value of which does not overlap with the normal values and the values less than 16% occur in iron deficiency and anaemia of chronic diseases [20]. Values less than 5% are found only in iron deficiency. Statistical analysis was carried out using ($P < 0.05$); one-way ANOVA test was used for comparison of hematological parameters. ANOVA (analysis of variance) showed significant P value between mean platelet volume (MPV) in females ($8.08 \, \mu m^3$) and males ($7.59 \, \mu m^3$), ($P < 0.05$) in iron deficiency anemia patients. Besides, the value of white blood cells (WBC) in males (10946.08/cmm) was significantly higher than that in females (9470.833/cmm) ($P < 0.05$). ANOVA showed statistical significance in hematological and biochemical parameters between IDA and the control group and anaemia due to other diseases. It has also showed that the role of TIBC in diagnosing IDA cannot be overemphasized. ANOVA also showed that anaemia with decrease in any two of the three biochemical parameters might have iron deficiency while anaemia with decrease in one of the three biochemical parameters did not have iron deficiency. This problem must be overemphasized by public health system, because of too easy and available treatment and nutrition education for people. Our people do not know which foods to eat and which foods help their health.

5. Conclusion

Iron deficiency anaemia in children is still considered a major health problem all over the world. This is because of long term effects on mental and cognitive skills and on immunity and general physical wellbeing. More recently, iron deficiency is suggested to be related to DNA damage. This prospective study conducted in Chattagram Maa-O-Shishu General Hospital and Medical College, Agrabad, Chittagong, from November 2010 to June 2011 showed that iron deficiency anaemia is one of the most common anemias and in 30.61% of anaemic patients the diagnosis was confirmed by decrease in three biochemical parameters.

Conflict of Interests

The authors hereby declare that they have no conflict of interests regarding this paper.

Acknowledgment

The authors thank Chattagram Maa-o-Shishu General Hospital, Chittagong, Bangladesh, and department of biochemistry and molecular biology for their logistic support and collaboration.

References

[1] W. Fowler, "Chlorosis-an obituary," *Annals of Medical History*, vol. 8, pp. 168–177, 1936.

[2] S. Ashwell, "Observations on chlorosis, and its complications," *Guy's Hospital Reports*, vol. 1, pp. 529–579, 1836.

[3] World Health Organization, *The World Health Report 1998-Life in the 21st Century: A Vision for All*, The World Health Report 1998: Life in the 21st Century a Vision for All; The World Health Report 1998: Life In The 21st Century a Vision for All, World Health Organization, Geneva, Switzerland, 1998.

[4] D. E. Scott and J. A. Pritchard, "Iron deficiency in healthy young college women," *The Journal of the American Medical Association*, vol. 199, no. 12, pp. 897–900, 1967.

[5] H. Takkunen, *Iron Deficiency in the Finnish Adult Population: An Epidemiological Survey from 1967 to 1972 Inclusive*, Munksgaard, 1976.

[6] L. Valberg, J. Sorbie, J. Ludwig, and O. Pelletier, "Serum ferritin and the iron status of *Canadians*," *Canadian Medical Association Journal*, vol. 114, no. 5, pp. 417–421, 1976.

[7] A. C. Looker, C. C. Johnston Jr., H. W. Wahner et al., "Prevalence of low femoral bone density in older U.S. women from NHANES III," *Journal of Bone and Mineral Research*, vol. 10, no. 5, pp. 796–802, 1995.

[8] A. C. Looker, P. R. Dallman, M. D. Carroll, E. W. Gunter, and C. L. Johnson, "Prevalence of iron deficiency in the United States," *The Journal of the American Medical Association*, vol. 277, no. 12, pp. 973–976, 1997.

[9] P. Hamedani, K. Z. Hashmi, and M. Manji, "Iron depletion and anaemia: prevalence, consequences, diagnostic and therapeutic implications in a developing Pakistani population," *Current Medical Research and Opinion*, vol. 10, no. 7, pp. 480–485, 1987.

[10] T. O. Scholl, "Iron status during pregnancy: setting the stage for mother and infant," *The American Journal of Clinical Nutrition*, vol. 81, no. 5, pp. 1218s–1222s, 2005.

[11] M. Vernet, "The transferrin receptor: its role in iron metabolism and its diagnosis utility," *Annales de Biologie Clinique*, vol. 57, no. 1, pp. 9–18, 1999.

[12] P. C. Elwood, W. E. Waters, W. J. W. Greene, P. Sweetnam, and M. M. Wood, "Symptoms and circulating haemoglobin level," *Journal of Chronic Diseases*, vol. 21, no. 9-10, pp. 615–628, 1969.

[13] L. D. Hamilton, C. J. Gubler, G. E. Cartwright, and M. M. Wintrobe, "Diurnal variation in the plasma iron level of man," *Experimental Biology and Medicine*, vol. 75, no. 1, pp. 65–68, 1950.

[14] D. F. Bainton, J. L. Ullyot, and M. G. Farquhar, "The development of neutrophilic polymorphonuclear leukocytes in human bone marrow," *The Journal of Experimental Medicine*, vol. 134, no. 4, pp. 907–934, 1971.

[15] L. H. Allen, "Pregnancy and iron deficiency: unresolved issues," *Nutrition Reviews*, vol. 55, no. 4, pp. 91–101, 1997.

[16] G. M. Brittenham, "Disorders of iron metabolism: iron deficiency and overload," *Hematology: Basic Principles And Practice*, vol. 3, pp. 397–428, 2000.

[17] B. E. Statland and P. Winkel, "Relationship of day to day variation of serum iron concentrations to iron binding capacity in healthy young women," *American Journal of Clinical Pathology*, vol. 67, no. 1, pp. 84–90, 1977.

[18] P. R. Dallman, "Diagnosis of anemia and iron deficiency: analytic and biological variations of laboratory tests," *The American Journal of Clinical Nutrition*, vol. 39, no. 6, pp. 937–941, 1984.

[19] J. H. Lee, J. S. Hahn, S. M. Lee, J. H. Kim, and Y. W. Ko, "Iron related indices in iron deficiency anemia of geriatric Korean patients," *Yonsei Medical Journal*, vol. 37, no. 2, pp. 104–111, 1996.

[20] S. K. Rai, T. Kubo, M. Nakanishi et al., "Status of soil-transmitted helminthic infection in Nepal," *The Journal of the Japanese Association for Infectious Diseases*, vol. 68, no. 5, pp. 625–630, 1994.

4

Prevalence of Anaemia and Evaluation of Transferrin Receptor (sTfR) in the Diagnosis of Iron Deficiency in the Hospitalized Elderly Patients: Anaemia Clinical Studies in Chile

Mauricio López-Sierra,[1] **Susana Calderón,**[1]
Jorge Gómez,[2] **and Lilian Pilleux**[1]

[1] *Hematology Unit, Institute of Medicine, Faculty of Medicine, Universidad Austral de Chile,
Bueras 1003 CP 5090000 Valdivia, Chile*
[2] *Institute of Public Health, Faculty of Medicine, Universidad Austral de Chile, Valdivia, Chile*

Correspondence should be addressed to Mauricio Lopez-Sierra, mlopezs@uach.cl

Academic Editor: Lodovico Balducci

Iron constitutes the most prevalent nutritional deficiency worldwide. In Chile, anaemia epidemiological data is scarce, evaluating mainly children and women. Our objective was to determine prevalence of anaemia in an inpatient elderly population (≥ 60 years) and assess the usefulness of sTfR levels analyzed by other authors as a good predictor in the differential diagnosis of iron deficiency anaemia and anaemia of chronic disease. *Method.* We studied medical patients admitted at Hospital of Valdivia (HV), Chile, in a 2month period. World Health Organization criteria were used for anaemia. *Results.* 391 patients were hospitalized, average age 62.5 years, 247 elderly and 99 of which had anaemia. Anaemia was normocytic in 88.8%, and we observed: low serum iron in 46.3%, low ferritin 10.1%, high TIBC 2%, low % transferrin saturation (Tsat) 40%, and high sTfR 25%. *Conclusions.* As a first figure known in Chile, the prevalence of anaemia in the elderly inpatient was 40.1%. Our findings encourage us to promote the implementation of sTfR determination in the clinical setting to analyze the state of erythropoiesis in patients with chronic diseases wich commonly occurs in elderly.

1. Introduction

Iron (Fe) is an essential metal ion for living beings; although it is the fourth most abundant mineral in the earth's crust, it is the most prevalent nutritional deficiency worldwide [1]. It participates in a variety of vital physiological processes such as oxygen transportation, energy production in the brain by cytochrome oxidase, enzymatic cofactor in the synthesis of neurotransmitters and myelin [2, 3]. The main consequence of iron deficiency is the generation of anaemia which allows us to estimate its prevalence in a given population indirectly by red blood cell counting. However, this approach has the limitation of including other aetiologies. The worldwide prevalence of iron deficiency is approximately 30%, resulting in close to 2 billion people with anaemia of this cause. In developing countries, the prevalence of anaemia among pregnant women and children under two years exceeds 50%

[4, 5]. In Chile, the epidemiological anaemia data is scarce and sectored, with values ranging from 5.1% in women [6] up to 36% in infants of low socioeconomic status [7].

The impact of iron deficiency occurs not only in the hematopoietic system and is more evident in the early stages of life affecting preschool children who suffer from behavioral and affective disorders [8], increased infection susceptibility, and pregnant women having increased risk of preterm delivery, low birth weight, and death in the newborn (NB). Children, especially premature NB children from mothers with iron deficiency, adolescent girls, and women of childbearing age [9, 10] represent the most vulnerable population for this deficiency because of their increased demand and/or physiological loss of Fe.

There is no epidemiological data available of iron deficiency in the elderly, but they are expected to have a higher prevalence of anaemia than in the general population, since longevity is associated with a variety of physiological dysfunctions, chronic and inflammatory diseases, and occasionally inadequate diet that lower reserves and availability of Fe. Clinical manifestations of anaemia in the elderly add to changes in sensory organs, increasing the risk of falls, with a decline in mobility and loss of autonomy [11] that results in an increase in health expenses.

When facing a patient with iron deficiency anaemia (IDA), the hematimetric and ferrokinetic classical standards can be altered by concomitant anaemia of chronic disease (ACD) secondary to infectious, neoplastic, or inflammatory diseases [12–15]. ACD is the consequence of the production of pro-inflammatory cytokines (IL1, 6, TNFα) [15] and some anti-inflammatory cytokines (IL-10) which induce the reticuloendothelial system to store Fe limiting its availability for erythropoiesis, decrease the half-life of erythrocytes, inhibit the production of erythropoietin (Epo) and decrease the sensitivity of erythroid precursors to Epo [16, 17]. Thus, ACD by itself results in hypoferremia and hyperferritinemia thereby complicating etiological diagnosis of patients with simultaneous IDA. Moreover, normal physiological levels of serum iron are difficult to establish in a population due to its circadian rhythm [18], technical limitations of the method, and frequent indication of ferrous salts [19].

In Fe deficiency, the decreased serum iron concentration leads to an increase in total capacity of iron binding (TIBC) and a decreased saturation of the iron transporter transferrin (Tsat). Ferritin (Ferr) and transferrin (Tf) have the disadvantage of being acute phase reactants with limited value in the differential diagnosis of ACD from IDA [20].

The above considerations justify efforts to design a highly sensitive and specific test to detect iron deficiency, ideally before the development of anaemia [21, 22]. Staining of the iron deposits in bone marrow (BM) remains as the gold standard, but it is an invasive technique. We assessed the use of soluble transferrin receptor (sTfR) [23, 24], present in the serum that can be easily quantified by conventional techniques and presents great potential for the distinction between IDA and ACD [24–26] highly necessary for the therapeutic treatment in the elderly. Its' concentration rises when there is marked lack of intracellular iron as the cell increases the number of receptors on its membrane [27, 28]. These parameters can eliminate the need of using BM aspirate to diagnose iron deficiency in some cases. However, it must be remembered that the sTfR commonly is ubiquitously expressed at low levels. Its expression can be elevated, in a variety of human cancers [29]. In addition to its role in iron metabolism it has been suggested that sTfR may play a role in cellular signaling and proliferation stimuli [30].

Our aim was to determine the prevalence of anaemia in a hospitalized elderly population and quantify the proportion that corresponds to iron deficiency using the ratio sTfR/logFerr as a gold standard diagnostic parameter, as other authors [21], in order to assess later its utility in the differential diagnosis of ACD with IDA in comparison to other ferrokinetic and hematological classical parameters for use in the future in elderly patients.

2. Patients and Methods

We studied all the patients who were admitted at the Internal Medicine Ward at HV, Chile, between October 31 and December 31, 2008. Prior to informed consent, they were asked to participate in this research protocol without compromising medical care for their condition. Identification data and sociodemographic variables were asked (age, sex, marital status, health insurance, urban or rural residence, and educational level), and the cause of their hospitalization was obtained from the medical history.

We defined as elderly adults those with age ≥60 years. We assessed the presence of anaemia through the first inpatient complete blood count (CBC) using the World Health Organization definition: Hemoglobin (Hb) <13 g/dL for males and 12 g/dL for women. Anaemia was considered microcytic when MCV was ≤80 fl, macrocytic ≥100 fl, and normocytic 81–99 fl. The severity of anaemia was considered to be severe: (Hb < 7 g/dL), moderate (Hb 7–9 g/dL) and mild (Hb 9–11 g/dL). Patients with anaemia were further for analyzed serum iron, serum ferritin, TIBC, Tsat and sTfR quantification. The techniques used in the study and their normal values according to the manufacturer are shown in Table 1.

The ratio sTfR/logFerr was calculated in patients with ferritin <30 ng/mL considering the value <1 as compatible with ACD, >2 as ACD associated with another etiology using the flowchart of Weiss and Goodnough [23]. Statistical analysis was expressed as mean ± SD or range of distribution if not distributed normally. Statistical calculations were performed with Epidat 3.1.

3. Results

During the study period, 391 patients were hospitalized, out of which 247 were over 60 years. Details of their sociodemographic variables are shown in Table 2. It was not possible to survey 44 patients because of their clinical features (confusion, dementia, etc.).

The patients hospitalized (n = 391) had an average hospitalization time of 6.3 days, with an average age of 62.5 years (15–95 years) of which a 63.15% were elderly. The CBC assessment revealed 99 elderly patients with anaemia according to the WHO criteria. This allowed us to calculate a prevalence of anaemia of 40.1% in the elderly inpatient population. In this population, the mean age was 73.2 years (60–90); the distribution by sex was 59.6% female and 40.4% male. The first three causes of hospitalization were in order of frequency: acute lung infection 12.5%, heart failure 10.2% and acute coronary syndrome with a 9.9%. Analysis of the haematological parameters revealed an anaemia distribution according to morphology of 88.8% normocytic, 9.1% microcytic and 2% macrocytic; and according to severity: severe 3% (Hb < 7 g/dL), moderate 25% (Hb 7–9 g/dL), mild 39% (Hb 9–11 g/dL), and of lower intensity 32% (Hb 11 to 12.9 g/dL). Ferrokinetic analysis revealed (see Figure 1) that serum iron was low in 50.5%, normal in 47.5%, and high in 2%; ferritin was low in 10.1%, normal in 52.5%, and high in 37.4%; TIBC was low in 73.5%, normal in 23.5%, and

TABLE 1: Techniques for ferrokinetics and haematological parameters and normal values according to manufacturer and iron deficiency criteria used in the study.

	Method	Manufacturer's normal value	Iron deficiency criteria
Serum iron	Iron liquicolor photometric colorimetric test for iron with lipid clearing	Men 59–148 ug/dL Women 37–145 ug/dL	Men < 59 ug/dL Women < 37 ug/dL
Total iron-binding capacity (TIBC)	TIBC test, iron saturation and aluminum oxide absorption method, human	250–370 ug/dL	>370 ug/dL
Ferritin (Ferr)	Electrochemiluminescence immunoassay. Roche, Elecsys 2010/modular analytics	30–300 ng/mL	<30 ng/mL
% Transferrin saturation (% Tsat)	TIBC test/iron liquicolor, human	20%–45% ref	<20%
Soluble transferrin receptor (sTfR)	Enzyme-linked quantikine IVD human sTfR immunoassay	8.7–28.1 nmol/L	>28,1 nmol/L
Ratio sTfR/log Ferritin (sTfR/log Ferr)		1-2	>2
MCV	SYSMEX. XE-alphaN automated hematology system roche,	80–99 fL	≤80 fL
CHCM	SYSMEX. XE-alphaN, automated hematology system roche,	32–36 ug/dL	≤32 ug/dL

TABLE 2: Main demographic variables of hospitalized patients, elderly and those elderly with anaemia.

	Total patients admitted	Elderly patients	Elderly patients with anaemia
Number of cases	391	247	99
Mean Age (years)	62.5	73	73.2
Residence			
Urban	280	180	65
Rural	95	60	27
Not available	16	7	6
Literacy			
Yes	288	161	46
No	47	41	20
Not available	56	45	33
Gender(%)			
Male	192	118	40
Female	199	129	59

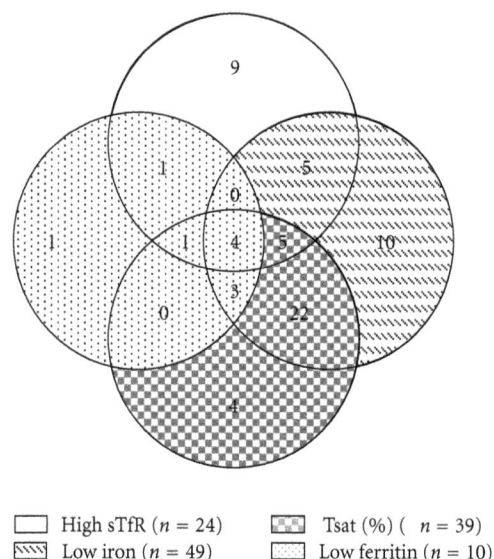

High sTfR ($n = 24$)   Tsat (%) ($n = 39$)
Low iron ($n = 49$)   Low ferritin ($n = 10$)

FIGURE 1: Schematic representation of the number of patients in each category according to their ferrokinetic tests results.

high in 2%, Tsat was low in 40.2%, normal in 44.8%, and high in 14.6%, and the sTfR quantification was low in 1%, normal in 74.3%, and high in 24.7%. Figure 1, illustrate the variability of the analyzes ferrokinetics present in the same group of patients (Elderly anaemic). Example: Serum iron was low in 50.5% ($n = 49$ patients) and 14 of them had high sTfR. Ferritin was low in 10.1% ($n = 10$) and 6 of them had high sTfR, %Tsat was low in 40.2% ($n = 39$) and 10 of them had high sTfR.

According to sTfR levels, patients were grouped into low 1%, normal 74%, and high 25%. Using the ferritin and sTfR/log Ferr values according to the algorithm suggested by Weiss [19], we concluded that there were 67% of ACD, 13.5% of IDA, 9.3% a combination of both, while 1.2% could not be

categorized. The statistical analysis comparing the sensitivity and specificity of the sTfR/LogFerr ratio versus the other ferrokinetic parameters (Serum iron, TIBC, Tsat, ferritin, sTfR) was obtained from receiver operating characteristic (ROC) curves (Figure 2). The following areas under the curve were obtained for serum iron 0.2487, Tsat 0.1938 and ferritin 0.1061. sTfR and TIBC areas under curve was better: 0.9609; 0.7538, respectively. But when comparing the areas under the curve of sTfR and TIBC, any of them is a better diagnostic support if we do not have other test (e.g.,: Perl's stain), since both have asymptotic significance less than 0.05. However, the confidence interval for TIBC test was significantly lower than sTfR, which was a statistically significant difference

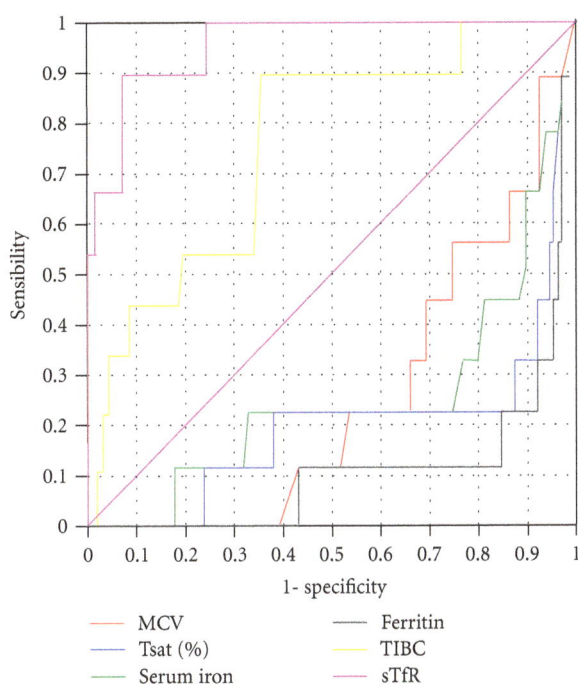

FIGURE 2: Receiver operating characteristic (ROC) curves for Serum iron, TIBC, Ferritin, % Tsat and sTfR for elderly patients with anaemia. sTfR/log Ferr ratio was considered the gold standard.

between the two areas under described under the ROC curves (χ^2 test of homogeneity $P = 0.0214$).

4. Conclusions

From an epidemiological point of view, the prevalence of anaemia was 40.1% for elderly hospitalized patients which is higher than that reported in other age groups in Chile and was unknown until now [6, 31, 32].

Our study confirms that sTfR quantification is a valid method to analyse the erythropoiesis in several diseases. To evaluate the clinical usefulness of sTfR in elderly patients for determining their iron deficiency status, receiver operating characteristic (ROC) curves were used, and the maximum discrimination cut-off point was calculated (see Figure 2). The sTfR was highly superior (sTfR area under ROC curve = 0.9609) to discriminate IDA from ACD in an adult patient population as compared to the classical ferrokinetics and haematological parameters. Ferrokinetic studies in the analyzed population were not useful for evaluating iron reserves and even were misleading in the diagnosis. A low ferritin concentration had been described as a good parameter for diagnosing iron deficiency anaemia [33] however, it only managed to predict 10% of patients with anaemia of this type in our study. The low Tsat was consistent with iron deficiency anaemia in 25%, but did not discriminate with ACD. This is consistent with the fact that transferrin, similar to ferritin, is an acute phase reactant which is elevated in inflammatory disorders [34], still both are widely used [19] in clinical practice due to the simpler technique and low cost.

Furthermore, low levels of transferrin or TIBC may be due to increased degradation rather than decreased synthesis, as a result of increased protein catabolism secondary to catabolic or antianabolic proinflammatory cytokines [35, 36]. Our study confirms that the analysis of different individual ferrokinetic parameters is of little use in patients with concomitant systemic diseases, which are especially prevalent in the elderly; see ROC curves and areas.

In elderly adults requiring hospitalization, ACD was the primary cause of anaemia constituting over 75% of cases, while only 10% were due to iron deficiency. Folic acid and/ or vitamin B12 deficiencies were not analyzed because it was beyond the scope of this study. Finally, the method of excellence to evaluate iron deposits remains bone marrow aspirate analysis with Perls stain constituting in some cases the only technique for diagnosing iron deficiency, however, this test cannot be performed routinely because it is invasive, expensive and slow [37, 38]. Our work shows that quantification of sTfR is more sensitive and specific for discriminating iron deficiency anaemia from anaemia associated with inflammatory events, consistent with work from others authors [21, 23, 39, 40], and will be a useful diagnostic tool for the future in our elderly patients. It is also necessary to note that most of the study population was admitted to the hospital primarily for cardiac diseases (29.22%), respiratory diseases (13.14%), and renal failure (6.17%). The latter is directly related to the generation of anemia by a low secretion of Epo, which must be considered when making the sTfR test if a patient with impaired renal function.

This sTfR/logFerr ratio gives us an inverse linear relationship of the iron stores state and has the advantage of combining the increase of one parameter (sTfR) and the decline of another (ferritin) [21, 41]. Our findings encourage us to promote the implementation of this determination (sTfR) in the clinical setting as was previously proposed [24, 26, 42], and high interest for the elderly adults. It is important to note that this method still requires international standardization in order to define normal ranges, which at the present time limits its routine clinical application [43].

Authors' Conribution

M. L-S. and L. P. responsible for the study design, performed the analysis, interpreted data, and wrote the manuscript; S. C. and L. P. obtained the patients data. J. G. performed the statistical analysis.

Conflict of Interests

The authors declare no competing financial interests.

Acknowledgments

This work has been supported by a Grant from the Colaboración Docente Asistencial Servicio de Salud Valdivia and Universidad Austral de Chile (COLDAS2007). Informed consent form was explained and applied.

References

[1] E. DeMaeyer and M. Adiels-Tegman, "The prevalence of anaemia in the world," *World Health Statistics Quarterly*, vol. 38, no. 3, pp. 302–316, 1985.

[2] B. T. Felt, J. L. Beard, T. Schallert et al., "Persistent neurochemical and behavioral abnormalities in adulthood despite early iron supplementation for perinatal iron deficiency anemia in rats," *Behavioural Brain Research*, vol. 171, no. 2, pp. 261–270, 2006.

[3] A. H. van Vliet, J. M. Ketley, S. F. Park, and C. W. Penn, "The role of iron in Campylobacter gene regulation, metabolism and oxidative stress defense," *FEMS Microbiology Reviews*, vol. 26, no. 2, pp. 173–186, 2002.

[4] E. Pollitt, *Malnutrition and Infection in the Classroom*, UNESCO, Paris, France, 1990.

[5] World Health Organization, *Report of WHO/UNICEF/UNU Consultation on Indicators and Strategies for Iron Deficiency and Anemia Programmer. Draft IDA REP.01*, WHO, Ginebra, Switzerland, 1994.

[6] Ministerio de Salud and Gobierno de Chile, "Encuesta Nacional de Salud," 2003, http://www.minsal.cl/.

[7] C. Artigas, L. González, C. Hidalgo, M. Vera, and S. Muñoz, "Prevalence of iron deficiency anemia in unweaned infants of Temuco: Chile," *Revista Chilena de Ciencias Médico-Biológicas*, vol. 7, no. 2, pp. 61–66, 1997.

[8] B. Lozoff, F. Corapci, M. J. Burden et al., "Preschool-aged children with iron deficiency anemia show altered affect and behavior," *Journal of Nutrition*, vol. 137, no. 3, pp. 683–689, 2007.

[9] J. M. Bourre, "Effects of nutrients (in food) on the structure and function of the nervous system: update on dietary requirements for brain. Part 1: micronutrients," *Journal of Nutrition, Health and Aging*, vol. 10, no. 5, pp. 377–385, 2006.

[10] J. M. Bourre, "Effects of nutrients (in food) on the structure and function of the nervous system: update on dietary requirements for brain. Part 2: macronutrients," *Journal of Nutrition, Health and Aging*, vol. 10, no. 5, pp. 386–399, 2006.

[11] "Anemias secondary to chronic disease and systemic disorder's," in *Wintrobe's Clinical Hematology*, chapter 47, Lippincott Williams & Wilkins, Baltimore, Md, USA, 2nd edition, 2004.

[12] E. R. Burns, S. N. Goldberg, C. Lawrence, and B. Wenz, "Clinical utility of serum tests for iron deficiency in hospitalized patients," *American Journal of Clinical Pathology*, vol. 93, no. 2, pp. 240–245, 1990.

[13] D. A. Lipschitz, "The anemia of chronic disease," *Journal of the American Geriatrics Society*, vol. 38, no. 11, pp. 1258–1264, 1990.

[14] J. M. Cash and D. A. Sears, "The anemia of chronic disease: spectrum of associated diseases in a series of unselected hospitalized patients," *American Journal of Medicine*, vol. 87, no. 6, pp. 638–644, 1989.

[15] B. B. Aggarwal, S. Shishodia, S. K. Sandur, M. K. Pandey, and G. Sethi, "Inflammation and cancer: how hot is the link?" *Biochemical Pharmacology*, vol. 72, no. 11, pp. 1605–1621, 2006.

[16] D. Yoon, Y. D. Pastore, V. Divoky et al., "Hypoxia-inducible factor-1 deficiency results in dysregulated erythropoiesis signaling and iron homeostasis in mouse development," *The Journal of Biological Chemistry*, vol. 281, no. 35, pp. 25703–25711, 2006.

[17] G. Noe, J. Augustin, S. Hausdorf, I. N. Rich, and B. Kubanek, "Serum erythropoietin and transferrin receptor levels in patients with rheumatoid arthritis," *Clinical and Experimental Rheumatology*, vol. 13, no. 4, pp. 445–451, 1995.

[18] A. S. Zhang and C. A. Enns, "Iron homeostasis: recently identified proteins provide insight into novel control mechanisms," *The Journal of Biological Chemistry*, vol. 284, no. 2, pp. 711–715, 2009.

[19] G. Weiss, "Pathogenesis and treatment of anaemia of chronic disease," *Blood Reviews*, vol. 16, no. 2, pp. 87–96, 2002.

[20] H. Tilg, H. Ulmer, A. Kaser, and G. Weiss, "Role of IL-10 for induction of anemia during inflammation," *Journal of Immunology*, vol. 169, no. 4, pp. 2204–2209, 2002.

[21] K. Punnonen, K. Irjala, and A. Rajamäki, "Serum transferrin receptor and its ratio to serum ferritin in the diagnosis of iron deficiency," *Blood*, vol. 89, no. 3, pp. 1052–1057, 1997.

[22] J. W. Choi, "Sensitivity, specificity, and predictive value of serum soluble transferrin receptor at different stages of iron deficiency," *Annals of Clinical and Laboratory Science*, vol. 35, no. 4, pp. 435–439, 2005.

[23] G. Weiss and L. T. Goodnough, "Anemia of chronic disease," *The New England Journal of Medicine*, vol. 352, no. 10, pp. 1011–1023, 2005.

[24] M. Markovic, N. Majkic-Singh, and V. Subota, "Usefulness of soluble transferrin receptor and ferritin in iron deficiency and chronic disease," *Scandinavian Journal of Clinical & Laboratory Investigation*, vol. 65, pp. 571–576, 2005.

[25] K. Thorstensen and I. Romslo, "The transferrin receptor: its diagnostic value and its potential as therapeutic target," *Scandinavian Journal of Clinical & Laboratory Investigation, Supplement*, vol. 215, pp. 113–120, 1993.

[26] E. Chua, J. E. Clague, A. K. Sharma, M. A. Horan, and M. Lombard, "Serum transferrin receptor assay in iron deficiency anaemia and anaemia of chronic disease in the elderly," *QJM: An International Journal of Medicine*, vol. 92, no. 10, pp. 587–594, 1999.

[27] Y. J. Shih, R. D. Baynes, B. G. Hudson, C. H. Flowers, B. S. Skikne, and J. D. Cook, "Serum transferrin receptor is a truncated form of tissue receptor," *The Journal of Biological Chemistry*, vol. 265, no. 31, pp. 19077–19081, 1990.

[28] R. D. Baynes, G. K. Reddy, Y. J. Shih, B. S. Skikne, and J. D. Cook, "Serum form of the erythropoietin receptor identified by a sequence- specific peptide antibody," *Blood*, vol. 82, no. 7, pp. 2088–2095, 1993.

[29] T. R. Daniels, T. Delgado, J. A. Rodriguez, G. Helguera, and M. L. Penichet, "The transferrin receptor part I: biology and targeting with cytotoxic antibodies for the treatment of cancer," *Clinical Immunology*, vol. 121, no. 2, pp. 144–158, 2006.

[30] B. Manger, A. Weiss, K. J. Hardy, and J. D. Stobo, "A transferrin receptor antibody represents one signal for the induction of IL 2 production by a human T cell line," *Journal of Immunology*, vol. 136, no. 2, pp. 532–538, 1986.

[31] P. Lira, A. Foradori, G. Grebe, and P. Vela, "Iron and folate deficiency in pregnant women at term," *Revista Medica de Chile*, vol. 112, no. 2, pp. 127–131, 1984.

[32] F. Mardones, A. Rioseco, M. Ocqueteau et al., "Anemia in pregnant women from the community of Puente Alto, Chile," *Revista Médica de Chile*, vol. 131, pp. 520–525, 2003.

[33] M. Munoz, J. A. Garcia-Erce, A. F. Remacha et al., "Disorders of iron metabolism. Part II: iron deficiency and iron overload," *Journal of Clinical Pathology*, vol. 64, no. 4, pp. 287–296, 2010.

[34] F. M. Torti and S. V. Torti, "Regulation of ferritin genes and protein," *Blood*, vol. 99, no. 10, pp. 3505–3516, 2002.

[35] M. T. Bertero and F. Caligaris-Cappio, "Anemia of chronic disorders in systemic autoimmune diseases," *Haematologica*, vol. 82, no. 3, pp. 375–381, 1997.

[36] A. N. Baer, E. N. Dessypris, and S. B. Krantz, "The pathogenesis of anemia in rheumatoid arthritis: a clinical and laboratory analysis," *Seminars in Arthritis and Rheumatism*, vol. 19, no. 4, pp. 209–223, 1990.

[37] G. Vreugdenhil, C. A. Baltus, H. G. van Eijk, and A. J. G. Swaak, "Anaemia of chronic disease: diagnostic significance of erythrocyte and serological parameters in iron deficient rheumatoid arthritis patients," *British Journal of Rheumatology*, vol. 29, no. 2, pp. 105–110, 1990.

[38] D. L. Witte, D. S. Angstadt, S. H. Davis, and R. D. Schrantz, "Predicting bone marrow iron stores in anemic patients in a community hospital using ferritin and erythrocyte sedimentation rate," *American Journal of Clinical Pathology*, vol. 90, no. 1, pp. 85–87, 1988.

[39] T. Chijiwa, K. Nishiya, and K. Hashimoto, "Serum transferrin receptor levels in patients with rheumatoid arthritis are correlated with indicators for anaemia," *Clinical Rheumatology*, vol. 20, no. 5, pp. 307–313, 2001.

[40] A. F. Remacha, M. P. Sarda, M. Parellada, J. Ubeda, and R. Manteiga, "The role of serum transferrin receptor in the diagnosis of iron deficiency," *Haematologica*, vol. 83, no. 11, pp. 963–966, 1998.

[41] B. S. Skikne, C. H. Flowers, and J. D. Cook, "Serum transferrin receptor: a quantitative measure of tissue iron deficiency," *Blood*, vol. 75, no. 9, pp. 1870–1876, 1990.

[42] M. M. Zorgati, R. Hafsia, A. Bahlous, S. Bahri, and S. Ben Ammar, "Soluble tranferrin receptor in the biological diagnosis of iron deficiency. Report of 24 cases," *La Tunisie Médicale*, vol. 87, no. 12, pp. 818–823, 2009.

[43] S. J. Thorpe, A. Heath, G. Sharp, J. Cook, R. Ellis, and M. Worwood, "A WHO Reference Reagent for the Serum Transferrin Receptor (sTfR): international collaborative study to evaluate a recombinant soluble transferrin receptor preparation," *Clinical Chemistry and Laboratory Medicine*, vol. 48, no. 6, pp. 815–820, 2010.

5

Intravenous Iron Therapy in Patients with Iron Deficiency Anemia: Dosing Considerations

Todd A. Koch,[1] Jennifer Myers,[2] and Lawrence Tim Goodnough[3]

[1]Luitpold Pharmaceuticals, Inc., Norristown, PA 19403, USA
[2]St. John's University, Jamaica, NY 11439, USA
[3]Department of Pathology and Medicine (Hematology), Stanford, CA 94305, USA

Correspondence should be addressed to Lawrence Tim Goodnough; ltgoodno@stanford.edu

Academic Editor: Bruno Annibale

Objective. To provide clinicians with evidence-based guidance for iron therapy dosing in patients with iron deficiency anemia (IDA), we conducted a study examining the benefits of a higher cumulative dose of intravenous (IV) iron than what is typically administered. *Methods.* We first individually analyzed 5 clinical studies, averaging the total iron deficit across all patients utilizing a modified Ganzoni formula; we then similarly analyzed 2 larger clinical studies. For the second of the larger studies (Study 7), we also compared the efficacy and retreatment requirements of a cumulative dose of 1500 mg ferric carboxymaltose (FCM) to 1000 mg iron sucrose (IS). *Results.* The average iron deficit was calculated to be 1531 mg for patients in Studies 1–5 and 1392 mg for patients in Studies 6-7. The percentage of patients who were *retreated* with IV iron between Days 56 and 90 was significantly ($p < 0.001$) lower (5.6%) in the 1500 mg group, compared to the 1000 mg group (11.1%). *Conclusions.* Our data suggests that a total cumulative dose of 1000 mg of IV iron may be insufficient for iron repletion in a majority of patients with IDA and a dose of 1500 mg is closer to the actual iron deficit in these patients.

1. Introduction

Iron is an essential element and its balance must be maintained for proper physiologic functioning. Blood loss, a major cause of iron deficiency, is highly prevalent (e.g., females with menses and patients with chronic occult gastrointestinal (GI) blood loss) and requires proper diagnosis and management [1–4]. Therapeutic management of IDA is focused primarily on repletion of iron stores [1–4]. While iron deficient individuals without inflammation may respond to oral iron therapy, administration of IV iron is beneficial in many patient populations, including those with inflammation (resulting, e.g., from kidney disease, heart failure, or rheumatological diseases), patients who cannot tolerate oral iron, and patients who are noncompliant with oral iron therapy [5–8]. Even under the best of circumstances, oral iron is not well tolerated, and patients are often nonadherent for a variety of reasons, including intolerable side effects and the need for multiple daily doses [9]. The frequently poor absorption of oral iron, moreover, can contribute to suboptimal patient response.

The hepcidin response in anemic patients having inflammatory conditions, such as inflammatory bowel disease (IBD), inhibits GI absorption of oral iron [10]. Moreover, hepcidin impacts iron homeostasis in patients with concurrent inflammation (e.g., repressed recycling of iron from the reticuloendothelial system and sequestration in bone marrow); this may limit both oral and IV iron supplementation and may serve to explain why such patients remain iron deficient despite multiple courses of therapy [6, 10, 11].

Cancer-related anemia (CRA) has multiple etiologies, including chemotherapy-induced myelosuppression, blood loss, functional iron deficiency, erythropoietin deficiency due to renal disease, and marrow involvement with tumor, among others. The most common treatment options for CRA include iron therapy, erythropoietic-stimulating agents (ESAs), and red cell transfusion. Safety concerns as well as restrictions and reimbursement issues surrounding ESA therapy for CRA have resulted in suboptimal treatment. Many believe that more routine use of IV iron for CRA and chemotherapy-induced anemia (CIA) is appropriate in view of existing

TABLE 1: Potential role of iron therapy in management of anemia [12].

Condition	Expected hepcidin levels	Iron parameters	Iron therapy strategies	Potential hepcidin therapy
Absolute iron deficiency anemia (IDA)	Low	Low TSAT and ferritin	PO or IV if poorly tolerated or malabsorbed	No
Functional iron deficiency (ESA therapy, CKD)	Variable, depending on ±CKD	Low TSAT, variable ferritin	IV	Antagonist (if hepcidin levels are not low)
Iron sequestration (anemia of inflammation (AI))	High	Low TSAT, normal-to-elevated ferritin	IV	Antagonist
Mixed anemia (AI/IDA or AI/functional iron deficiency)	Variable	Low TSAT, low-to-normal ferritin	IV*	Antagonist (if hepcidin levels are not low)

TSAT = transferrin saturation; PO = oral; IV = intravenous; CKD = chronic kidney disease; ESA = erythropoiesis-stimulating agent.
*Mixed anemia is a diagnosis of exclusion without a therapeutic trial of iron.
From [12].

evidence. Oncology patients whose CIA is treated with ESAs, furthermore, respond better to IV iron therapy than to oral supplementation [7, 13–19].

Table 1 illustrates various conditions where IV iron therapy may be warranted.

Despite beneficial effects in a wide range of patients, administration of IV iron may generate oxidative stress and other inflammatory changes, and the risk-benefit profile of IV iron continues to undergo evaluation in renal dialysis patients [20, 21], as well as patients with anemia due to other chronic diseases [22]. The long-term effects of IV iron preparations will require further study in relevant clinical settings, [23] as will the long-term deleterious effects of allogeneic blood transfusions [24–26].

IV iron preparations currently approved in the US are listed in Table 2 [8, 10, 27–36]. Beginning with the first iron dextran product introduced, the recommended cumulative replacement dose for many of these products has been approximately 1000 mg of iron [29–35].

A patient's total body iron deficit can be calculated using the Ganzoni formula (total iron dose = [actual body weight × (15-actual Hb)] × 2.4 + iron stores) [32]. Because many view this formula as inconvenient, it is not consistently used in clinical practice [37]. Although use of the Ganzoni formula is ideally the best way to select dose, it is impractical, partly because product labels state specific dosing regimens. In typical clinical practice, doses are more efficiently chosen based on approved product labels and local protocols, and only in the Dexferrum (iron dextran injection, USP) and INFeD (iron dextran injection, USP) prescribing information is a weight and Hb-based table available to calculate a patient's total iron requirement utilizing similar formula. There are also only a limited number of clinical practice guidelines regarding the use of a total cumulative repletion dose of IV iron in IDA patients, and, as mentioned above, the FDA-approved labeling for many IV iron products recommends a total cumulative dose of approximately 1000 mg. Currently, there is no consensus regarding the most appropriate iron deficit repletion dosing in patients with IDA, partly because

the iron dosing selected for virtually all trials has been based largely on clinical judgment, clinical guidelines in nephrology, or best estimates from past results. In this retrospective study, we systematically explored the iron deficit in patients who received IV iron in clinical studies and examined the potential benefits (i.e., normalization of Hb and time to retreatment with IV iron) of a higher cumulative dose of IV iron than what is typically administered, with the goal of providing clinicians with practical, evidence-based guidance for determining iron dosing requirements in a wide range of patients with IDA.

2. Materials and Methods

In this study, we used the same population recruited from previous clinical trials [38–44]. These studies adhered to US federal regulations and were performed in accordance with the Declaration of Helsinki and lastly protocols and informed consent forms were approved by local or national institutional review boards. All participants in these studies provided written informed consent. Patient records/information were anonymized and deidentified prior to analysis.

In Studies 1–5 (summarized below), each patient's iron deficit (mg) had been originally calculated and dose of iron administered, according to a modified Ganzoni formula: subject weight in kg × [15-current Hb g/dL] × 2.4 + 500, as specified in each study protocol. The Ganzoni formula had been modified for use in these studies to help alleviate any potential for iron overload in subjects who had a transferrin saturation (TSAT) >20% and ferritin >50 ng/mL at study entry. For these subjects, a conservative estimate was made, and the additional 500 mg from the formula to replete iron stores was not added to the total iron requirement. Each study administered IV iron (ferric carboxymaltose, FCM) as a total cumulative dose to randomized patients based upon the iron deficit so calculated. In analyzing each study, we utilized the baseline iron deficits for each patient using the same method and then averaged the total iron deficit across patients. These clinical studies examined IDA in postpartum

TABLE 2: Current FDA-approved intravenous iron preparations [8, 10, 27–36].

Trade name	Dexferrum (iron dextran injection, USP)	INFeD (iron dextran injection, USP)	Ferrlecit (sodium ferric gluconate complex in sucrose injection)	Venofer (iron sucrose injection, USP)	Feraheme (ferumoxytol)	Injectafer (ferric carboxymaltose injection)
Manufacturer	American Regent, Inc.	Actavis Pharma, Inc.	Sanofi-Aventis	American Regent, Inc.	AMAG Pharmaceuticals	American Regent, Inc.
Test dose	Yes	Yes	No	No	No	No
Black box warning	Yes	Yes	No	No	Yes	No
FDA-approved indications	Iron deficiency where oral iron administration is unsatisfactory or impossible	Iron deficiency where oral iron administration is unsatisfactory or impossible	Iron deficiency anemia in adult and pediatric CKD patients receiving hemodialysis and receiving ESAs	IDA in adult and pediatric patients with non-dialysis-dependent, hemodialysis dependent, and peritoneal dialysis-dependent CKD	IDA in adult patients with CKD	IDA in adult patients who have intolerance to oral iron or have had unsatisfactory response to oral iron or adult patients with non-dialysis-dependent CKD
Total cumulative dose	Dependent on patient's total iron requirement	Dependent on patient's total iron requirement	1000 mg	1000 mg	1020 mg	1500 mg

CKD = chronic kidney disease; ESA = erythropoiesis-stimulating agent; IDA = iron deficiency anemia.
American Regent, Inc., is the human drug division of Luitpold Pharmaceuticals, Inc., Shirley, NY.

TABLE 3: Average calculated iron deficit dose in clinical Studies 1–5.

Study	Patient population	Calculated mean iron deficit based on the modified Ganzoni formula* (mg)	Standard deviation	Number of patients
(1) van Wyck et al., 2007 [38]	Postpartum	1458	330	182
(2) van Wyck et al., 2009 [39]	Heavy uterine bleeding	1608	383	251
(3) Seid et al., 2008 [40]	Postpartum	1539	351	143
(4) Barish et al., 2012 [41]	IDA various etiologies	1520	342	348
(5) Hussain et al., 2013 [42]	IDA various etiologies	1508**	359	161
Overall mean		1531	NC	1085

IDA = iron deficiency anemia; NC = not calculated.
*Patients randomized to receive IV iron based on a calculated iron deficit.
**Including all randomized patients.
Data on file, Luitpold Pharmaceuticals, Inc.

patients, patients with heavy uterine bleeding (HUB), non-dialysis-dependent chronic kidney disease (NDD-CKD), GI disorders, and other underlying conditions.

Following are short descriptions of each study:

(1) Comparison of the safety and efficacy of IV iron (FCM) and oral iron (ferrous sulfate) in patients with postpartum anemia ($N = 361$) [38], NCT00396292.

(2) Comparison of the safety and efficacy of IV iron (FCM) and oral iron (ferrous sulfate) in the treatment of IDA secondary to HUB ($N = 477$) [39], NCT00395993.

(3) Comparison of the safety and efficacy of IV iron (FCM) and oral iron (ferrous sulfate) in the treatment of postpartum patients ($N = 291$) [40], NCT00354484.

(4) Comparison of the safety and tolerability of IV iron (FCM) and standard medical care (oral and IV iron) in treating IDA of various etiologies ($N = 708$) [41], NCT00703937.

(5) Comparison of the safety and tolerability of IV iron (FCM) and iron dextran in treating IDA of various etiologies ($N = 160$) [42], NCT00704028.

Following review of Studies 1–5, two larger studies (6 and 7) that utilized 1500 mg IV iron (as specified in the protocols) were examined. Although the modified Ganzoni formula was *not* specified in the protocols to determine dose requirements in these 2 studies, we did apply the formula to determine each patient's baseline iron deficit in a separate retrospective *post hoc* analysis of each study. We then averaged the total iron deficit across patients. Additionally, Study 7 compared the safety and efficacy of 1500 mg of IV iron (as FCM) to 1000 mg of IV iron (as iron sucrose [IS]) examining any potential efficacy or safety difference between the two dosing regimens.

A short summary of Studies 6 and 7 follows:

(6) Comparison of 1500 mg IV iron (FCM) with oral iron and IV iron standard of care (SoC) therapy (as determined by the investigator) in patients with IDA of various etiologies who had an unsatisfactory

response to oral iron or were deemed inappropriate for oral iron [43], NCT00982007.

(7) Comparison of the safety and efficacy of 1500 mg (FCM) to 1000 mg of IV iron (IS) in patients with IDA and NDD-CKD [44], NCT00981045.

Statistical Analysis. Baseline iron deficits in each clinical study were calculated for all subjects who were randomized to receive IV iron. In Study 5 [42], iron deficits were calculated for all subjects, as the comparator (iron dextran) was also dosed based on the modified Ganzoni formula and was summarized with descriptive statistics. For the iron deficit calculations performed for Studies 6 and 7, all subjects in the Safety Population were included. The iron deficits were averaged and the standard deviation was generated.

For Study 7, the Safety Population consisted of all subjects who received a dose of randomized treatment. The intent-to-treat (ITT) population for evaluating all efficacy endpoints consisted of all subjects from the Safety Population who received at least 1 dose of randomized study medication and had at least 1 postbaseline Hb assessment. Treatment assignments were analyzed according to the actual treatment received. The differences between 1500 mg and 1000 mg for time-to-event variables in Study 7 were assessed with the point estimate and 95% CI for the hazard ratio calculated from a Cox proportional hazards model. Treatment group differences were assessed using the Cox proportional hazards model with treatment as a fixed factor. In addition, p values for treatment differences were provided from the log-rank test. Time-to-event variables are displayed descriptively as Kaplan-Meier curves.

All statistical tests were *post hoc* with no adjustment to type I error for multiple comparisons.

3. Results

The average total iron deficits for patients in the 7 cited trials are summarized in Tables 3 and 4. The overall average total iron deficit in the initial 5 clinical trials was 1531 mg (Table 3). Total iron requirements among patients in each cohort in Studies 6 and 7 are summarized in Table 4. In Study 6, the average calculated iron deficit (Cohorts 1 and 2) was 1496 mg.

TABLE 4: Average calculated iron deficit dose in clinical Studies 6 and 7.

Study	Patient population	Treatment group	Calculated mean iron deficit based on the modified Ganzoni formula (mg)	Standard deviation	Number of patients	Total mean
Study 6	IDA of various etiologies	Cohort 1 (A): 1500 mg IV iron	1340	356	246	1496 mg
		Cohort 1 (B): oral iron	1344	360	253	
		Cohort 2 (C): 1500 mg IV iron	1600	446	252	
		Cohort 2 (D): IV SoC	1703	482	245	
Study 7 (REPAIR-IDA)	NDD-CKD	1500 mg IV iron	1355	401	1275	1352 mg
		1000 mg IV iron	1349	403	1285	
Overall mean			1392	NC	3556	

IDA = iron deficiency anemia; NDD-CKD = non-dialysis-dependent chronic kidney disease; SoC = standard of care; NC = not calculated.
Data on file, Luitpold Pharmaceuticals, Inc.

TABLE 5: Retreatment between Days 56–90 in clinical Study 7 (Safety Population).

	1500 mg IV iron ($n = 1276$)	1000 mg IV iron ($n = 1285$)	p value
N (%) patients retreated	71 (5.6%)	142 (11.1%)	$p < 0.001$

Data on file, Luitpold Pharmaceuticals, Inc.

TABLE 6: Hb >12 g/dL and end of treatment (Day 56) from clinical Study 7 (ITT population).

	1500 mg IV iron ($n = 1249$)	1000 mg IV iron ($n = 1244$)	p value
N (%) patients with Hb >12.0 g/dL	265 (24.4%)	169 (15.6%)	$p = 0.001$

Hb = hemoglobin; ITT = intent-to-treat.
Data on file, Luitpold Pharmaceuticals, Inc.

TABLE 7: Subjects with Hb >11 g/dL, 12 g/dL, or Hb change ≥1 g/dL in Study 7 anytime from randomization to end of study (Safety Population).

	1500 mg IV iron ($n = 1276$)	1000 mg IV iron ($n = 1244$)	Hazard ratio (95% CI)
N (%) of patients with Hb >11 g/dL	557 (56.1%)	504 (51.1%)	1.15 (1.02–1.30)
N (%) of patients with Hb >12 g/dL	358 (28.6%)	251 (20.0%)	1.44 (1.23–1.70)
N (%) of patients with Hb change ≥1 g/dL	610 (48.7%)	513 (41.0%)	1.27 (1.13–1.43)

Hb = hemoglobin.
Data on file, Luitpold Pharmaceuticals, Inc.

In Study 7, the average calculated iron deficit for patients receiving either 1500 mg or 1000 mg was 1352 mg. Overall, the average total iron deficit for clinical Studies 6 and 7 was 1392 mg.

In Study 7, study participants were randomized to receive either two 750 mg doses of IV iron (FCM) 7 days apart or IS 200 mg administered in up to 5 infusions over 14 days. The primary efficacy endpoint was the mean change in Hb from baseline to highest reported Hb (from baseline to Day 56). Patients were followed up for safety to Day 120. The mean total dose of iron received was 1464 mg in the 1500 mg group and 963 mg in the 1000 mg group. Mean baseline Hb values were 10.31 g/dL for the 1500 mg group and 10.32 g/dL for the 1000 mg group.

In this study, the mean increase in Hb overall was 1.13 g/dL in the 1500 mg group and 0.92 g/dL in the 1000 mg group (95% CI, 0.13–0.28), meeting the prespecified endpoint of noninferiority of 1500 mg to 1000 mg. Additionally, as evidenced by the 95% CI not including 0, 1500 mg was superior to 1000 mg in increasing Hb.

The proportion of patients in the 1500 mg group who were *retreated* with IV iron between Days 56 and 90 (Safety Population) was significantly ($p < 0.001$) lower, 71/1276 (5.6%), than the 142/1285 (11.1%) patients who required retreatment in the 1000 mg group (Table 5). Figure 1 displays the time from Day 56 to additional IV iron when comparing 1500 mg to 1000 mg.

Post hoc analyses of patients with Hb >12 g/dL at end of treatment (Day 56) and time to first Hb >11 g/dL and >12 g/dL and Hb increase ≥1 g/dL were conducted. The proportion of patients with Hb >12 g/dL at the end of treatment (baseline to Day 56) was 265/1249 in the 1500 mg group (24.4%) and 169/1244 in the 1000 mg group (15.6%), $p = 0.001$ (Table 6).

Patients who received 1500 mg IV iron were also more likely to achieve Hb >11 g/dL, Hb >12 g/dL, or an increase in Hb ≥1 g/dL compared with those receiving 1000 mg (Table 7).

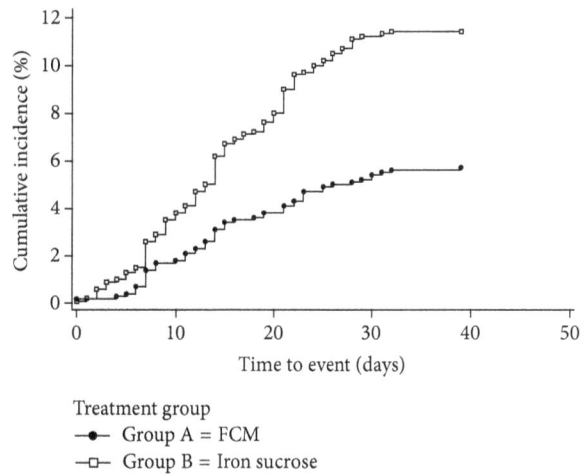

FIGURE 1: The time to additional intravenous (IV) iron after Day 56 comparing 1500 mg to 1000 mg IV iron in the Safety Population of Study 7. Data on file, Luitpold Pharmaceuticals, Inc.

Furthermore, the times to first Hb >11 g/dL and >12 g/dL and to Hb increases ≥1 g/dL were all statistically significantly shorter for the 1500 mg group than for the 1000 mg group ($p = 0.013$, $p < 0.001$, and $p < 0.001$, resp.). Figure 2 presents the Kaplan-Meier analysis for time to first Hb >12 g/dL.

The 1500 mg total cumulative dose had a similar safety profile to that of 1000 mg of IS, demonstrating that 50% more iron in the form of FCM can be administered while maintaining a safety profile comparable to that of IS [44].

4. Discussion

In the US, it has become common practice to administer a cumulative dose of approximately 1000 mg of IV iron (in

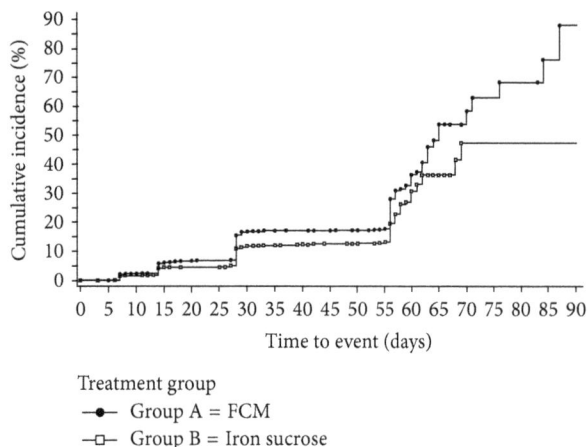

FIGURE 2: The time from randomization to first hemoglobin >12 g/dL in patients who received 1500 mg IV iron and patients who received 1000 mg from Study 7, $p < 0.001$. Day 56 is the last study visit, and at the discretion of the investigator, patients were allowed to be retreated with additional IV iron between Days 56 and 90. Data on file, Luitpold Pharmaceuticals, Inc.

divided doses) for the treatment of IDA. This is due, in large part, to the use of IV iron in nephrology. Both the Kidney Disease Outcomes Quality Initiative (KDOQI), initially developed in 1996, and the more recent Kidney Disease: Improving Global Outcomes (KDIGO) practice guidelines provide recommendations for the treatment of IDA utilizing IV iron. In the randomized controlled trials reviewed to develop the guidelines, a cumulative dose of 1000 mg of IV iron was utilized [45, 46]. Although that has now become the standard therapeutic dose for iron deficiency of various etiologies in light of a wealth of safety and efficacy data, it may not provide repletion of iron that is sufficient to alleviate the iron deficient state, thereby necessitating retreatment or creating the potential for a subtherapeutic response.

Despite these recommendations, in many clinical situations the treatment of IDA with IV iron has not been limited to a cumulative dose of 1000 mg. In oncology patients, for example, the National Comprehensive Cancer Network (NCCN) states that if the calculated dose exceeds 1000 mg, the remaining dose may be given after 4 weeks if the Hb response is inadequate [47].

Additionally, in two randomized controlled trials involving IV iron supplementation in oncology patients, a total of up to 3000 mg iron was administered in weekly doses of 100 mg [48]. In another prospective, randomized, controlled trial, patients with chemotherapy-related anemia received cumulative doses of IV iron ranging from 1000 to 3000 mg [7].

Guidelines for the management of IDA in inflammatory bowel disease (IBD), moreover, recommend IV iron as the preferred route of administration and state that anemic IBD patients rarely present with total iron deficits below 1000 mg. These guidelines recommend use of the Ganzoni formula to estimate iron replacement needs, and in controlled trials, up to 3600 mg of iron sucrose has been administered safely (up

to TSAT >50%) [49]. A 2011 review by Gozzard [50] further highlights numerous clinical situations requiring doses of IV iron above a cumulative dose of 1000 mg. Congruent with evidence reported in the international IBD guidelines, the article states that cumulative doses up to 3600 mg of IV iron may be administered safely in these patients. The review also suggests that higher doses of IV iron may overcome impaired iron absorption associated with hepcidin blockade in this patient population. In another multiple-dose, phase II/III study of IDA patients with GI disorders, mean total cumulative doses of 1800 mg IV iron were administered [51]. Clinical evidence also indicates that iron requirements of 1000 to 1500 mg or higher may be required in patients with NDD-CKD to attain target ferritin and Hb levels, up to 1600 mg may be required in obstetric patients, and as much as 2000 mg may be needed in patients with heavy or abnormal menstrual bleeding [50].

To help determine the optimal means of administering these higher doses, it is important to note that the degradation kinetics, and therefore the safety, of parenteral iron products are directly related to the molecular weight and stability of the iron complex [52–56].

Complexes can be generally classified as labile or robust (kinetic variability, i.e., how fast the ligands coordinated to the iron can be exchanged) and weak or strong (thermodynamic variability, i.e., how strongly the ligands are bound to the iron and thus how much energy is required to dissociate a ligand from the iron) or any intermediate state [52]. The reactivity of each complex correlates inversely with its molecular weight; larger complexes are less prone to release significant amounts of labile iron or react directly with transferrin [53, 54]. Type I complexes such as iron dextran preparations (INFeD Dexferrum) or FCM (Injectafer) have a high molecular weight and a high structural homogeneity and thereby deliver iron from the complex to transferrin in a regulated way via macrophage endocytosis and subsequent controlled export [52, 55]. They also bind iron tightly as nonionic polynuclear iron(III) hydroxide and do not release large amounts of iron ions into the blood. Such complexes can be administered intravenously and are clinically well tolerated even when administered at high doses. For less stable iron complexes, the maximum single doses are significantly lower and the administration times are drastically longer [54, 56].

FCM is a stable type I polynuclear iron(III) hydroxide carbohydrate complex that prevents the partial release of iron to serum ferritin observed with IS, allowing administration of high doses, since this iron is available only via reticuloendothelial processing [37, 57, 58]. FCM can be administered as a single 750 mg dose via a slow IV push injection over 7.5 minutes or as an IV infusion over at least 15 minutes. The second dose is administered at least 7 days later for a recommended cumulative dose of 1500 mg iron [36]. Use of high doses reduces the number of infusions, enabling the possibility of cost reductions compared to multiple administrations [59–62].

In our study, a modified Ganzoni formula was used to calculate total iron deficits in patients from 5 clinical studies involving FCM. After analyzing each study individually, we found the overall average iron deficit in those trials to be 1531 mg, suggesting that patients having IDA of various etiologies may benefit from a higher cumulative dose of IV iron than what is typically administered in clinical practice utilizing most of the currently available IV iron formulations.

Using the same modified Ganzoni formula, total iron deficits were also calculated in our *post hoc* analyses of the 2 larger studies (6 and 7) involving patients with IDA secondary to numerous underlying disorders, including HUB, GI diseases, and CKD. In Study 6, the average calculated iron deficit was 1496 mg. In Study 7, the average calculated iron deficit for patients receiving either 1500 mg IV iron, as FCM, or 1000 mg of IS was 1352 mg. The lower figure may be due to higher baseline ferritin and TSAT values in the CKD population, as 29% of the patients did not have the 500 mg of iron stores included in their iron deficit when it was calculated using the modified Ganzoni formula. Overall, the average calculated iron deficit in patients from Studies 6 and 7 was 1392 mg.

Data from Study 7 reinforced the benefits of higher IV iron dosing such that significantly fewer patients who received a total cumulative dose of 1500 mg of iron required IV iron retreatment during the follow-up period (Days 56–90) than those who received a total cumulative dose of 1000 mg. In addition, patients who received 1500 mg of iron achieved their first Hb >11 g/dL and >12 g/dL and a ≥1 g increase in Hb faster than those who received 1000 mg. This finding suggests that patients given 1000 mg may not be receiving a full repletion dose of iron compared to those given 1500 mg. Study 6 was not similarly analyzed because of confounders (i.e., small sample size and lack of consistent dosing for comparators). Despite patients in Cohort D (IV SoC) of that study having the highest mean calculated iron deficit (1703 mg), the mean amount of iron they received was paradoxically only 812 mg. This discrepancy between deficit and treatment in patients who received IV SoC may be due, in part, to convenience factors associated with the IV SoC dosing available to the investigators during the study, as well as the lack of practical guidance for determining iron dosing requirements.

In a study that compared the Ganzoni calculated dose to a simplified dose regimen, it was found that adherence was higher with the simplified dosing and resulted in better efficacy outcomes [59]. As a result, standard of care in Europe has moved from the Ganzoni calculation to a simple dosing scheme. In the US, most of the IV iron has a simple dosing scheme and the Ganzoni formula is not utilized as frequently, our study suggests that the simplified dosing scheme most often utilized may not fully replete the iron stores of the majority of patients.

Although the results of our study suggest that a total cumulative dose of IV iron greater than 1000 mg may be appropriate for many patients with IDA (we are aware of no similar published analyses), there are some limitations to consider. Parts of our analyses were retrospective in nature, and further prospective research will be needed to establish the long-term efficacy and safety of these higher total cumulative doses of IV iron. The population analyzed from Study 7 was limited to patients with CKD. Other etiologies of IDA may respond differently in relation to IV iron. In addition, most of the studies that evaluated the Ganzoni formula included patients with IDA resulting

from a variety of disease states. Also while, to the author's knowledge significant efficacy differences between similar cumulative doses of the various IV iron products have not been demonstrated, a future prospective study comparing various doses of the same product in a homogenous patient population would remove any product or population related bias that may have occurred in our study. It may be beneficial to observe whether higher or lower total cumulative doses of the same IV iron are more efficacious for patients with specific IDA etiologies.

5. Conclusions

Our study suggests that a total cumulative dose of 1000 mg of IV iron may be insufficient for iron repletion in the majority of patients with IDA and that a dose of 1500 mg is closer to the actual iron deficit in these patients. Additionally, 1500 mg of iron resulted in a more rapid, robust Hb response, allowed more patients to reach target Hb levels, and required a longer mean time to retreatment with additional IV iron compared to 1000 mg of iron. Our analysis and review of the literature suggest that 1500 mg of IV iron is more suitable for iron repletion in many patients with IDA compared to the commonly utilized dose of 1000 mg of IV iron. Further studies to confirm appropriate dose requirements in various patient populations are warranted.

Conflict of Interests

Lawrence Tim Goodnough is a consultant for Luitpold Pharmaceuticals, Inc. Jennifer Myers was an employee of Luitpold Pharmaceuticals, Inc. Todd A. Koch is an employee of Luitpold Pharmaceuticals, Inc.

Acknowledgments

The authors would like to thank David Morris, Ph.D. degree, for statistical input during the preparation of this paper, Andy He, PharmD, for publication management, and Aesculapius Consulting, Inc., for the editorial services.

References

[1] L. T. Goodnough, "The new age of iron: evaluation and management of iron-restricted erythropoiesis," *Seminars in Hematology*, vol. 46, no. 4, pp. 325–327, 2009.

[2] B. Annibale, G. Capurso, A. Chistolini et al., "Gastrointestinal causes of refractory iron deficiency anemia in patients without gastrointestinal symptoms," *The American Journal of Medicine*, vol. 111, no. 6, pp. 439–445, 2001.

[3] P. L. Acher, T. Al-Mishlab, M. Rahman, and T. Bates, "Iron-deficiency anaemia and delay in the diagnosis of colorectal cancer," *Colorectal Disease*, vol. 5, no. 2, pp. 145–148, 2003.

[4] D. Raje, H. Mukhtar, A. Oshowo, and C. Ingham Clark, "What proportion of patients referred to secondary care with iron deficiency anemia have colon cancer?" *Diseases of the Colon and Rectum*, vol. 50, no. 8, pp. 1211–1214, 2007.

[5] M. Auerbach, J. A. Pappadakis, H. Bahrain, S. A. Auerbach, H. Ballard, and N. V. Dahl, "Safety and efficacy of rapidly

administered (one hour) one gram of low molecular weight iron dextran (INFeD) for the treatment of iron deficient anemia," *American Journal of Hematology*, vol. 86, no. 10, pp. 860–862, 2011.

[6] L. T. Goodnough, E. Nemeth, and T. Ganz, "Detection, evaluation, and management of iron-restricted erythropoiesis," *Blood*, vol. 116, no. 23, pp. 4754–4761, 2010.

[7] M. Auerbach, H. Ballard, J. R. Trout et al., "Intravenous iron optimizes the response to recombinant human erythropoietin in cancer patients with chemotherapy-related anemia: a multicenter, open-label, randomized trial," *Journal of Clinical Oncology*, vol. 22, no. 7, pp. 1301–1307, 2004.

[8] M. Auerbach, "Ferumoxytol as a new, safer, easier-to-administer intravenous iron: yes or no?" *The American Journal of Kidney Diseases*, vol. 52, no. 5, pp. 826–829, 2008.

[9] J. Bonnar, A. Goldberg, and J. A. Smith, "Do pregnant women take their iron?" *The Lancet*, vol. 1, no. 7592, pp. 457–458, 1969.

[10] G. Weiss and L. T. Goodnough, "Anemia of chronic disease," *The New England Journal of Medicine*, vol. 352, no. 10, pp. 1011–1059, 2005.

[11] N. C. Andrews, "Anemia of inflammation: the cytokine-hepcidin link," *Journal of Clinical Investigation*, vol. 113, no. 9, pp. 1251–1253, 2004.

[12] L. T. Goodnough and A. Shander, "Current status of pharmacologic therapies in patient blood management," *Anesthesia & Analgesia*, vol. 116, no. 1, pp. 15–34, 2013.

[13] D. H. Henry, N. V. Dahl, M. Auerbach, S. Tchekmedyian, and L. R. Laufmane, "Intravenous ferric gluconate significantly improves response to epoetin alfa versus oral iron or no iron in anemic patients with cancer receiving chemotherapy," *Oncologist*, vol. 12, no. 2, pp. 231–242, 2007.

[14] M. Hedenus, G. Birgegard, P. Nasman et al., "Addition of intravenous iron to epoetin beta increases hemoglobin response and decreases epoetin dose requirement in anemic patients with lymphoproliferative malignancies: a randomized multicenter study," *Leukemia*, vol. 21, no. 4, pp. 627–632, 2007.

[15] L. Bastit, A. Vandebroek, S. Altintas et al., "Randomized, multicenter, controlled trial comparing the efficacy and safety of darbepoetin alfa administered every 3 weeks with or without intravenous iron in patients with chemotherapy-induced anemia," *Journal of Clinical Oncology*, vol. 26, no. 10, pp. 1611–1618, 2008.

[16] A. Gafter-Gvili, D. P. Steensma, and M. Auerbach, "Should the ASCO/ASH guidelines for the use of intravenous iron in cancer- and chemotherapy-induced anemia be updated?" *Journal of the National Comprehensive Cancer Network*, vol. 12, no. 5, pp. 657–664, 2014.

[17] J. A. Gilreath, D. D. Stenehjem, and G. M. Rodgers, "Diagnosis and treatment of cancer-related anemia," *American Journal of Hematology*, vol. 89, no. 2, pp. 203–212, 2014.

[18] M. Auerbach, A. S. Liang, and J. Glaspy, "Intravenous iron in chemotherapy and cancer-related anemia," *Community Oncology*, vol. 9, no. 9, pp. 289–295, 2012.

[19] J. D. Rizzo, M. Brouwers, P. Hurley, J. Seidenfeld, M. R. Somerfield, and S. Temin, "American Society of Clinical Oncology/American Society of Hematology clinical practice guideline update on the use of epoetin and darbepoetin in adult patients with cancer," *Journal of Oncology Practice*, vol. 6, no. 6, pp. 317–320, 2010.

[20] D. S. Silverberg, A. Iaina, G. Peer et al., "Intravenous iron supplementation for the treatment of the anemia of moderate to severe chronic renal failure patients not receiving dialysis," *American Journal of Kidney Diseases*, vol. 27, no. 2, pp. 234–238, 1996.

[21] R. S. Hillman and P. A. Henderson, "Control of marrow production by the level of iron supply," *Journal of Clinical Investigation*, vol. 48, no. 3, pp. 454–460, 1969.

[22] R. L. Jurado, "Iron, infections, and anemia of inflammation," *Clinical Infectious Diseases*, vol. 25, no. 4, pp. 888–895, 1997.

[23] K. Bishu and R. Agarwal, "Acute injury with intravenous iron and concerns regarding long-term safety," *Clinical Journal of the American Society of Nephrology*, supplement 1, pp. S19–S23, 2006.

[24] L. T. Goodnough, J. H. Levy, and M. F. Murphy, "Concepts of blood transfusion in adults," *The Lancet*, vol. 381, no. 9880, pp. 1845–1854, 2013.

[25] D. R. Spahn and L. T. Goodnough, "Alternatives to blood transfusion," *The Lancet*, vol. 381, no. 9880, pp. 1855–1865, 2013.

[26] L. T. Goodnough, "Blood management: transfusion medicine comes of age," *The Lancet*, vol. 381, no. 9880, pp. 1791–1792, 2013.

[27] A. Shander, R. K. Spence, and M. Auerbach, "Can intravenous iron therapy meet the unmet needs created by the new restrictions on erythropoietic stimulating agents?: report from the Society for the Advancement of Blood Management 2008 Annual Meeting," *Transfusion*, vol. 50, no. 3, pp. 719–732, 2010.

[28] M. Auerbach, L. T. Goodnough, D. Picard, and A. Maniatis, "The role of intravenous iron in anemia management and transfusion avoidance," *Transfusion*, vol. 48, no. 5, pp. 988–1000, 2008.

[29] G. M. Chertow, P. D. Mason, O. Vaage-Nilsen, and J. Ahlmén, "Update on adverse drug events associated with parenteral iron," *Nephrology Dialysis Transplantation*, vol. 21, no. 2, pp. 378–382, 2006.

[30] Dexferrum [package insert], American Regent, Shirley, NY, USA, 2008.

[31] INFeD, *Package Insert*, Watson Pharma, Morristown, NJ, USA, 2009.

[32] A. M. Ganzoni, "Intravenous iron-dextran: therapeutic and experimental possibilities," *Schweizerische Medizinische Wochenschrift*, vol. 100, no. 7, pp. 301–303, 1970.

[33] American Regent, *Venofer [Package Insert]*, American Regent, Shirley, NY, USA, 2012.

[34] Ferrlecit, *Package Insert*, Sanofi-Aventis US, Bridgewater, NJ, USA, 2011.

[35] Feraheme [package insert], AMAG Pharmaceuticals, Lexington, Mass, USA, 2015.

[36] American Regent, *Injectafer [Package Insert]*, American Regent, Shirley, NY, USA, 2013.

[37] S. Kulnigg, S. Stoinov, V. Simanenkov et al., "A novel intravenous iron formulation for treatment of anemia in inflammatory bowel disease: the ferric carboxymaltose (FERINJECT) randomized controlled trial," *The American Journal of Gastroenterology*, vol. 103, no. 5, pp. 1182–1192, 2008.

[38] D. B. van Wyck, M. G. Martens, M. H. Seid, J. B. Baker, and A. Mangione, "Intravenous ferric carboxymaltose compared with oral iron in the treatment of postpartum anemia: a randomized controlled trial," *Obstetrics and Gynecology*, vol. 110, no. 2, pp. 267–278, 2007.

[39] D. B. van Wyck, A. Mangione, J. Morrison, P. E. Hadley, J. A. Jehle, and L. T. Goodnough, "Large-dose intravenous ferric carboxymaltose injection for iron deficiency anemia in heavy

uterine bleeding: a randomized, controlled trial," *Transfusion*, vol. 49, no. 12, pp. 2719–2728, 2009.

[40] M. H. Seid, R. J. Derman, J. B. Baker, W. Banach, C. Goldberg, and R. Rogers, "Ferric carboxymaltose injection in the treatment of postpartum iron deficiency anemia: a randomized controlled clinical trial," *American Journal of Obstetrics & Gynecology*, vol. 199, no. 4, pp. 435.e1–435.e7, 2008.

[41] C. F. Barish, T. Koch, A. Butcher, D. Morris, and D. B. Bregman, "Safety and efficacy of intravenous ferric carboxymaltose (750 mg) in the treatment of iron deficiency anemia: two randomized, controlled trials," *Anemia*, vol. 2012, Article ID 172104, 9 pages, 2012.

[42] I. Hussain, J. Bhoyroo, A. Butcher, T. A. Koch, A. He, and D. B. Bregman, "Direct comparison of the safety and efficacy of ferric carboxymaltose versus iron dextran in patients with iron deficiency anemia," *Anemia*, vol. 2013, Article ID 169107, 10 pages, 2013.

[43] J. E. Onken, D. B. Bregman, R. A. Harrington et al., "A multicenter, randomized, active-controlled study to investigate the efficacy and safety of intravenous ferric carboxymaltose in patients with iron deficiency anemia," *Transfusion*, vol. 54, no. 2, pp. 306–315, 2014.

[44] J. E. Onken, D. B. Bregman, R. A. Harrington et al., "Ferric carboxymaltose in patients with iron-deficiency anemia and impaired renal function: the REPAIR-IDA trial," *Nephrology Dialysis Transplantation*, vol. 29, no. 4, pp. 833–842, 2014.

[45] National Kidney Foundation. KDOQI, "Clinical practice guidelines and clinical practice recommendations for anemia in chronic kidney disease," *American Journal of Kidney Diseases*, vol. 47, supplement 3, pp. S1–S145, 2006.

[46] Kidney Disease: Improving Global Outcomes (KDIGO) Anemia Work Group, "KDIGO clinical practice guideline for anemia in chronic kidney disease," *Kidney International Supplements*, vol. 2, no. 4, pp. S279–S335, 2012.

[47] National Comprehensive Cancer Network (NCCN), *Clinical Practice Guidelines in Oncology. Cancer- and Chemotherapy-Induced Anemia. Version 2*, NCCN, 2015.

[48] M. Aapro, A. Österborg, P. Gascón, H. Ludwig, and Y. Beguin, "Prevalence and management of cancer-related anaemia, iron deficiency and the specific role of I.V. iron," *Annals of Oncology*, vol. 23, no. 8, pp. 1954–1962, 2012.

[49] C. Gasche, A. Berstad, R. Befrits et al., "Guidelines on the diagnosis and management of iron deficiency and anemia in inflammatory bowel diseases," *Inflammatory Bowel Diseases*, vol. 13, no. 12, pp. 1545–1553, 2007.

[50] D. Gozzard, "When is high-dose intravenous iron repletion needed? Assessing new treatment options," *Drug Design, Development and Therapy*, no. 5, pp. 51–60, 2011.

[51] P. Geisser and V. Rumyantsev, "Pharmacodynamics and safety of ferric carboxymaltose: a multiple-dose study in patients with iron-deficiency anaemia secondary to a gastrointestinal disorder," *Arzneimittelforschung*, vol. 60, no. 6, pp. 373–385, 2010.

[52] R. R. Crichton, B. Danielson, and P. Geisser, *Iron Therapy with Special Emphasis on Intravenous Administration*, UNI-MED, Bremen, Germany, 4th edition, 2008.

[53] B. G. Danielson, "Structure, chemistry, and pharmacokinetics of intravenous iron agents," *Journal of the American Society of Nephrology*, vol. 15, no. 2, pp. S93–S98, 2004.

[54] P. Geisser, M. Baer, and E. Schaub, "Structure/histotoxicity relationship of parenteral iron preparations," *Drug Research*, vol. 42, no. 12, pp. 1439–1452, 1992.

[55] S. Beshara, H. Lundqvist, J. Sundin et al., "Pharmacokinetics and red cell utilization of iron(III) hydroxide-sucrose complex in anaemic patients: a study using positron emission tomography," *British Journal of Haematology*, vol. 104, no. 2, pp. 296–302, 1999.

[56] P. Geisser and S. Burckhardt, "The pharmacokinetics and pharmacodynamics of iron preparations," *Pharmaceutics*, vol. 3, no. 1, pp. 12–33, 2011.

[57] M. Malone, C. Barish, A. He, and D. Bregman, "Comparative review of the safety and efficacy of ferric carboxymaltose versus standard medical care for the treatment of iron deficiency anemia in bariatric and gastric surgery patients," *Obesity Surgery*, vol. 23, no. 9, pp. 1413–1420, 2013.

[58] K. A. Lyseng-Williamson and G. M. Keating, "Ferric carboxymaltose: a review of its use in iron-deficiency anaemia," *Drugs*, vol. 69, no. 6, pp. 739–756, 2009.

[59] R. Evstatiev, P. Marteau, T. Iqbal et al., "FERGIcor, a randomized controlled trial on ferric carboxymaltose for iron deficiency anemia in inflammatory bowel disease," *Gastroenterology*, vol. 141, no. 3, pp. 846.e2–853.e2, 2011.

[60] X. Calvet, M. À. Ruíz, A. Dosal et al., "Cost-minimization analysis favours intravenous ferric carboxymaltose over ferric sucrose for the ambulatory treatment of severe iron deficiency," *PLoS ONE*, vol. 7, no. 9, Article ID e45604, 2012.

[61] F. Gomollón and J. P. Gisbert, "Current management of iron deficiency anemia in inflammatory bowel diseases: a practical guide," *Drugs*, vol. 73, no. 16, pp. 1761–1770, 2013.

[62] A. A. Khalafallah and A. E. Dennis, "Iron deficiency anaemia in pregnancy and postpartum: pathophysiology and effect of oral versus intravenous iron therapy," *Journal of Pregnancy*, vol. 2012, Article ID 630519, 10 pages, 2012.

6

Iron Deficiency Anemia in Adult Onset Still's Disease with a Serum Ferritin of 26,387 μg/L

Sheetal Patel,[1] Seyed Monemian,[2] Ayesha Khalid,[1] and Harvey Dosik[3, 4]

[1] Department of Internal Medicine, New York Methodist Hospital, 506 Sixth Street, Brooklyn, NY 11215, USA
[2] Division of Hematology-Oncology, Department of Internal Medicine, New York Methodist Hospital, 506 Sixth Street, Brooklyn, NY 11215, USA
[3] Division of Hematology, Department of Internal Medicine, New York Methodist Hospital, 506 Sixth Street, Brooklyn, NY 11215, USA
[4] Weill Cornell Medical College of Cornell University, 1300 York Avenue, New York, NY 10065, USA

Correspondence should be addressed to Sheetal Patel, sheetal306@gmail.com

Academic Editor: Aurelio Maggio

Serum ferritin rises in the anemia of chronic inflammation reflecting increased iron storage and other changes mediated by inflammation. When iron deficiency coexists, the ferritin may not always decline into the subnormal range. We describe the rare interaction of iron deficiency with the extreme hyperferritinemia characteristic of adult onset Still's disease. The combination has clinical relevance and allows deductions about the presence of serum ferritin at 26,387 μg/L despite obvious iron depletion. The diagnosis of iron deficiency anemia was delayed and became fully obvious when her Still's disease remitted and serum ferritin decreased to 6.5 μg/L. The coexistence of iron deficiency should be considered when evaluating a patient with anemia of chronic inflammation even when the ferritin level is elevated several hundredfold. Further insights on ferritin metabolism in Still's disease are suggested by the likelihood that the patient's massive hyperferritinemia in the acute phase of Still's disease was almost entirely of the iron-free apoferritin form.

1. Introduction

In the anemia of chronic inflammation, iron metabolism is disturbed and the serum ferritin usually rises moderately, achieving mean levels such as 300–400 μg/L [1]. In this setting, it has become clear that ferritin criteria often must be relaxed to allow the recognition of coexisting iron deficiency in patients who have chronic inflammation [2, 3]. Indeed, ferritin levels less than 100 μg/L may be viewed with suspicion in a patient with inflammatory disease [4]. We describe an extreme manifestation of this situation in a patient with the massive hyperferritinemia of adult onset Still's disease. This illustrates the need for diagnostic flexibility in special disorders, and it provides further insight into the likelihood that ferritin metabolism is both qualitatively and quantitatively disturbed in Still's disease to an unusual extent.

2. Case Report

A 38-year-old Haitian woman was admitted to the hospital with a five-day history of evanescent salmon-colored maculopapular rash, generalized fatigue, and joint stiffness worsening. Associated symptoms included high spiking fevers, nausea, vomiting, and decreased appetite. She denied weight loss, infectious contacts, or recent travel.

Two weeks earlier, she had visited our emergency department (ED) twice. On the first visit, she had a similar salmon-colored rash on her neck, legs, and forearm and was given diphenhydramine. Several days later, she visited the ED because of generalized fatigue and joint stiffness, mainly involving both knees, elbows, and wrists. She was again discharged receiving acetaminophen this time. The patient's joint stiffness, generalized fatigue, and rash persisted, however. Additionally, she developed very high fevers, which now mandated her admission to the hospital.

TABLE 1: Hematological data.

| | Hospitalization | | | | | |
	Day 0**	Day 6	Day 7	Day 10	6 months later[†]	10 months later
Hgb g/dL (12–16)*	10.3	9.2	8.9	9.3	9.2	11.9
MCV fl (80–94)*	67	68	68	70	70	81
Ferritin μg/L (13–150)*	26,387	1,365	1,095	835	6.5	35
Iron μg/dL (45–160)*	49				14	48
TIBC μg/dL (240–450)*	215				306	244
Iron saturation % (20–55)*	23%				5%	20%

**Adult onset Still's disease was diagnosed and methylprednisolone treatment started.
[†]Treatment was started for iron deficiency anemia.
*Normal ranges are shown in parentheses.

Her past history was otherwise unremarkable. However, she had also been having heavy menstrual periods, averaging 7 days per cycle for the past several years. She described a craving for cornstarch and clay since her last pregnancy 5 years ago. She denied blood in her stool and had never been tested for parasites while in Haiti. There was no family history of anemia or bleeding disorders.

Her physical examination revealed posterior cervical lymphadenopathy and a maculopapular rash involving the neck. Furthermore, warmth and tenderness of the wrist, elbows, and ankle joints were appreciated. The stool was negative for occult blood.

Pertinent laboratory values on admission were a low hemoglobin (Hgb) (10.3 g/dL), low MCV (67 fl), normal platelet count (272 k/uL), mildly elevated white blood cell count (10.3 k/uL), high RDW (18.3%), and low absolute reticulocyte count (14.2 k/uL). C-reactive protein (139 mg/L) and erythrocyte sedimentation rate (79 mm/hr) were markedly elevated. A comprehensive metabolic panel was normal except for marginally elevated serum aspartate transaminase (72 u/L). Antinuclear antibody (ANA) and rheumatoid factor (RF) were negative. An extensive workup for rheumatologic and infectious processes was done and found to be negative. The serum ferritin level was found to be 26,387 μg/L (normal 13–150 μg/L). Serum iron was 49 μg/dL, total iron binding capacity 215 μg/dL, and iron saturation 23%.

The patient's high grade fevers with persistent rash led to a diagnosis of adult onset Still's disease by Yamaguchi's criteria [5], and her marked hyperferritinemia was compatible with the diagnosis. Subsequently, she was given intravenous methylprednisolone with good response. As her fever subsided, the serum ferritin level initially declined steeply within 6 days and then steadily decreased (Table 1). Her anemia at that time was attributed to her inflammation. She was discharged with tapering doses of oral prednisone.

At her scheduled visit to a hematologist six months later, there was complete resolution of her inflammatory symptoms. Her laboratory data now showed a serum ferritin of 6.5 ng/mL (Table 1). Her Hgb was 9.2 g/dL, MCV 70 fl, serum iron 14 ug/dL, total iron binding capacity 306 ug/dL, and iron saturation 5%. A hemoglobin electrophoresis was normal (Hgb A 97.5%, Hgb A2 2.5%) excluding β-thalassemia. These laboratory values now indicated obvious iron deficiency anemia, for which she was subsequently treated with ferrous sulfate 325 mg three times a day. When seen 4 months later after starting iron therapy, her blood count and iron studies had returned to normal and her pica resolved (Table 1).

3. Discussion

Anemia of chronic inflammation features a network of intracellular absorptive and plasma iron changes that are mediated by hepcidin. Ferritin is often moderately elevated (Table 2) reflecting the fact that increased iron is retained in intracellular stores causing serum ferritin to rise as an acute phase reactant [6–9]. In the presence of coexisting iron deficiency anemia, the serum ferritin often remains modestly elevated despite the iron depletion. In the setting of anemia of chronic inflammation, extra leeway is often allowed when assessing serum ferritin levels if a diagnosis of superimposed iron deficiency anemia is suspected [10].

Our patient is unique because of a heretofore undescribed partial masking of coexisting iron deficiency anemia by the extreme hyperferritinemia which is typical for adult onset Still's disease [11]. Although multiple biomarkers such as C-reactive protein reflect the systemic inflammatory nature of Still's disease, none are specific for it. Serum ferritin is considered a useful diagnostic and disease activity marker for Still's disease, however. The serum ferritin levels are usually higher than in any other autoimmune or inflammatory disease and very high levels between 3,000–30,000 μg/L are not uncommon (Table 2) [12]. A cutoff for ferritin levels of 1,000 μg/L has been used to indicate Still's disease in many studies [12, 13].

Despite the extreme initial hyperferritinemia of 26,387 μ/L, iron deficiency anemia was eventually recognized in our patient. Her iron-deficiency anemia had likely been present for many years as she described pica (which is not unusual in iron deficient women) for the past 5 years. A longstanding microcytosis, with an MCV as low as 67, anisocytosis with a high RDW, and a history of menorrhagia, give further credence to a diagnosis of coexisting iron deficiency anemia. Only after her Still's disease was put in remission did her serum ferritin achieve the subnormal levels diagnostic for iron deficiency anemia.

TABLE 2: Ferritin levels in published surveys of inflammatory conditions.

Diagnosis	Ferritin (μg/L)*	
	Range	Mean ± SD
Rheumatoid arthritis [6]		90 ± 123
Inflammatory bowel disease ($n = 45$) [7]	(34–650)	
SLE ($n = 128$) [6]		436 ± 1,186
Dermatomyositis/polymyositis ($n = 9$) [8]		1,097 ± 1,827
Acute hepatitis ($n = 5$) [8]		1,347 ± 861
Hemophagocytic syndrome ($n = 7$) [8]		8,485 ± 8,388
Autoimmune hepatitis ($n = 1$) [8]		11,262
Adult onset still's disease ($n = 9$) [9]	(400–27,000)	13,910 ± 3,640

* Mean ± SD.
n = Number of patients reported.

Although iron metabolism is complicated and many details of the qualitative ferritin changes in inflammatory disease are still unknown and we saw the patient only after her Still's disease and extreme hyperferritinemia resolved, a few observations may be noted that are relevant to the changes, their interaction with iron deficiency anemia, and how they might be modified in the extreme example of adult onset Still's disease.

Using the formula equating serum ferritin with iron stores in the normal state (1 μg/L of serum ferritin = 8–10 mg of storage iron), our patient would be calculated to have 211 g of storage iron [14]. Yet this is clearly impossible even in persons with typical anemia of chronic inflammation, in whom the equation probably requires variable but modest modification. In Still's disease, even without iron deficiency, the equation obviously does not hold. In our patient with coexisting iron deficiency anemia and thus no available iron stores, it becomes clear that the extreme elevation of ferritin bears no relationship to body iron stores whatsoever. It is highly likely that her ferritin was virtually devoid of iron.

Ferritin normally consists of H and L isoforms. The H form is found in the heart, and the L form is found in the liver and formed during inflammation by the histiocyte-macrophage system. The L isoform holds less iron and is likely the form increased by cytokine-mediated ferritin release in Still's disease [11]. Ferritin glycosylation is also abnormal in patients with Still's disease. Glycosylation typically serves many roles, such as transport and protection of serum ferritin from proteolytic enzymes [13]. Healthy patients have 50–80% of their total serum ferritin glycosylated and this fraction falls to 20–50% in patients with inflammatory conditions [13, 15]. Whether our unique patient's serum ferritin has consisted even more disproportionately of the L isoform, was exclusively apoferritin, and had even more abnormal ferritin glycosylation than usual in Still's disease is unknown because we did not see her until her serum ferritin was nearly undetectable.

To our knowledge, this is the first documented case report of iron deficiency anemia in Still's disease with such an elevated ferritin. However, based on the usual predominance of Still's disease in women of menstruating age, one would wonder whether this is a more common phenomenon that is often undiagnosed. It is worthwhile for physicians to bear this in mind and look for clues such as disproportionate degree of microcytosis when evaluating patients with Still's disease.

References

[1] J. Prchal, "Anemia of chronic diease," in Williams Hematology, M. A. Lichtman, T. J. Kipps, K. Kaushansky, E. Beutler, U. Seligsohn, and J. Prchal, Eds., pp. 566–567, McGraw Hill Medical, New York, NY, USA, 7th edition, 2006.

[2] M. A. Knovich, J. A. Storey, L. G. Coffman, S. V. Torti, and F. M. Torti, "Ferritin for the clinician," Blood Reviews, vol. 23, no. 3, pp. 95–104, 2009.

[3] D. Coyne, "Iron indices: what do they really mean?" Kidney International, vol. 69, pp. S4–S8, 2006.

[4] E. Beutler, A. V. Hoffbrand, and J. D. Cook, "Iron deficiency and overload," Hematology, pp. 40–61, 2003.

[5] M. Yamaguchi, A. Ohta, T. Tsunematsu et al., "Preliminary criteria for classification of adult Still's disease," Journal of Rheumatology, vol. 19, no. 3, pp. 424–430, 1992.

[6] M. K. Lim, C. K. Lee, Y. S. Ju et al., "Serum ferritin as a serologic marker of activity in systemic lupus erythematosus," Rheumatology International, vol. 20, no. 3, pp. 89–93, 2001.

[7] A. B. R. Thomson, R. Brust, M. A. M. Ali, M. J. Mant, and L. S. Valberg, "Iron deficiency in inflammatory bowel disease. Diagnostic efficacy of serum ferritin," Digestive Diseases and Sciences, vol. 23, no. 8, pp. 705–709, 1978.

[8] Y. Kirino, M. Takeno, M. Iwasaki et al., "Increased serum HO-1 in hemophagocytic syndrome and adult-onset Still's disease: use in the differential diagnosis of hyperferritinemia," Arthritis Research & Therapy, vol. 7, no. 3, pp. R616–R624, 2005.

[9] N. Akritidis, Y. Giannakakis, and L. Sakkas, "Very high serum ferritin levels in adult-onset Still's disease," British Journal of Rheumatology, vol. 36, no. 5, pp. 608–609, 1997.

[10] L. Hallberg, C. Bengtsson, L. Lapidus, G. Lindstedt, P. A. Lundberg, and L. Hulten, "Screening for iron deficiency: an analysis based on bone-marrow examinations and serum ferritin determinations in a population sample of women," British Journal of Haematology, vol. 85, no. 4, pp. 787–798, 1993.

[11] W. Wang, M. A. Knovich, L. G. Coffman, F. M. Torti, and S. V. Torti, "Serum ferritin: past, present and future," Biochimica et Biophysica Acta, vol. 1800, no. 8, pp. 760–769, 2010.

[12] V. Bagnari, M. Colina, G. Ciancio, M. Govoni, and F. Trotta, "Adult-onset Still's disease," *Rheumatology International*, vol. 30, no. 7, pp. 855–862, 2010.

[13] B. Fautrel, "Ferritin levels in adult Still's disease: any sugar?" *Joint Bone Spine*, vol. 69, no. 4, pp. 355–357, 2002.

[14] M. Tarek Elghetany and K. Banki, "Erythrocytic disorders," in *Henry's Clinical Diagnosis and Management by Laboratory Methods*, R. McPherson and M. Pincus, Eds., p. 506, Saunders Elsevier, Philadelphia, Pa, USA, 21st edition, 2007.

[15] B. Fautrel, G. Le Moël, B. Saint-Marcoux et al., "Diagnostic value of ferritin and glycosylated ferritin in adult onset Still's disease," *Journal of Rheumatology*, vol. 28, no. 2, pp. 322–329, 2001.

7

Effects of Iron Deficiency on Cognitive Function in School Going Adolescent Females in Rural Area of Central India

Sarika More,[1] V. B. Shivkumar,[2] Nitin Gangane,[2] and Sumeet Shende[3]

[1] Department of Pathology, Sri Lakshmi Narayana Institute of Medical Sciences, Osudu, Kudapakkam Post, Villanur Communie, Pondicherry 605502, India
[2] Department of Pathology, Mahatma Gandhi Institute of Medical Sciences, Sevagram, Maharashtra, India
[3] Department of Forensic Medicine, Sri Lakshmi Narayana Institute of Medical Sciences, Pondicherry 605502, India

Correspondence should be addressed to Sarika More; dr.sarikamore@rediffmail.com

Academic Editor: Eitan Fibach

Iron deficiency anemia is most common nutritional deficiency disorder in India and remains a formidable health challenge. Girls in the period of later school age and early adolescence are prone to develop iron deficiency. Iron deficiency leads to many non-hematological disturbances which include growth and development, depressed immune function in infants; reduces physical work capacity; decreases the cognitive function in both infants and adolescents. Present study was done to know the prevalence of iron deficiency in both the anemic and non anemic school going adolescent girls, to assess the effect of iron deficiency on cognitive functions in anemic iron deficient and non-anemic iron deficient school girls in a village school situated in central India. *Methods.* A secondary school having girl students in the age group of 12–15 years studying in sixth to ninth standard was selected. Serum ferritin concentration was estimated by ELISA. For assessing the cognitive function mathematics score, one multi-component test for memory, attention and verbal learning and Intelligent Quotient scores of the students were used. *Results.* Scholastic Performance, IQ and Scores of Mental balance, Attention & Concentration, Verbal Memory and Recognition were decreased in iron deficient girls, both anemic and non anemic as compared to the non iron deficient girls.

1. Introduction

Iron deficiency is the third greatest global health risk after obesity and unsafe sex [1]. Anemia resulting from iron deficiency affects approximately 2 billion people or 34% of the world population [2]. Iron deficiency anemia most severe stage of iron deficiency (defined as a low hemoglobin concentration with iron deficiency) was found in 3% of the adolescent females in the United State of America [3].

Iron deficiency has both physiologic and pathologic causes. Physiologic causes relate to the greater iron demands during periods of growth and development whereas pathologic causes refer to iron losses secondary to a chronic medical condition. In general, iron deficiency results when iron demands by the body are not met by iron absorption. Thus, iron deficiency can result from inadequate intake, impaired absorption, increased requirements, and chronic blood loss.

More than half of the world's undernourished population lives in India [4] and half of Indian children and women are malnourished [5]. Apart from overall poverty and lower literacy rate the health status of women in India reflects gender discrimination from birth [6]. Intrafamilial food distribution, where the males are privileged with high quality nutritious food and the females are deprived of it, is seen in India. Moreover, early and frequent reproductive cycling and presence of reproductive tract infections in adolescent girls lead to iron deficiency anemia [7]. Among females, menstrual blood loss becomes an issue and heavy loss (>80 mL/month) is a significant risk factor. Menstrual blood loss averages about 20 mg of iron per month and in some individuals be as high as 58 mg [8]. In spite of increased iron needs many adolescent girls have iron intake of only 10-11 mg/day, resulting in approximately 1 mg of absorption of iron. About three fourth of adolescent females do not meet the dietary requirements [8].

Iron deficiency is a systemic condition which has many non ematological consequences, which occurs in relation to its severity, like decreased physical work capacity [9], decreased athletic performance [10], lowered indurations [11], depressed immune function [12], decreased scholastic performance, compromised growth and development, and increased risk of pregnancy complication including prematurity and total growth retardation and impaired cognitive function [13–15].

In present study, effort has been made to assess the effect of iron deficiency on cognitive functions in anemic iron deficient and in nonanemic iron deficient school going adolescent girls in a village school.

2. Materials and Methods

The present study was carried out in the Department of Pathology, MGIMS, Sevagram, India from July 2007 to September 2009. Approval was obtained from the Institutional Ethics Committee for the study.

2.1. Selection of Subjects. A secondary school in the neighborhood, having girl students in the age group of 12–15 years studying in sixth to ninth standard was selected. Necessary permission was taken from the school authority and girls were explained in detail about the study in the school assembly. Participation in the screening programme was voluntary. An explanatory letter and consent form was given to all the girls. Written consent was obtained from parents or guardian for participation in the screening as all participants were minor. Participants completed a questionnaire asking for significant family, medical and menstrual history, parent education, and their dietary habits.

2.2. Method of Screening. Screening for anemia and iron deficiency was done by (1) complete blood count: done by automatic cell counter, that is, Coulter for hemoglobin concentration. (2) estimation of serum ferritin concentration was done by ELISA. For this recommended protocol by the kit used was followed. Established age adjusted values for hemoglobin and serum ferritin were used.

The participants after screening were divided into three groups.

(1) *Group I*—participants who were anemic (Hb < 12 gm%) and iron deficient (serum ferritin less than 12 μg/L).

(2) *Group II*—participants who were nonanemic (Hb $\geq$ 12 gm%) and iron deficient (serum ferritin less than 12 μg/L).

(3) *Group III*—participants who were nonanemic (Hb $\geq$ 12 gm%) and noniron deficient (serum ferritin levels of 12 μg/L or more).

2.3. Method of Assessing the Cognitive Function. After dividing the participants into three groups, that is, anemic iron deficient (group I), nonanemic iron deficient (group II), and nonanemic noniron deficient (group III), for assessing the cognitive function mathematics score, one multicomponent test for memory, attention and verbal learning, and intelligent quotient (IQ) scores of the students was used.

2.3.1. Scholastic Assessment (Mathematics Score). For assessment of scholastic performance, the mathematics score obtained in the final term examination was noted from the report card. The score obtained were from total 100 marks.

2.3.2. Multicomponent Test (MCT) for Verbal Learning, Memory, and Attention. Multicomponent test of the three groups was assessed after randomization by using PGI test—(Dr. N. N. Wig & Dr. Dwarka Prasad) for testing memory attention and verbal learning [16] Both participants and the investigators were unaware of the group assignment.

PGI test—(Dr. N. N. Wig & Dr. Dwarka Prasad), consisted of the following ten subtests: (I) remote memory, (II) recent memory, (III) mental balance, (IV) attention and concentration, (V) delayed recall, (VI) immediate memory, and (VII) verbal retention for similar pairs, (VIII) verbal retention with dissimilar pairs, (IX) visual retention, and (X) recognition.

2.3.3. For Intelligent Quotient (IQ) Assessment. For assessing the intelligent quotient of the girl student's, Bhatia battery performance test—(Dr. C. M. Bhatia) for intelligent quotient (I.Q) was used, which includes two subtest Kohl's block design and Pass along test [17].

All these tests were selected because these have Indian norms and are constructed and standardized in India. *Statistical analysis*: the data was analyzed with SPSS (version 16) statistical software. One-way ANOVAs test (Table 2) and test of significance for comparison of two sample means (Tables 3 and 4) were applied; P value and mean and standard deviation were calculated.

2.4. Results. Out of total 110 girl students in the age group of 12–15 years, consent was obtained from 103 students to participate in the study. Subsequently 100 students were tested for hemoglobin concentration, serum ferritin, and cognitive function. (3 students refused to give blood for test.)

63 of 100 girl students had hemoglobin levels less than 12 gm% and 37 had hemoglobin levels above 12 gm%. Thus, prevalence of anemia in school going adolescent girls was 63%. The overall mean hemoglobin in the study was 11.66 $\pm$ 1.27 g/dL.

Out of the 63 girl students who had anemia, 56 girls (56%) had Hb values between 10 and 12 gm%, 5 girls (5%) had Hb values between 7 and 10 gm%, and rest of the 2 girls (2%) had Hb values below 7 gm%. Thus, mild anemia (Hb 10–12 gm%) was present in 56% of the study subjects, moderate anemia (Hb 7–10 gm%) in 5%, and severe anemia (Hb < 7 gm%) was present in only 2% of the study subjects.

Serum ferritin was done in 100 girl students between the age group of 12–15 years, 67 were iron deficient (serum ferritin <12 μg/L). So the prevalence of iron deficiency was 67%.

Out of 63 girls who were anemic, 50 girls had reduced serum ferritin. Since the total number of students was 100

TABLE 1: Number of students in different groups, mean serum ferritin, and hemoglobin levels.

Groups	Number of students	Mean serum ferritin (μg/L)	Mean hemoglobin levels (gm%)
Anemic iron deficient (group I)	50	8.458	11.01
Nonanemic iron deficient (group II)	17	10.02	12.61
Nonanemic noniron deficient (group III)	20	25.275	12.975

TABLE 2: The mean mathematics score of the girl students in different groups.

Groups	Mean mathematics score $\pm$ SD
Anemic iron deficient (group I) ($n = 50$)	47.76 $\pm$ 8.26
Nonanemic iron deficient (group II) ($n = 17$)	52.64 $\pm$ 9.88
Nonanemic noniron deficient (group III) ($n = 20$)	62.15 $\pm$ 5.93

SD: Standard deviation.

thus, the prevalence of iron deficiency anemia was 50% and rest of the 13 girls who were anemic, the cause of anemia was other than iron deficiency (see Table 1). To know the probable cause of anemia in these 13 girls who were anemic but were not iron deficient, further investigation in the form of peripheral smear examination, reticulocyte count, and electrophoresis was done. Sickle cell trait was found in 4 out of the 13 students, 1 was sickle cell disease, 1 was thalassemia minor, and 7 were macrocytic anemia probably due to vitamin B12 and folic acid deficiency; hence, they were excluded from the study.

For assessing the cognitive function, mathematics score, one multicomponent test for verbal learning, attention and memory, and IQ scores was used. For assessing the scholastic performance, the mathematics scores obtained in the final term examination was noted from the report card. The scores obtained were from a total of 100 marks. Mean mathematic score calculated for three groups.

The difference in mathematics score was highly significant (P value < 0.0001) between nonanemic noniron deficient (group III) and anemic iron deficient (group I), it was significant (P value 0.001) between nonanemic noniron deficient (group III) and nonanemic iron deficient (group II).

Multicomponent test (MCT) of verbal learning, attention, memory and IQ scores of all the three groups was assessed after randomization. Tests were administered under the guidance of trained research assistant of the Department of Psychological Medicine. The person who was assessing the tests was unaware of the group assignment.

The difference in scores of mental balance between the nonanemic noniron deficient (group III) and anemic iron deficient (group I) was significant (P value < 0.0001) and also the scores of mental balance differed significantly (P value 0.002) between the nonanemic noniron deficient (group III) and nonanemic iron deficient (group II). The difference in scores of attention and concentration was significant (P value < 0.0001) between non anemic noniron deficient (group III) and anemic iron deficient (group I). And the nonanemic iron deficient (group II) and nonanemic noniron deficient

(group III) also showed statistically significant (P value 0.004) difference in scores of attention and concentration.

Non anemic non iron deficient (group III) and anemic iron deficient (group I) when compared for scores of Verbal Retention for Similar Pairs showed significant difference (P value < 0.0001), and on comparing the scores of Verbal Retention for Similar Pairs between the non-anemic iron deficient (group II) and non anemic non iron deficient (group III) the difference was also statistically significant (P value 0.004).

The difference in scores of verbal retention for dissimilar pairs between the anemic iron deficient (group I) and nonanemic iron deficient (group III) was statistically significant (P value 0.004) and also between the nonanemic iron deficient (group II) and nonanemic noniron deficient (group III) showed statistically significant difference (P value 0.045).

The scores of recognition between the anemic iron deficient (group I) and nonanemic iron deficient (group III) showed significant difference (P value 0.032), similarly the difference in scores of recognition between the nonanemic iron deficient (group II) and nonanemic iron deficient (group III) were statistically significant (P value 0.04).

For assessing the intelligent quotient (IQ) of the girl students two test, that is, Kohl's block design test and Pass along test were used. After obtaining the test quotient (TQ) from these two tests the IQ was calculated.

The IQ levels differed significantly between nonanemic noniron deficient (group III) and anemic iron deficient (group I) with P value < 0.0001 and also between nonanemic noniron deficient (group III) and nonanemic iron deficient (group II) (P value 0.003).

Thus, the cognitive function scores which included the mathematics score, multicomponent test scores, and IQ scores were less in iron deficient both anemic and nonanemic groups (group I and II) than the noniron deficient nonanemic group (group III).

3. Discussion

Although all the features of cognition are important but verbal learning and attention and concentration along with memory are particularly more important for academic performance.

3.1. Scholastic Assessment (Mathematics Scores). In present study, iron deficient both anemic and nonanemic students had scored less in mathematics than the normal non iron deficient students. This is in accordance to the study done by Prestonjee [18] wherein iron deficient adolescents both

TABLE 3: The mean multicomponent test (MCT) scores in the three different groups.

Test	Anemic iron deficient (group I) $N = 50$ (Mean $\pm$ SD)	Nonanemic iron deficient (group II) $N = 17$ (Mean $\pm$ SD)	Nonanemic noniron deficient (group III) $N = 20$ (Mean $\pm$ SD)
Recent memory	4.98 ± 0.14	5 ± 0	4.95 ± 0.22
Remote memory	5.82 ± 0.52	5.88 ± 0.48	5.6 ± 0.75
Mental balance	1.66 ± 0.55	2.05 ± 0.74	2.7 ± 0.47
Attention and concentration	11.28 ± 3.83	13.76 ± 3.41	16.2 ± 2.06
Delayed recall	8.28 ± 1.48	8.48 ± 1.85	8.9 ± 1.07
Immediate recall	1.78 ± 0.73	1.82 ± 0.72	1.9 ± 0.78
Verbal retention for similar pairs	4.1 ± 0.64	4.23 ± 0.83	4.9 ± 0.30
Verbal retention for dissimilar pairs	4.3 ± 0.67	4.35 ± 0.49	4.8 ± 0.41
Visual retention	2.36 ± 1.13	2.41 ± 1.46	2.85 ± 1.34
Recognition	7.7 ± 1.84	7.87 ± 1.66	8.95 ± 2.39
Total test scores	52.26 ± 5.73	55.82 ± 6.12	61.75 ± 4.92

SD: Standard deviation.

TABLE 4: The mean scores in Kohl's block design, pass along test, and mean IQ score.

Groups	Kohl's block design	Pass along test	Test quotient (TQ)	Mean intelligent quotient ($\pm$SD)
Anemic iron deficient (group I)	11.86	12.76	193.06	96.6 ($\pm$7.28)
Nonanemic iron deficient (group II)	12.82	15.47	205.17	102.61 ($\pm$6.33)
Nonanemic noniron deficient (group III)	14.4	16.9	215.65	107.82 ($\pm$4.95)

SD: Standard deviation.

anemic and non anemic had lower mathematics score compared with adolescent with normal iron status. Similarly Sungthong et al. [19] observed that the school performance including Thai language and mathematics score were less in iron deficient children than in non iron deficient children in a study done on school children in Thailand.

3.2. Multicomponent Test for Verbal Learning, Memory, and Attention.

Multicomponent test of verbal learning, attention, and memory of all the three groups was assessed after randomization. The overall total score was less in iron deficient both anemic and nonanemic groups than noniron deficient nonanemic group.

Similar findings were also seen in scores of mental balance and verbal retention for similar and dissimilar pairs. There was no difference in score of recent and remote memory, delayed and immediate recall, and visual retention subsets between iron deficient (group I and II) and noniron deficient (group III).

The findings suggest that iron deficiency, even in the absence of anemia causes decrease in at least some aspect of cognitive functioning.

The present findings are in accordance with the findings of a randomized trial done by Bruner et al. [20] on nonanemic iron deficient adolescent girls in four Baltimore high schools in USA, where baseline cognitive function was assessed.

The investigators then randomly assigned these girls to either placebo or oral ferrous sulphate treatment for 8 weeks. The girls treated with ferrous sulphate had improved scores in verbal learning and memory compared to the scores of girls who were given placebo. Similar observation was also seen in the study done by Seshadri et al. [21] in India who showed beneficial effect of iron therapy on cognitive function of anemic children of various age. In anemic adolescent girls of 8–15 years of age group on iron therapy there was improvement in the scores of attention, memory, and concentration than those girls who were given placebo. A study done in Vadodara, India by Sen, and Kanani present evidence from a controlled intervention trial that iron and folic acid supplementation in children aged between 9 and 13 years leads to modest (1.5 to 2 units on a scale of 100) but significant improvement in the various cognitive tests [22].

3.3. Intelligent Quotient Assessment.

The difference of mean IQ scores between iron deficient both anemic and nonanemic groups (I and II) and nonanemic noniron deficient was statistically significant.

Pollitt et al. [23], Soemantri et al. [24], and Sunthong et al. [19] also reported low IQ scores in iron deficient subjects compared to the noniron deficient subjects. This is in accordance with present study findings.

4. Conclusion

The findings of the present study are iron deficient school going adolescent females both anemic and nonanemic had low scholastic performance in the form of low mathematics score and low scores in verbal learning, attention, mental balance, and recognition component of multicomponent test along with low IQ scores than their noniron deficient comparers. Iron deficiency independently leads to decreased cognitive scores. Iron deficiency without anemia is the initial stage and as the iron deficiency increases anemia manifests. The cognitive scores were lowest in the iron deficient anemic (group I). In iron deficient without anemia it was slightly more than group I but much less than group III, that is, nonanemic noniron deficient subjects. Prevalence of anemia was 63% while prevalence of iron deficiency anemia in present study was 50%.

There is need to initiate programme for supplementation of iron and folic acid to school going adolescent girls for the prevention of hematological and nonhematological consequences of iron deficiency with government and private organizational efforts.

Conflict of Interests

The authors declare there is no conflict of interests.

References

[1] A. M. Rosenthal, "WHO names top 10 health risks," *Environmental Health Perspectives*, vol. 111, no. 9, article A456, 2003.

[2] J. R. Boccio and I. Ventkatesh, "Iron deficiency causes, consequences and stratification to overcome the nutritional problem," *Biological Trace Element Research*, vol. 94, no. 1, pp. 1–31, 2003.

[3] Centre for disease control and prevention, "Recommendations to prevent and control iron deficiency in the United States," *Morbidity & Mortality Weekly Report*, vol. 47, no. RR-3, pp. 1–29, 1998.

[4] T. Ganz, "Hepcidin, a key regulator of iron metabolism and mediator of anemia of inflammation," *Blood*, vol. 102, no. 3, pp. 783–788, 2003.

[5] K. Krishnaswami, "Counrty profile: India. Nutritional disorders—old and changing," *The Lancet*, vol. 351, pp. 1268–1269, 2000.

[6] S. Kumar, "India health survey finds too many women and children in poor health," *The Lancet*, vol. 356, no. 9244, p. 1830, 2000.

[7] S. Kishor, "Gender differentials in child mortality: a review of the evidence," in *Women's Health in India: Risk and Vulnerability*, M. Das Gupta, L. C. Chen, and T. N. Krishnan, Eds., pp. 19–54, Bombay Oxford University Press.

[8] J. L. Beard, "Iron biology in immune function, muscle metabolism and neuronal functioning," *Journal of Nutrition*, vol. 131, no. 2, pp. 568S–580S, 2001.

[9] A. Sen and S. J. Kanani, "Deleterious functional impact of anemia on young adolescent school girls," *Indian Pediatrics*, vol. 43, no. 3, pp. 219–226, 2006.

[10] T. W. Rowland, M. B. Deisroth, G. M. Green, and J. F. Kelleher, "The effect of iron therapy on the exercise capacity of nonanemic iron-deficient adolescent runners," *American Journal of Diseases of Children*, vol. 142, no. 2, pp. 165–169, 1988.

[11] S. S. Basta, S. Soekirman, D. Karyadi, and N. S. Scrimshaw, "Iron deficiency anemia and the productivity of adult males in Indonesia," *American Journal of Clinical Nutrition*, vol. 32, no. 4, pp. 916–925, 1979.

[12] P. R. Dallman, "Iron deficiency & immune response," *The American Journal of Clinical Nutrition*, vol. 47, pp. 496–501, 1988.

[13] J. Beard, W. Green, L. Miller, and C. Finch, "Effect of iron-deficiency anemia on hormone levels and thermoregulation during cold exposure," *The American Journal of Physiology*, vol. 247, no. 1, part 2, pp. R114–R119, 1984.

[14] M. J. Murray, A. B. Murray, M. B. Murray, and C. J. Murray, "The adverse effect of iron repletion on the course of certain infections," *British Medical Journal*, vol. 2, no. 6145, pp. 1113–1115, 1978.

[15] E. Pollitt and R. L. Leibel, "Iron deficiency and behavior," *Journal of Pediatrics*, vol. 88, no. 3, pp. 372–381, 1976.

[16] C. M. Bhatia, *Performance Test of Intelligence under Indian Conditions*, London Oxford University Press, 1955.

[17] J. S. Halterman, J. M. Kaczorowski, C. A. Aligne, P. Auinger, and P. G. Szilagyi, "Iron deficiency and cognitive achievement among school-aged children and adolescents in the United States," *Pediatrics*, vol. 107, no. 6, pp. 1381–1386, 2001.

[18] D. M. Prestonjee, *Third Handbook of Psychological and Social Instrument*, 1997.

[19] R. Sungthong, L. Mo-suwan, and V. Chongsuvivatwong, "Effects of haemoglobin and serum ferritin on cognitive function in school children," *Asia Pacific Journal of Clinical Nutrition*, vol. 11, no. 2, pp. 117–122, 2002.

[20] A. B. Bruner, A. Joffe, A. K. Duggan, J. F. Casella, and J. Brandt, "Randomised study of cognitive effects of iron supplementation in non-anaemic iron-deficient adolescent girls," *The Lancet*, vol. 348, no. 9033, pp. 992–996, 1996.

[21] S. Seshadri, T. Gopaldas, T. Walter, and A. Heywood, "Impact of iron supplementation on cognitive functions in preschool and school-aged children: the Indian experience," *American Journal of Clinical Nutrition*, vol. 50, no. 3, pp. 675–686, 1989.

[22] A. Sen and S. J. Kanani, "Impact of iron-folic acid supplementation on cognitive abilities of school girls in Vadodara," *Indian Pediatrics*, vol. 46, no. 2, pp. 137–143, 2009.

[23] E. Pollitt, P. Hathirat, N. J. Kotchabhakdi et al., "Iron deficiency and educational achievement in Thailand," *American Journal of Clinical Nutrition*, vol. 50, no. 3, pp. 687–697, 1989.

[24] A. G. Soemantri, E. Pollitt, and I. Kim, "Iron deficiency anemia and educational achievement," *American Journal of Clinical Nutrition*, vol. 42, no. 6, pp. 1221–1228, 1985.

8

Trace Element Status (Iron, Zinc, Copper, Chromium, Cobalt, and Nickel) in Iron-Deficiency Anaemia of Children under 3 Years

Maria Georgieva Angelova,[1] **Tsvetelina Valentinova Petkova-Marinova,**[2]
Maksym Vladimirovich Pogorielov,[3] **Andrii Nikolaevich Loboda,**[4] **Vania Nedkova**
Nedkova-Kolarova,[2] **and Atanaska Naumova Bozhinova**[1]

[1] *Department of Chemistry and Biochemistry & Physics and Biophysics, University of Medicine-Pleven,*
 1 Kliment Ohridski Street, 5800 Pleven, Bulgaria
[2] *Department of Pediatrics, University of Medicine-Pleven, 1 Kliment Ohridski Street, 5800 Pleven, Bulgaria*
[3] *Department of Hygiene and Ecology, Sumy State University, Medical Institute, 31 Sanatornaya Street, Sumy 40007, Ukraine*
[4] *Department of Pediatrics with Medical Genetics, Sumy State University, Medical Institute, 31 Sanatornaya Street, Sumy 40007, Ukraine*

Correspondence should be addressed to Maria Georgieva Angelova; angelovamg@abv.bg

Academic Editor: Aurelio Maggio

Aim. To determine trace element status and aetiologic factors for development of trace elements deficiencies in children with iron-deficiency anaemia (IDA) aged 0 to 3 years. *Contingent and Methods.* 30 patients of the University Hospital, Pleven, Bulgaria—I group; 48 patients of the Sumy Regional Child's Clinical Hospital, Sumy, Ukraine—II group; 25 healthy controls were investigated. Serum concentrations of iron, zinc, copper, chromium, cobalt, and nickel were determined spectrophotometrically and by atomic absorption spectrophotometry. *Results.* Because the obtained serum levels of zinc, copper, and chromium were near the lower reference limits, I group was divided into IA and IB. In IA group, serum concentrations were lower than the reference values for 47%, 57%, and 73% of patients, respectively. In IB group, these were within the reference values. In II group, results for zinc, cobalt, and nickel were significantly lower ($P < 0.05$), and results for copper were significantly higher in comparison to controls higher in comparison to controls. *Conclusion.* Low serum concentrations of zinc, copper, cobalt, and nickel were mainly due to inadequate dietary intake, malabsorption, and micronutrient interactions in both studied groups. Increased serum copper in II group was probably due to metabolic changes resulting from adaptations in IDA. Data can be used for developing a diagnostic algorithm for IDA.

1. Introduction

Under conditions of iron-deficiency anaemia (IDA), a host of metabolic changes representing adaptation mechanisms for maximizing iron delivery for erythropoiesis occur [1, 2]. There are close relations between the metabolism of different trace elements including iron based on antagonistic or synergistic interactions [3, 4]. One of known links is at the level of common intestinal transporters for iron and other divalent metals. Upregulation of their expression induced by iron deficiency (ID) predisposes to metabolic imbalances and

respective changes in trace element status [1, 2]. Another known link is at the level of metal-storage proteins, metallothioneins, which bind different metals, thus acting in their storage and detoxification [5–7].

Interactions of different trace elements with iron determine the relationship between changes in trace element status in the organism and development of IDA. Increases in content of antagonistic to iron trace elements, such as cobalt, zinc, copper, chromium, and calcium, which impair iron absorption or its physiological impact, can lead to development of IDA. Deficiencies of synergistic to iron trace elements implicated in iron metabolism or processes of haematopoiesis, such as copper, chromium, nickel, sodium, and potassium, can contribute substantially to the aetiology of IDA [4].

Only 35–55% of cases of IDA in children are solely due to iron deficiency and others are associated with changes in status of multiple trace elements.

In our study, we use serum trace element concentrations as markers of trace element status in the organism.

Results published from different researchers on status of trace elements in IDA are various and often conflicting.

Most of the researchers have discovered lower serum zinc levels in subjects with IDA in comparison to nonanaemic subjects [8–11], but others have not found significant differences in serum zinc between IDA subjects and healthy controls [12–14].

In studies on copper content in serum and blood, higher [8–10, 12, 15] and lower levels [16, 17] as well as levels without significant differences [13, 14] have been discovered in subjects with ID and anaemia in comparison to nonanaemic and iron-adequate subjects. Both low and high serum copper concentrations have been observed in a subset of anaemic participants in a study of Knovich et al. [18].

Although chromium is considered synergistic to iron [4] and some researchers have found lower concentrations in blood of anaemic patients when compared to control subjects [17], it is known as an antagonistic competition between trivalent chromium and trivalent iron for binding to apotransferrin [4, 19]. On the basis of this interaction, Lukaski et al. have suggested adverse effect of high-dose and long-term chromium supplementation on iron metabolism and status in adults [20].

Cobalt and nickel are essential trace elements with significant impact on the processes of haematopoiesis—stimulation of erythropoietin production and haemoglobin synthesis [21]. Lower concentrations of nickel have been observed in blood of anaemic children as compared to healthy controls [17]. Higher concentrations of cobalt have been found in blood at low body iron stores [2].

Our literature search shows that many researchers do not explain changes in trace element status with mechanisms for transport and storage.

The aim of the study is to determine trace element status, aetiologic factors, and mechanisms for development of trace elements deficiencies in children with IDA from 0 to 3 years of age.

2. Clinical Contingent and Methods

Our investigation comprises 78 patients from 0 to 3 years of age with clinical and laboratory signs of IDA. 30 children-patients are of the University Hospital, Medical University, Pleven, Bulgaria—I group, and 48 are patients of the Sumy Regional Child's Clinical Hospital, Sumy, Ukraine—II group. Comparison group includes 25 healthy children at the same age.

Anaemia was defined according to the criteria adopted by the WHO. Haemoglobin level below 110 g/L and haematocrit

value below 0.33 l/l were used as diagnostic limits of anaemia. In I group of patients, measures of iron status, especially serum iron concentrations below 8.0 μmol/L and transferrin saturation (TS) below 16%, and low red cell indices were used to identify that anaemia was due to ID [22]. Percent TS was calculated as a ratio of serum iron and total iron-binding capacity (TIBC)—serum iron/TIBC × 100. Serum ferritin values were used as indicators for iron deficiency in II group.

All children were enrolled in the study after informed consent from their parents or guardians. Ethical approval was obtained from the Institutional research ethics committees.

A parental questionnaire was provided to collect information about feeding patterns.

Fasting venous blood samples were obtained for analysis in the morning from all children into sterile tubes untreated with heparin, EDTA, citrate, and so forth. After two hours standing and centrifugation at 3500 rpm for 10 minutes, blood serum was separated. The serum samples were put in closed plastic laboratory vessels and stored at −18°C until trace element analysis.

In I group, serum content of trace elements iron, zinc, copper, and chromium was determined spectrophotometrically: ferrozine method [23] for serum iron and total iron-binding capacity by COBAS INTEGRA 400 (Roche) analyzer, spectrophotometric methods using GIESSE diagnostics (Italy) tests for serum zinc and AUDIT diagnostics (Ireland) tests for serum copper, and spectrophotometric method [24] with our modifications for serum chromium. Serum concentrations of zinc, copper, and chromium were determined by a spectrophotometer DR2800 (Hach Lange, Germany).

The serum ferritin levels were determined by ELISA using a kit of reagents "UBI MAGIVEL FERRITIN" produced by "United Biotech Inc." (USA).

Haematological parameters, such as haemoglobin (Hb), haematocrit (Ht), red blood cell (erythrocyte) count (RBC), and the red cell indices, mean corpuscular volume (MCV), mean corpuscular haemoglobin (MCH), mean corpuscular haemoglobin concentration (MCHC), and red cell distribution width (RDW) were examined by analyzer MIKROS—18 (ABX). The reticulocyte count was determined by microscopic examination of a peripheral blood smear stained with a supravital dye.

Serum trace element concentrations and haematological parameters in I group of patients were compared to their respective reference values indicated in Table 1.

In II group, the content of trace elements iron, zinc, copper, cobalt, and nickel in blood serum and erythrocytes was determined by atomic absorption spectrophotometry (AAS) on a spectrophotometer C-115 M1 (JSC "Selmi," Ukraine) [25, 26]. All results from trace element analysis and investigated haematological parameters in II group of patients were compared to healthy controls. Content of trace elements in blood serum and erythrocytes in comparison group was determined by AAS.

Statistical data processing was performed using Excel (Microsoft Corporation, Redmond, WA), Statgraphics Plus (Manugistics, Rockville, MD), and Statistica 6.1

TABLE 1: Haematological parameters and content of trace elements in blood serum of children with IDA.

Parameter	Reference values		I group with IDA ($n = 30$)	II group with IDA ($n = 48$)	Comparison group ($n = 25$)
	Mean [27, 28]	−2 SD [27, 28]			
Haemoglobin (g/L)	120	105	90.23 ± 11.09	89.79 ± 1.23	119.15 ± 2.41
Haematocrit (L/L)	0.36	0.33	0.279 ± 0.029	0.301 ± 0.004	0.3442 ± 0.006
RBC (×10^{12} cells/L)	4.5	3.7	4.41 ± 0.65	3.58 ± 0.05	4.07 ± 0.12
Rtc (Ğ)	10 [28]	—	—	5.5 ± 0.87	7.86 ± 0.98
MCV (fL)	78	70	64.3 ± 9.87	74.66 ± 1.08	82.52 ± 1.17
MCH (pg)	27	23	20.93 ± 4.17	24.77 ± 0.39	29.82 ± 0.56
MCHC (g/L)	330	300	322.67 ± 18.16	323.47 ± 4.34	365.17 ± 3.6
RDW (%)	1.5–15 [29]		15.58 ± 1.56	—	—
Iron (μmol/L)	8.0–24.0 [30]		4.43 ± 1.21	9.23 ± 0.86	22.92 ± 1.83
Zinc (μmol/L)	11.1–19.5 [5, 31]		11.22 ± 4.40	11.02 ± 1.79	17.96 ± 1.06
Copper (μmol/L)	11.0–24.0 [6, 32]		11.81 ± 4.39	23.80 ± 0.76	16.50 ± 0.71
Chromium (μmol/L)	0.95–9.5 [33]		0.83 ± 0.69	—	—
Cobalt (μmol/L × 10^{-3})	0.00–15.25 [34]		—	5.74 ± 0.76	9.16 ± 0.61
Nickel (μmol/L × 10^{-3})	1.70–10.22 [35]		—	8.99 ± 0.868	14.35 ± 1.09

(StatSoft, USA). All values were expressed as mean ± standard deviation (SD). Student's t-test and Wilcoxon's test were used to evaluate differences between study groups. Statistically significant differences were indicated by P values < 0.05.

3. Results

Clinical manifestations of IDA in all children were demonstrated by the presence of sideropenic and anaemic syndromes.

Anaemic syndrome is manifested by such symptoms as pallor of skin and mucous membranes, fatigue and faintness, tachycardia, and systolic murmur. In a number of patients apathy, drowsiness, or conversely, excessive irritability, and emotional lability were observed due to decreased oxygen delivery to the brain [36] and deficiency of iron which has been shown to play a key role in brain functions [22].

Manifestations of hyposiderosis were due to deficiency of iron-containing enzymes. Dryness of skin, changes in hair—fragility, and dim color were observed; signs of angular stomatitis and atrophic glossitis were also found. Most children suffered from loss of appetite. A number of patients had a syndrome of muscular hypotonia. In some of the patients with IDA increased size of the liver and spleen was observed due to extramedullary haematopoiesis (Figures 1(a) and 1(b)).

Results of investigated clinical laboratory indicators in patients with IDA, comparison group, and the respective reference values are presented in Table 1.

All haematological parameters in anaemic children exhibited changes in accordance with the presence of IDA. Mean value of serum iron in I group of patients with IDA was found to be lower than the reference values–4.43 ± 1.21 μmol/L (Table 1, Figure 2(a)), and along with the low transferrin saturation (TS)–6.23 ± 2.65%, indicated presence of ID. In II group, serum ferritin content was found to be 9.42 ± 0.75 ng/mL which is significantly lower (P < 0.001) in comparison to healthy controls –38.67 ± 4.18 ng/mL.

Mean values of serum zinc, copper, and chromium in I group were all near the lower limits of the reference ranges (Table 1, Figure 2(a)). In II group of patients with IDA, mean serum iron, zinc, cobalt, and nickel concentrations were found to be significantly lower, and mean serum copper level was found to be significantly higher in comparison to their respective controls (Table 1, Figure 2(b)) with reliability level P < 0.05.

In I group, results for serum levels of zinc, copper, and chromium (Table 1, Figure 2(a)) enable to divide examined patients into two groups for each of the investigated trace elements (Figure 3).

Patients with serum trace elements concentrations lower than the reference values—serum zinc 7.29 ± 2.54 μmol/L, copper 8.6 ± 1.46 μmol/L, and chromium 0.47 ± 0.14 μmol/L, are included in IA group. For each of the investigated trace elements, the number of patients in this group constitutes 47% ($n = 14$), 57% ($n = 17$), and 73% ($n = 22$) of total number of children with IDA in I group.

Patients with serum trace elements concentrations within the reference values—serum zinc 14.65 ± 2.21 μmol/L, copper 16.0 ± 3.2 μmol/L, and chromium 1.83 ± 0.61 μmol/L, are included in IB group. For each of the investigated trace elements, the number of patients in this group includes 53% ($n = 16$), 43% ($n = 13$), and 27% ($n = 8$) of total number of participants with IDA in I group.

There are statistically significant differences between IA and IB groups (P < 0.001).

Examination of trace element content in erythrocytes showed significantly lower values for all investigated trace elements in patients with IDA in comparison to control subjects (Table 2).

(a)

(b)

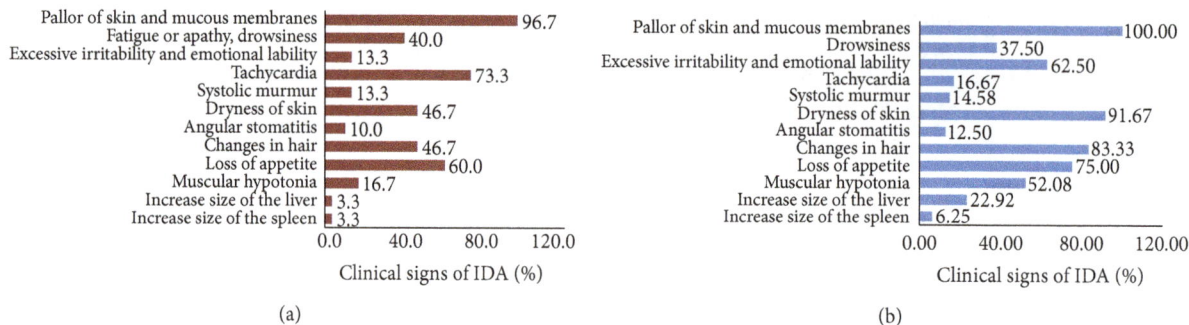

FIGURE 1: Clinical signs of IDA in I group (a) and II group (b).

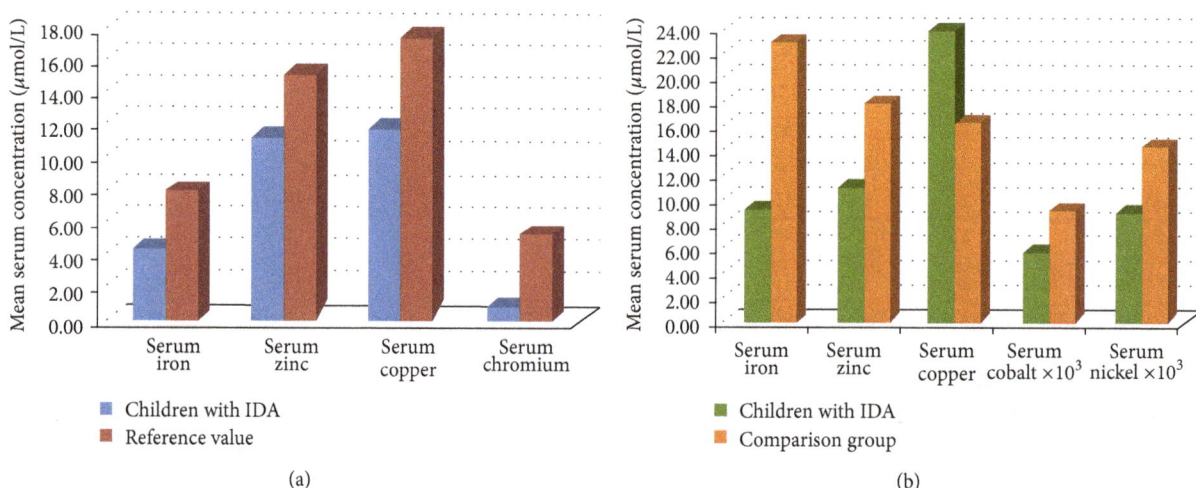

(a)

(b)

FIGURE 2: Serum concentrations of trace elements in I group (a) and II group (b) of children with IDA.

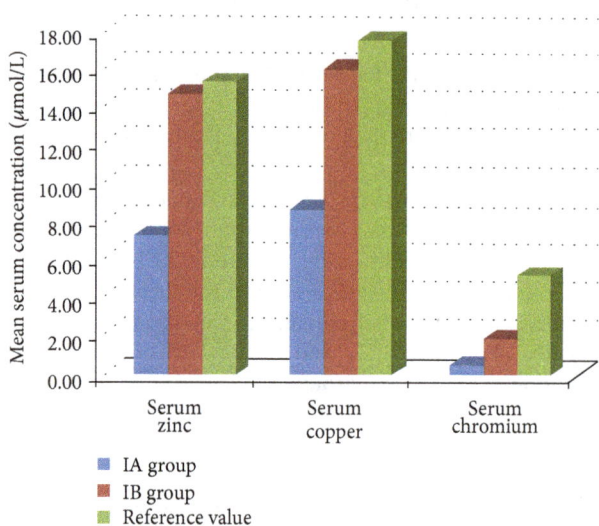

FIGURE 3: Serum concentrations of zinc, copper, and chromium among IA group and IB group of children with IDA.

4. Discussion

Under conditions of IDA, trace element status in the organism is largely influenced by metabolic interactions between

TABLE 2: Content of trace element in erythrocytes in children with IDA and healthy controls.

Trace element content (μg/mg ash)	II group with IDA ($n = 48$)	Comparison group ($n = 25$)
Iron*	15.58 ± 1.13	31.56 ± 1.65
Zinc*	0.208 ± 0.013	0.260 ± 0.012
Copper*	0.176 ± 0.016	0.271 ± 0.039
Cobalt*	0.0316 ± 0.0023	0.0411 ± 0.0034
Nickel*	0.0330 ± 0.0023	0.0500 ± 0.0034

*Reliability level $P < 0.05$.

trace elements, some of which result from adaptation mechanisms for maximizing iron delivery for erythropoiesis [1, 2, 22]. Nutrition, physiologic features in different life periods, and underlying pathological conditions also affect trace element status. It has been shown that children in infancy and early childhood are particularly susceptible to deficiencies of iron and zinc, and copper deficiency occurs mainly in infancy. This vulnerability is due to increased requirements for rapid growth which are frequently not met by the diet [6, 17, 22, 36, 37].

IDA often shows association with low serum zinc levels, as well as zinc deficiency states [8–10]. In our study, obtained values for serum zinc in patients with IDA were also lower in comparison to reference values and controls (Figures 2(b) and 3(a)). These changes in zinc status are frequently explained by coexisting deficiencies of iron and zinc due to common dietary sources of both micronutrients and decreasing their intestinal absorption by the same dietary factors [9, 11].

Lower serum levels than the reference values were also obtained for copper among most patients in I group (57%, $n = 17$).

In our research, we found a number of factors associated with low serum concentrations of zinc and copper in children with IDA.

In 20% of children with IDA from I group, there was a history of preterm birth or low birth weight which are important contributing factors for zinc and copper deficiencies because of the inadequate prenatal stores and elevated requirements for growth [6, 38].

Association between short duration of breast-feeding, exclusive cow's milk feeding and low serum levels of zinc was observed in 57.14% of patients in IA group. Association between the same dietary factors and low serum levels of copper was observed in 64.7% of patients in IA group. This relationship may probably be due to the lower zinc and copper bioavailability from cow's milk in comparison to human milk and the low copper content of cow's milk [5–7, 38, 39].

Malabsorption due to cow's milk protein-induced enteropathy may be regarded as a factor for development of micronutrient deficiencies in 10% of patients with IDA [5, 6, 18, 37].

Low serum concentrations of zinc and copper in some of the investigated children may be attributed to the inadequate consumption of foods with high bioavailability of zinc and copper—meat, poultry, and fish, which are important dietary sources of zinc and copper in children's diet [5, 15, 39, 40]. Other dietary factor is the early introduction and high intake of flour-based foods containing the inhibitors of zinc and copper absorption phytates [7, 17]. These dietary factors were observed in 78.6% of patients with low serum levels of zinc and in 76.47% of patients with low serum levels of copper from I group.

The proposed mechanisms explaining low serum zinc and copper levels in some of the investigated children are antagonistic interactions between zinc and copper within the enterocyte [7]. Impaired intestinal absorption of zinc is observed under conditions of high intake of copper attributed to competitive antagonism between both metals for absorption sites in the gastrointestinal tract [3, 5].

In relatively high dietary intake of zinc, production of metal-binding proteins metallothioneins in intestinal mucosa is induced. As metallothioneins have a greater affinity for copper than zinc, this is followed by sequestration of high proportion of dietary copper in a stable copper-metallothionein complex in intestinal mucosal cells—"mucosal block" in copper transport, reduction in copper absorption, and increased copper excretion [5, 7].

Low serum concentrations of zinc and copper, which we found in investigated children, may be considered as contributing factors for IDA due to known synergistic interactions of both trace elements with iron—participation of zinc in haemoglobin synthesis and its essentiality in erythropoiesis [7, 41], and implication of copper-containing enzymes ceruloplasmin and hephaestin, ferrochelatase and cytochrom-c oxidase in iron metabolism, formation of haemoglobin, and mechanisms of hematopoiesis [4, 6, 7, 42]. Studies in animals and humans have found that copper deficiency can lead to ID [1, 4] and IDA [6, 7, 43].

It is difficult to identify factors explaining relatively high serum levels of zinc found in some patients with IDA from IB group, as well as their relationship with development of IDA. Some studies have shown that nutritional deficiency of iron enhances the intestinal absorption of zinc suggesting the divalent metal transporter 1 (DMT1) as a common absorptive pathway for both metals and physiological basis for such an interaction [44]. Although zinc is considered antagonistic to iron [4] on the basis of absorptive competition, conflicting results have been obtained in studies evaluating effect of zinc on iron absorption, and DMT1 has been postulated as an unlikely site for competitive antagonism [7].

Discovering significantly higher serum copper in II group of patients with IDA in comparison to healthy controls and relatively high serum copper in a part of IB group may be considered as a consequence of adaptation mechanisms in ID intended to maximize iron delivery for erythropoiesis [1]. There are data for upregulating the duodenal iron transporter DMT1 which is also a physiologically relevant copper transporter and the Menkes copper ATPase (MNK protein, Atp7a) on the basolateral membrane of enterocytes under low iron conditions [1, 2, 13].

It has been shown that increased copper absorption induced by ID might contribute to IDA [12] due to known antagonistic competition between copper and iron at the level of DMT1 [4, 8]. Moreover, higher serum copper concentrations are related to high levels of serum ceruloplasmin which, because of the antagonism with zinc, lowers zinc to copper (Zn : Cu) ratio. This is known to increase hemolysis and peroxidation of erythrocytes and thereby promotes anemia [7, 43]. Therefore, higher serum levels of copper in II group of patients and relatively high although in the reference range serum levels of copper in IB group may be considered as an important contributing factor for IDA.

In addition, imbalance of erythrocyte and serum copper was observed in II group of children with IDA with significant increase of its concentration in the blood serum, but copper deficiency in red blood cells (Table 2). It is known that erythrocyte deficiency of copper impairs incorporation of iron into the haem structure [43].

The serum concentrations of chromium were found to be lower than the reference values in 73% of children with IDA in I group. Other researchers [17] have also discovered significantly lower concentrations of chromium in blood of anaemic patients when compared to control subjects. Chromium is considered synergistic to iron and its deficiency can lead to ID [4]. For the rest 27% of patients with IDA in I group, serum chromium concentrations within the reference values were found. This is explained by the fact that besides being synergistic, chromium can be antagonistic to iron due to competition for binding to apotransferrin. Significantly reduced uptake of iron by serum transferrin has been observed in the presence of chromium [4, 19]. Therefore, in these children, serum chromium levels found may be associated with negative influence of chromium on iron metabolism, thus contributing to the aetiology of IDA.

Both cobalt and nickel mean serum concentrations in our study were found to be significantly lower in children with IDA than healthy controls ($P < 0.05$). Cobalt and nickel play important roles in the processes of erythropoiesis. It has been shown that both metals stimulate erythropoietin production by activation of the transcription factor hypoxia-inducible factor 1α (HIF-1α). Cobalt influences DNA synthesis accelerating maturation of erythroid stem cells and stimulates haemoglobin synthesis [21, 45]. Nickel is considered synergistic to iron by promoting its intestinal absorption and nickel deficiency can lead to ID and anaemia [4, 17, 46]. Therefore, deficiencies of both trace elements might be a contributing factor for development of IDA in our study.

However, it is difficult to identify the contribution factors explaining these results because although serum levels of cobalt and nickel were found to be lower than the control subjects, they were within the reference values. It has been shown that the intestinal absorption of iron, cobalt, and nickel is mediated by a common transport mechanism, DMT1 [2, 47], which is known to be upregulated by ID [2, 13]. It has been found, however, that transport capacity for cobalt and nickel was lower than the iron because of a higher binding constant and lower exchange rate for both metals as compared with iron. This probably not only results in suppressed duodenal uptake of iron but also explains lower levels of cobalt and nickel which we observed in children with IDA [21].

We also found that dietary factors and malabsorption may be regarded as associated with lower serum concentrations of cobalt and nickel in our patients with IDA. Important dietary sources of cobalt are animal tissues or products, such as meat, eggs, and dairy products, which were found to be scarce in the diet of the children with IDA. High dietary intake of cow's milk, frequently observed in children of infancy and early childhood, and found as a common dietary pattern in our patients with IDA, does not obligatory provide sufficient intake of cobalt because of the known geochemical cobalt deficiency. As cow's milk has low nickel content and contains factors inhibiting nickel absorption, cow's milk-based dietary patterns observed in our study may be a possible reason for lower serum levels of nickel discovered. Intestinal malabsorption, found in certain patients with IDA, is also known as contributing to low cobalt and nickel content in the organism [48–50].

5. Conclusion

Through the present study including investigation of trace element status, we expand the aetiology of IDA. Data obtained can be used for developing a diagnostic algorithm for IDA.

Low serum trace element concentrations of zinc, copper, cobalt, and nickel, mainly due to inadequate dietary intake,

malabsorption problems, and trace element interactions, were found in both studied groups (I and II groups) of children with IDA.

Profiles of trace elements iron and zinc in blood serum do not differ in the two examined groups by the means of two analytical methods applied. Increased serum concentrations of copper in II group in comparison to control subjects are probably due to metabolic changes resulting from adaptation mechanisms in IDA.

Dietary insufficiencies of micronutrients, as well as low concentrations of trace elements in blood serum, are common in children with IDA under 3 years of age. However, mechanisms for metabolic interactions between trace elements based on transport and storage molecules are not clearly investigated yet. Micronutrient deficiency in patients with IDA can lead to the formation of so-called related functional iron deficiency. In this case, it is considered that molecular mechanisms provided by trace elements responsible for iron absorption and transport and further included in haem structure are probably impaired. This could lead to low efficiency of the monotherapy by iron supplements.

High prevalence of nutrition-related disorders in trace element status under conditions of IDA indicates the need to develop and implement appropriate intervention strategies for prevention and control of micronutrient deficiencies—supplementation, fortification, and dietary diversification/modification.

Conflict of Interests

The authors declare that there is no conflict of interests regarding the publication of this paper.

Acknowledgments

This study was performed with financial support from the Medical University, Pleven, Bulgaria, and Sumy State University, Ukraine.

References

[1] P. N. Ranganathan, Y. Lu, L. Jiang, C. Kim, and J. F. Collins, "Serum ceruloplasmin protein expression and activity increases in Iron-deficient rats and is further enhanced by higher dietary copper intake," *Blood*, vol. 118, no. 11, pp. 3146–3153, 2011.

[2] E. Bárány, I. A. Bergdahl, L.-E. Bratteby et al., "Iron status influences trace element levels in human blood and serum," *Environmental Research*, vol. 98, no. 2, pp. 215–223, 2005.

[3] J. W. Choi and S. K. Kim, "Relationships of lead, copper, zinc, and cadmium levels versus hematopoiesis and Iron parameters in healthy adolescents," *Annals of Clinical and Laboratory Science*, vol. 35, no. 4, pp. 428–434, 2005.

[4] D. L. Watts, "The nutritional relationships of Iron," *Journal of Orthomolecular Medicine*, vol. 3, no. 3, pp. 110–116, 1988.

[5] World Health Organization, "Environmental health criteria 221: Zinc," Tech. Rep., World Health Organization, Geneva, Switzerland, 2001.

[6] World Health Organization, "Environmental health criteria 200: Copper," Tech. Rep., World Health Organization, Geneva, Switzerland, 1998.

[7] M. Olivares, E. Hertrampf, and R. Uauy, "Copper and zinc interactions in anemia: a public health perspective," in *Nutritional Anemia*, K. Kraemer and M. B. Zimmermann, Eds., pp. 99–109, Sight and Life Press, Basel, Switzerland, 2007.

[8] M. Wajeunnesa, N. Begum, S. Ferdousi, S. Akhter, and S. B. Quarishi, "Serum Zinc and Copper in Iron deficient adolescents," *Journal of Bangladesh Society of Physiologist*, vol. 4, no. 2, pp. 77–80, 2009.

[9] M. K. Gürgöze, A. Ölcücü, A. D. Aygün, E. Taskin, and M. Kilic, "Serum and hair levels of Zinc, Selenium, Iron, and Copper in children with Iron-deficiency anemia," *Biological Trace Element Research*, vol. 111, no. 1–3, pp. 23–29, 2006.

[10] A. Ece, B. S. Uyanik, A. Işcan, P. Ertan, and M. R. Yiğitoğlu, "Increased serum Copper and decreased serum Zinc levels in children with Iron deficiency anemia," *Biological Trace Element Research*, vol. 59, no. 1–3, pp. 31–39, 1997.

[11] C. R. Cole, F. K. Grant, E. D. Swaby-Ellis et al., "Zinc and Iron deficiency and their interrelations in low-income African American and Hispanic children in Atlanta," *American Journal of Clinical Nutrition*, vol. 91, no. 4, pp. 1027–1034, 2010.

[12] S. Turgut, A. Polat, M. Inan et al., "Interaction between anemia and blood levels of Iron, Zinc, Copper, Cadmium and Lead in children," *Indian Journal of Pediatrics*, vol. 74, no. 9, pp. 827–830, 2007.

[13] S. Turgut, S. Hacioğlu, G. Emmungil, G. Turgut, and A. Keskin, "Relations between Iron deficiency anemia and serum levels of Copper, Zinc, Cadmium and Lead," *Polish Journal of Environmental Studies*, vol. 18, no. 2, pp. 273–277, 2009.

[14] A. A. Hegazy, M. M. Zaher, M. A. Abd El-Hafez, A. A. Morsy, and R. A. Saleh, "Relation between anemia and blood levels of Lead, Copper, Zinc and Iron among children," *BMC Research Notes*, vol. 3, article 133, 2010.

[15] V. De la Cruz-Gongora, B. Gaona, S. Villalpando, T. Shamah-Levy, and R. Robledo, "Anemia and Iron, Zinc, Copper and Magnesium deficiency in Mexican adolescents: National Health and Nutrition Survey 2006," *Salud Publica Mex*, vol. 54, no. 2, pp. 135–145, 2012.

[16] S. S. Gropper, D. M. Bader-Crowe, L. S. McAnulty, B. D. White, and R. E. Keith, "Non-anemic Iron depletion, oral Iron supplementation and indices of Copper status in college-aged females," *Journal of the American College of Nutrition*, vol. 21, no. 6, pp. 545–552, 2002.

[17] F. Shah, T. G. Kazi, H. I. Afridi et al., "Evaluation of status of trace and toxic metals in biological samples (scalp hair, blood, and urine) of normal and anemic children of two age groups," *Biological Trace Element Research*, vol. 141, no. 1–3, pp. 131–149, 2011.

[18] M. A. Knovich, D. Il'yasova, A. Ivanova, and I. Molnár, "The association between serum Copper and anaemia in the adult Second National Health and Nutrition Examination Survey (NHANES II) population," *British Journal of Nutrition*, vol. 99, no. 6, pp. 1226–1229, 2008.

[19] M. Ani and A. A. Moshtaghie, "The effect of chromium on parameters related to Iron metabolism," *Biological Trace Element Research*, vol. 32, pp. 57–64, 1992.

[20] H. C. Lukaski, W. W. Bolonchuk, W. A. Siders, and D. B. Milne, "Chromium supplementation and resistance training: effects on body composition, strength, and trace element status of men," *American Journal of Clinical Nutrition*, vol. 63, no. 6, pp. 954–965, 1996.

[21] P. Maxwell and K. Salnikow, "HIF-1: an Oxygen and metal responsive transcription factor," *Cancer Biology and Therapy*, vol. 3, no. 1, pp. 29–35, 2004.

[22] World Health Organization, *Iron Deficiency Anemia: Assessment, Prevention, and Control—A Guide for Program Managers*, World Health Organization, Geneva, Switzerland, 2001.

[23] L. L. Stookey, "Ferrozine—a new spectrophotometric reagent for Iron," *Analytical Chemistry*, vol. 42, no. 7, pp. 779–781, 1970.

[24] R. Soomro, M. J. Ahmed, and N. Memon, "Simple and rapid spectrophotometric determination of trace level chromium using bis (salicylaldehyde) orthophenylenediamine in nonionic micellar media," *Turkish Journal of Chemistry*, vol. 35, no. 1, pp. 155–170, 2011.

[25] F. W. Sunderman Jr., A. Marzouk, M. C. Crisostomo, and D. R. Weatherby, "Electrothermal atomic absorption spectrophotometry of nickel in tissue homogenates," *Annals of Clinical and Laboratory Science*, vol. 15, no. 4, pp. 299–307, 1985.

[26] B. Brzozowska and T. Zawadzka, "Atomic absorption spectrophotometry method for determination of Lead, Cadmium, Zinc and Copper in various vegetable products," *Roczniki Panstwowego Zakladu Higieny*, vol. 32, no. 1, pp. 9–15, 1981.

[27] C. Brugnara, "Refernce values in infancy and childhood," in *Nathan and Oski's Hematology of Infancy and Childhood*, S. H. Orkin and D. G. Nathan, Eds., p. 1774, Elsevier Saunders, 7th edition, 2009.

[28] B. Glader, "The anemias," in *Nelson Textbook of Pediatrics*, R. M. Kliegman, R. E. Behrman, H. B. Jenson, and B. F. Stanton, Eds., p. 2003, Elsevier Saunders, Philadelphia, Pa, USA, 18th edition, 2007.

[29] N. C. Andrews, C. K. Ullrich, and M. D. Fleming, "Disorders of Iron metabolism and sideroblastic anemia," in *Nathan and Oski's Hematology of Infancy and Childhood*, S. H. Orkin and D. G. Nathan, Eds., Elsevier Saunders, 7th edition, 2009.

[30] G. Hetet, I. Devaux, N. Soufir, B. Grandchamp, and C. Beaumont, "Molecular analyses of patients with hyperferritinemia and normal serum Iron values reveal both L ferritin IRE and 3 new ferroportin (slc11A3) mutations," *Blood*, vol. 102, no. 5, pp. 1904–1910, 2003.

[31] M. A. Akl, "Spectrophotometric and AAS determinations of trace zinc(II) in natural waters and human blood after preconcentration with phenanthraquinone monophenylthiosemicarbazone," *Analytical Sciences*, vol. 17, no. 4, pp. 561–564, 2001.

[32] R. S. Gibson, *Principles of Nutritional Assessment*, Oxford University, New York, NY, USA, 2nd edition, 2005.

[33] J. B. Mason, "Chapter 237: vitamins, trace minerals, and other micronutrients," in *Cecil Medicine*, L. Goldman and D. Ausiello, Eds., Elsevier Saunders, Philadelphia, Pa, USA, 23rd edition, 2007.

[34] D. E. Leavelle, Ed., *Mayo Medical Laboratories Interpretive Handbook: Interpretive Data for Diagnostic Laboratory Tests*, The Laboratories, Rochester, Vt, USA, 2001.

[35] World Health Organization, "Environmental health criteria 108: Nickel," Tech. Rep., World Health Organization, Geneva, Switzerland, 1991.

[36] R. J. Stoltzfus, L. Mullany, and R. E. Black, "Iron deficiency anaemia," in *Comparative Quantification of Health Risks. Global and Regional Burden of Disease Attribution To Selected Major Risk Factors*, M. Ezzati, A. D. Lopez, A. Rodgers, and C. J. L. Murray, Eds., pp. 164–165, World Health Organization, Geneva, Switzerland, 2004.

[37] I. Voskaki, V. Arvanitidou, H. Athanasopoulou, A. Tzagkaraki, G. Tripsianis, and A. Giannoulia-Karantana, "Serum Copper and Zinc levels in healthy Greek children and their parents," *Biological Trace Element Research*, vol. 134, no. 2, pp. 136–145, 2010.

[38] International Zinc Nutrition Consultative Group (IZiNCG), K. H. Brown, J. A. Rivera et al., "International Zinc Nutrition Consultative Group (IZiNCG) technical document #1. Assessment of the risk of zinc deficiency in populations and options for its control," *Food and Nutrition Bulletin*, vol. 25, no. 1, supplement 2, pp. S99–S203, 2004.

[39] M. Kaji and Y. Nishi, "Growth and minerals: Zinc," *Growth, Genetics & Hormones (GGH)*, vol. 22, no. 1, pp. 1–10, 2006.

[40] A. Taylor, E. W. Redworth, and J. B. Morgan, "Influence of diet on Iron, Copper, and Zinc status in children under 24 months of age," *Biological Trace Element Research*, vol. 97, no. 3, pp. 197–214, 2004.

[41] R. S. Gibson, Y. Abebe, S. Stabler et al., "Zinc, gravida, infection, and Iron, but not vitamin B-12 or folate status, predict hemoglobin during pregnancy in Southern Ethiopia," *Journal of Nutrition*, vol. 138, no. 3, pp. 581–586, 2008.

[42] M. Olivares and R. Uauy, "Copper as an essential nutrient," *American Journal of Clinical Nutrition*, vol. 63, no. 5, pp. 791S–796S, 1996.

[43] B. A. Hayton, H. E. Broome, and R. C. Lilenbaum, "Copper deficiency-induced anemia and neutropenia secondary to intestinal malabsorption," *American Journal of Hematology*, vol. 48, no. 1, pp. 45–47, 1995.

[44] R. J. Cousins and R. J. McMahon, "Integrative aspects of Zinc transporters," *Journal of Nutrition*, vol. 130, no. 5, pp. 1384S–1387S, 2000.

[45] Y. Gluhcheva, V. Atanasov, J. Ivanova, and M. Mitewa, "Cobalt-induced changes in the spleen of mice from different stages of development," *Journal of Toxicology and Environmental Health A*, vol. 75, no. 22-23, pp. 1418–1422, 2012.

[46] M. Anke, B. Groppel, H. Kronemann, and M. Grün, "Nickel—an essential element," *IARC Scientific Publications*, no. 53, pp. 339–365, 1984.

[47] M. Muñoz, I. Villar, and J. A. García-Erce, "An update on Iron physiology," *World Journal of Gastroenterology*, vol. 15, no. 37, pp. 4617–4626, 2009.

[48] B. Glader, "Anemias of inadequate production," in *Nelson Textbook of Pediatrics*, R. M. Kliegman, R. E. Behrman, H. B. Jenson, and B. F. Stanton, Eds., p. 2013, Elsevier Saunders, Philadelphia, Pa, USA, 18th edition, 2007.

[49] "FAO/WHO expert consultation on human vitamin and mineral requirements," in *Human Vitamin and Mineral Requirements*, Food and Nutrition Division FAO, Rome, Italy, 2001.

[50] A. D. Sharma, "Low nickel diet in dermatology," *Indian Journal of Dermatology*, vol. 58, no. 3, pp. 240–247, 2013.

9

Uptake of Non-Transferrin Iron by Erythroid Cells

Eugenia Prus and Eitan Fibach

Department of Hematology, Hadassah-Hebrew University Medical Center, Ein-Kerem, P.O. Box 12000, Jerusalem 91120, Israel

Correspondence should be addressed to Eitan Fibach, fibach@yahoo.com

Academic Editor: Antonis Kattamis

Most of the iron in the plasma is bound to transferrin (Tf) and is taken up by cells through their surface Tf receptors (TfRs). Under pathological conditions of iron-overload, the plasma iron which is in excess of the binding capacity of Tf is present as non-Tf-bound iron. We probed the uptake of non-Tf iron and its consequences on the oxidative status of peripheral RBC and reticulocytes as well as developing erythroid precursors grown in vitro. The cells were exposed to ferrous ammonium sulfate under Tf-supplemented and Tf-free conditions. Using flow cytometry techniques, we found that both the TfR-deficient mature RBC and their TfR-containing precursors at all stages of maturation can take up non-Tf iron that accumulates as redox-active labile iron and generates reactive oxygen species. Such a mechanism may account for ineffective erythropoiesis of developing precursors in the bone marrow and for the shortening of the lifespan of mature RBCs in the circulation.

1. Introduction

Most of the iron in the plasma is bound to transferrin (Tf) which serves as a carrier protein that mediates the uptake of iron by cells through their surface Tf receptor-1 (TfR) [1]. Intracellularly, iron is released from Tf following a decrease in endosomal pH and is then transported across the endosomal membrane by DMT1 (also known as Nramp2) [2]. Under pathological conditions of iron-overload, plasma iron which is in excess of the binding capacity of Tf is present as non-Tf bound iron (NTBI) [3]. This chemically ill-defined iron and its redox potent labile plasma iron (LPI) can be taken up by cells in vital organs via several pathways and be responsible for the major pathological consequences of iron-overload [4].

In erythroid cells, while most of the iron is in the form of hemoglobin (Hb), some iron is in the form of labile iron [5]. It has a redox potential and generates reactive oxygen species (ROS) which leads to cytotoxic effects [6]. We have previously reported that the labile iron pool (LIP), also termed labile cellular iron (LCI), is increased in RBCs under conditions of iron overload, such as in the case of chronic anemias associated with blood transfusions [7]. Increased LIP in RBCs may be the result of abnormal iron turnover in developing precursors (due to increased

uptake from iron-overloaded plasma, diminished utilization because of reduced Hb production, or degradation of unstable Hb). In addition, RBCs may take up NTBI from their environment (the plasma). Iron uptake by RBCs and reticulocytes (retics) has been previously demonstrated in various model systems using radiolabeled iron [8–11]. But, the results have been disputed because the experiments were carried out in artificial media containing high sucrose. In the present study, we probed the uptake of non-Tf iron by various erythroid cells. We utilized a novel flow cytometry methodology [12] to measure the uptake of iron and the generation of ROS by peripheral blood RBCs and retics in their autologous plasma as well as by human developing erythroid precursors grown in vitro. The results showed that both the TfR-deficient mature RBCs and the TfR-bearing erythroid precursors at all stages of maturation can take up non-Tf iron. This uptake was associated with increased LIP and ROS generation. Such a mechanism may account for the hematological consequences of iron-overload—ineffective erythropoiesis and short lifespan of RBCs in the circulation.

2. Methods

2.1. Blood Cells and Erythroid Cultures. Normal human peripheral RBCs, obtained in heparin-containing tubes, were used in all experiments, unless otherwise stated. Some experiments were performed with RBCs obtained from thalassemic mice. The founders of the mouse colony were obtained from Dr. S. Rivella, Weill Medical College of Cornell University, NY, NY. Heterozygotes (Hbb$^{th3/+}$) mice exhibit severe anemia (7 to 9 g/dL Hb), abnormal RBCs morphology, splenomegaly, and hepatic iron deposition [13]. Animals were bred at the animal facility of Hadassah—Hebrew University Medical Center. The research was approved by the Hadassah—Hebrew University Medical Center Human Experimentation Review Board and the Animal Ethics Committee. All human participants gave written informed consent.

Erythroid cultures were initiated by growing human peripheral blood mononuclear cells in a two-phase liquid culture system as previously described in [14, 15]. In short, cells were first cultured in alpha medium supplemented with 10% fetal calf serum and 10% conditioned medium obtained from cultures of the human 5637 bladder carcinoma cell line and 1 μg/mL cyclosporin A (phase I). After 7 days, nonadherent cells were harvested, washed and suspended in phase II medium, containing alpha medium, 30% fetal calf serum, 1% bovine serum albumin, 10 μM β-mercaptoethanol, 1.5 mM glutamine, 10 μM dexamethasone, 5 ng/ml stem cell factor and 1 U/ml human recombinant erythropoietin. Hb-containing cells were scored by staining with benzidine dihydrochloride [15].

2.2. Iron and Chelators. Ferrous ammonium sulfate (FAS) (Sigma, St. Louis, MO) was freshly dissolved for each experiment in water to 1 mM. Human holotransferrin (90% saturated) was purchased from Biological Industries (Beit-Hemek, Israel) and added to cells at 300 μg/mL. Deferiprone (L1) (Apotex, Weston, ON, Canada) was freshly dissolved in water to 20 mM and added at 50 μM.

2.3. Measurements of Iron Uptake and ROS Generation. Iron uptake was measured as previously described in [12]. For measurement of cytoplasmic LIP cells were loaded for 15 min at 37°C with calcein acetoxymethyl ester (CA-AM) (Sigma-Aldrich, St. Louis, MO) (1 μM for RBCs and retics, and 0.5 μM for cultured cells). CA-AM enters viable cells and becomes fluorescent upon hydrolysis by esterases; its fluorescence is quenched by binding of LIP [16–19]. Mitochondrial LIP was measured by staining cultured cells with 1 μM rhodamine B-[(1,10-phenanthrolin-5-yl)-aminocarbonyl] benzyl ester (RPA, Squarix biotechnology, Marl, Germany) for 20 min at 37°C as previously described in [12].

ROS were measured by staining with 0.1 mM 2′–7′-dichlorofluorescin diacetate (DCF, Sigma) for 15 min at 37°C [20]. Upon crossing the membrane, this compound undergoes deacetylation by intracellular esterases, producing a nonfluorescent compound that is trapped inside the cells. Its oxidation by ROS produced a highly fluorescent compound—2′–7′-dichlorofluorescine (CA) [21].

2.4. Flow Cytometry. Cell fluorescence was analyzed by a flow cytometer (FACS-calibur^R, Becton-Dickinson, Immunofluorometry systems, Mountain View, CA) as previously described in [12]. A 488-nm argon and 635-nm red diode lasers were used for excitation. At least 20,000 cells were analyzed using logarithmic amplification for the fluorescence signal height and linear amplification for forward light scatter and side light scatter. "Threshold" was set on forward light scatter to exclude cell debris, microparticles and platelets. In some experiments, blood cells were stained simultaneously with CA or DCF and an allophycocyanin-(APC-) conjugated anti-CD71 antibody (Becton-Dickinson, San Jose, CA) for 15 min at 37°C. Cells were gated as CD71$^+$ (retics) and CD71$^-$ (RBCs), and the green fluorescence (CA or DCF) of each population was measured. Mitochondrial LIP was measured in cultured erythroid cells stained with RPA. The arithmetic Mean Fluorescence Intensities (MFI) were calculated by the CellQuest^R software (Becton-Dickinson). For each experiment, unstained cells served as controls; their MFI was <10. The statistical significance was calculated using the two-sample Student's t-test for differences in means $P < .05$ was considered significant.

3. Results

The flow cytometry methodology for measuring iron uptake and ROS generation in RBCs and retics is illustrated in Figure 1. Blood cells were diluted in PBS, labeled with an APC-conjugated anti-CD71 antibody and either CA-AM or DCF, washed with PBS, diluted in their autologous plasma, and incubated with or without FAS (20 μM for 1 hr). Figures 1(a) and 1(b) demonstrate FSC × CD71 dot plots of RBCs (CD71$^-$) and retics (CD71$^+$), respectively. Figures 1(c) and 1(d) show histogram distributions of both populations with respect to CA- and DCF-fluorescence, respectively. Cells incubated without iron showed a much higher basal CA-fluorescence (MFI−Fe 1450 versus 810) and DCF-fluorescence (1003 versus 315) in retics compared to RBCs (Figures 1(e) and 1(f)). Iron uptake resulted in a decrease in the CA-fluorescence (Figure 1(e)) and an increase in the DCF-fluorescence (Figure 1(f)). The data for each population were reported as the percent change in the MFI following incubation with FAS, calculated as percentage of the basal fluorescence [100 × (MFI − Fe − MFI + Fe)/(MFI − Fe)]. In the representative experiment shown in Figure 1, the change in the CA-MFI was 14.9% for RBCs and 20.7% for retics (Figure 1(e)). The change in the DCF-MFI was 34.9% for RBCs and 35.2% for retics (Figure 1(f)).

Using this methodology, we studied the time- and dose-related effects (Figures 2(a) and 2(b), resp.) of iron uptake by RBCs and retics. Iron uptake was detected as early as 1 min after addition of FAS. It was faster in retics than in RBCs; in RBCs it plateaued after 45 min, whereas in retics it continued to increase for 3 hrs, reaching 6.8-fold higher levels than in RBCs. In both RBCs and retics, iron uptake was dose dependent; it was detected at 1 μM FAS and increased up to 20 μM. Iron uptake was associated with increased ROS

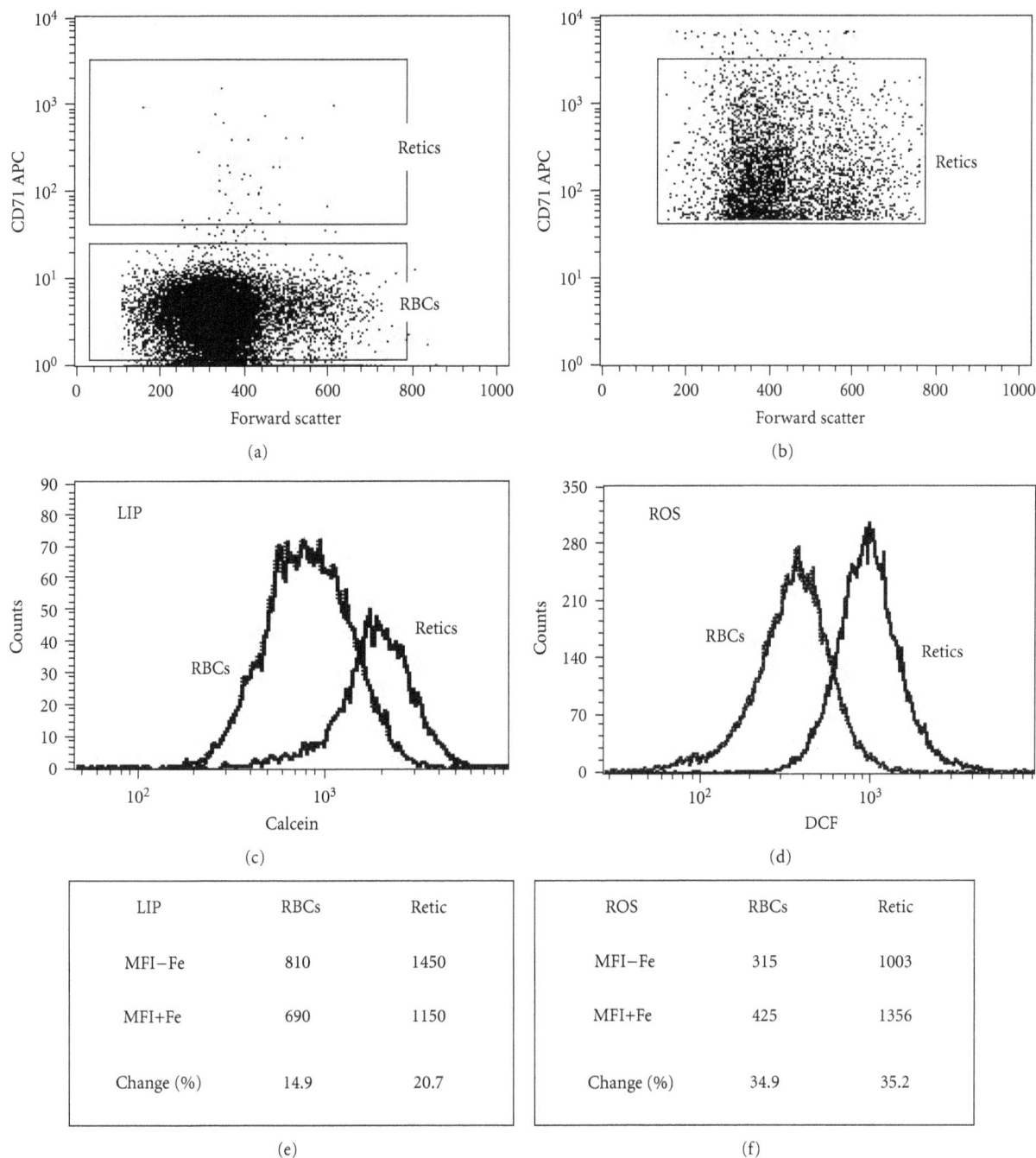

FIGURE 1: Flow cytometry measurement of iron uptake and reactive oxygen species (ROS) generation in RBCs and reticulocytes. Normal peripheral blood cells were diluted (5×10^6/ml) in PBS, stained with CA-AM or DCF and an APC-conjugated anti-CD71 antibody. Following washing with PBS, they were resuspended in their autologous plasma and then incubated with (+Fe) or without ($-$Fe) 20μM FeSO$_4$ for 1 hr. (a) A FSC $\times$ CD71 dot-plot, showing the gates for RBCs (CD71$^-$) and reticulocytes (retics) (CD71$^+$). (b) A FSC $\times$ CD71 dot-plot of events acquired in the retic gate. (c, d) Histogram distributions of both populations with respect to CA- and DCF-fluorescence, respectively. (e, f) Summaries of the results obtained in each population following incubation with and without Fe. The MFIs and the percent change in the MFIs of each population incubated with and without Fe, calculated per the basal fluorescence (MFI$-$Fe) are indicated.

generation during the first 15–30 min in both RBCs and in retics (Figures 2(c) and 2(d)).

Normal plasma contains unsaturated Tf, therefore some of the iron added in these experiments became bound to Tf. Since mature RBCs are devoid of TfR [22], their iron uptake is necessarily Tf independent. To substantiate this point and to determine whether such a mechanism is operative also in retics, iron uptake was measured in parallel in Tf-containing (autologous plasma) and Tf-free media. The results showed that iron uptake was slower in plasma (2.5-fold in RBCs and

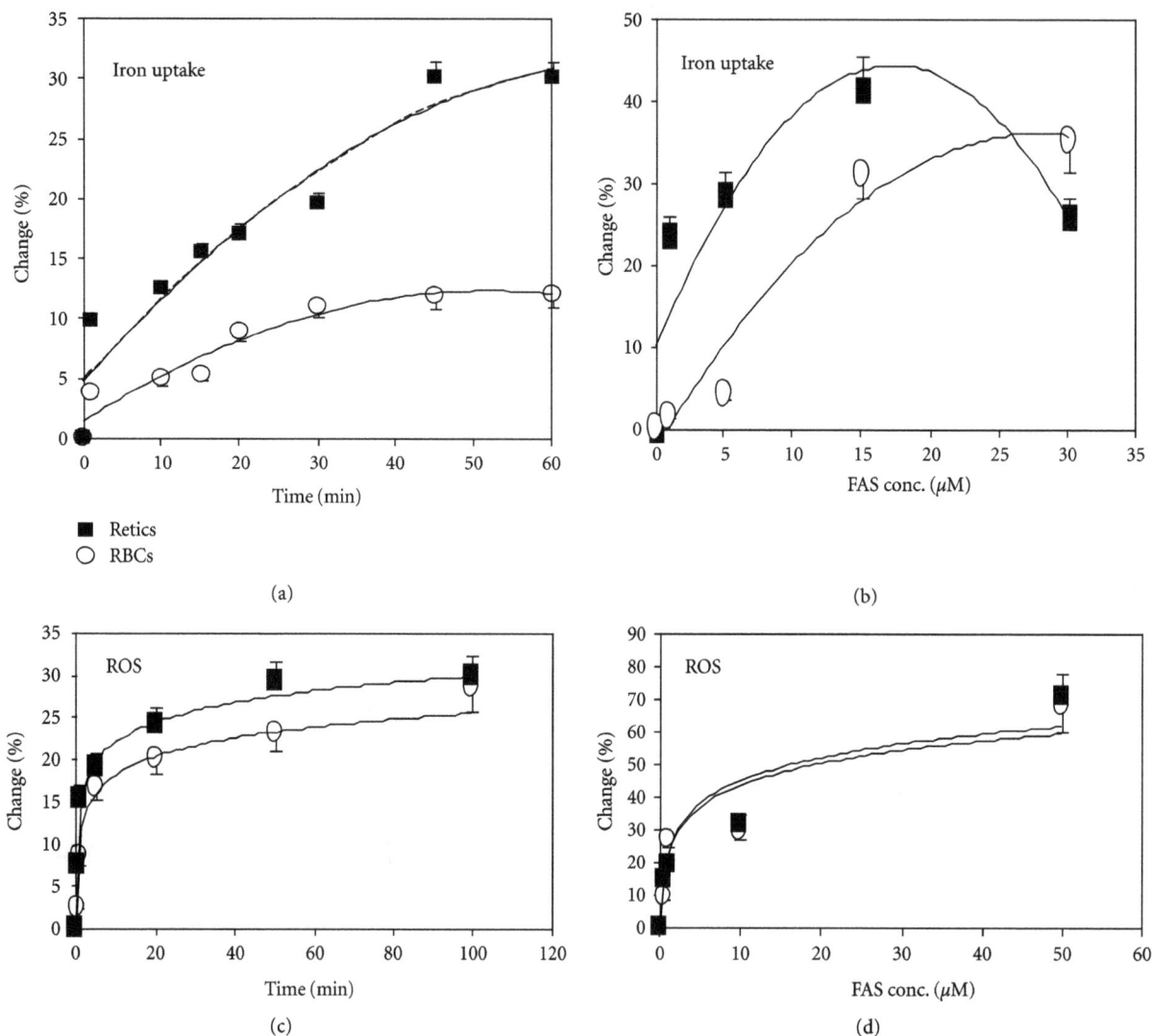

FIGURE 2: Time- and dose-related iron uptake and ROS generation by RBCs and reticulocytes. Normal peripheral blood cells were labeled, suspended in their autologous plasma and incubated with or without FeSO$_4$ (FAS) as described in the legends to Figure 1. (a, c) Labeled cells were incubated with or without 20 μM FAS for the indicated durations. (b, d) Labeled cells were incubated with the indicated concentrations of FAS for 1 hr. The results of iron uptake (a, b) and ROS generation (c, d) in RBCs ($\circ$) and retics ($\blacksquare$) are expressed as the percent (%) change (mean $\pm$ SD, $N = 4$) in the MFIs following incubation with and without Fe, calculated per the MFI$-$Fe.

2-fold in retics, both $P < .01$) and indicated that both cells take up iron by a Tf-independent mechanism.

In order to probe the nature of the incoming iron, CA-loaded RBCs were exposed to 20 μM FAS in PBS, washed, and then further incubated with or without the cell-permeable iron-chelator-L1 (50 μM for 1 hr). The results showed a 33% ($P = .005$) increase in the CA-MFI following incubation with L1, similar to the fluorescence of iron-untreated cells. The ability of L1 to overcome the iron-mediated quenching of CA, most probably by binding and thus removing iron from its complex with CA, fulfils the operational definition of the incoming iron as LIP [12].

To establish the pathological significance of non-Tf iron uptake, we used blood from heterozygotes (Hbb$^{th3/+}$) mice, a mouse model of β-thalassemia, which suffer from

iron-overload [13]. CA-loaded normal mouse RBCs were incubated for 1 hour in plasma derived either from normal or thalassemic mice. The results showed lower CA-MFI of RBCs incubated in thalassemic plasma by 10$\pm$2% ($P = .005$), indicating increased LIP than the same RBCs incubated in normal plasma. These results suggest that in thalassemia, continuous, Tf-independent, uptake of iron from the plasma might have a significant effect on the RBCs LIP content.

To determine the ability of developing erythroid precursors to take up iron in a Tf-independent pathway, cultured erythroid precursors were harvested on days 7-8 of phase II cultures, loaded with CA, washed, and resuspended in phase II medium (containing 30% serum) or in PBS and incubated for 1 or 2 hrs with different concentrations of FAS. The results (Figure 3(a)) indicated enhanced iron uptake in PBS than in serum-containing medium (P = .001). Tf-independent iron uptake in PBS was associated with increased ROS generation as reflected by DCF fluorescence (Figure 3(b)). In another set of experiments, the CA-loaded cells were washed, and resuspended in PBS supplemented with or without Tf (300 μg/mL) and incubated for 1–3 hrs with different concentrations of FAS (Figure 3(c)). The results showed that in the presence of Tf, iron uptake was slower, but after 3 hrs, at the higher concentrations of FAS (20–50 μM), the intracellular iron reached a comparable level to that of cells incubated without Tf.

When erythroid precursors from day 6 phase II cultures were washed and incubated in PBS with 20 μM FAS for 1 hr, they demonstrated not only an increased cytoplasmic LIP but also a significant increase (P = .001) in mitochondrial LIP, assayed by the change in the fluorescence of a mitochondrial-specific probe (RPA), and in ROS (Figure 4(a)).

The effect of non-Tf iron on development of erythroid cells was demonstrated by adding various concentrations of FAS to day 6 phase II cultures. Counting Hb-containing cells after 3 days indicated a significant decrease (FAS = 100 μM versus FAS = 0, P < .001) by the addition of iron (Figure 4(b)).

4. Discussion

The labile iron pool (LIP) is considered the main cause of malfunctioning of vital organs (e.g., heart, liver, endocrine glands) of patients with iron-overload [3, 23]. Increased LIP may be deleterious to erythroid cells as well; it may be involved in increased apoptosis of developing precursors in the bone marrow (ineffective erythropoiesis) [24] and in shortening of the lifespan of mature RBCs due to extravascular hemolysis. The cytotoxic effects of LIP are probably mediated by increased generation of ROS and the resultant state of oxidative stress [25, 26]. In thalassemia, where iron overload is caused by enhanced iron absorption in the gastrointestinal track [27] and by frequent blood transfusions, we have shown that LIP is high in RBCs and retics, as well as in immature developing erythroid precursors, compared to their normal counterparts [7].

Increased LIP in RBCs may be the result of leftover of unused iron in precursors due to increased uptake (from iron-overloaded plasma), diminished utilization because of reduced Hb production, or degradation of unstable Hb. In addition, RBCs may take up iron from their environment, especially when the amount of iron in the plasma exceeds the binding capacity of Tf. Since mature RBCs are devoid of TfR [22], this uptake is necessarily of non-Tf iron.

In the present study we probed the uptake of non-Tf iron supplied as FAS and its consequences on ROS generation in normal human peripheral blood RBCs and retics as well as in their precursors grown in vitro. The incoming iron and the ROS generation were measured by flow cytometry of cells loaded with fluorescent probes, CA or DCF, respectively. Iron uptake resulted in a decrease in CA-fluorescence while ROS generation resulted in an increase in DCF-fluorescence. The results were expressed as the percent change in the

MFI of iron-treated cells compared to untreated cells. Dual staining with CA or DCF and APC-conjugated antibodies to TfR (CD71) permitted simultaneous analysis of RBCs (TfR-negative cells) and retics (TfR-bearing cells). The results indicated that iron uptake by RBCs and retics was dose- and time dependent. It was detected at FAS concentrations as low as 1 μM and increased at higher concentrations. The uptake was faster and reached higher levels in retics than in RBCs. The ability of the incoming iron to bind and quench the fluorescence of CA indicated its labile, chelatable nature. Indeed, when the potent, cell permeable iron-chelator, deferiprone (L1), was added to FAS-treated cells it increased the CA-fluorescence to levels of FAS-untreated cells.

The results also showed that iron uptake by both cell types was associated with an enhanced ROS generation, which was ameliorated by L1. The latter results are in agreement with our previous report that in vitro treatment of iron-overloaded thalassemic RBCs with clinically used iron-chelators, including L1, decreased their LIP as well as ROS [28].

In the present study, iron uptake was first analyzed by exposing peripheral blood cells to FAS in their autologous plasma. Normal plasma, however, contains unsaturated Tf; some of the added iron in these experiments could, therefore, bind to and delivered by Tf. Since mature RBCs are devoid of TfR [22], their iron uptake was necessarily Tf independent. To study whether Tf-independent iron uptake was also operative in TfR-carrying retics, we exposed the cells to FAS in parallel in Tf-containing (autologous plasma) and in Tf-free (PBS) media. The results showed slower iron uptake in plasma than in PBS and indicated those both RBCs and retics take up iron by Tf-independent mechanisms. These results are in agreement with previous data that normal mouse retics acquire non-Tf iron at rates much higher than that at which iron is taken up physiologically from Tf [29]. These results and our present data suggest that in iron-overload, when non-Tf iron is present in the serum, the levels of Tf-receptors do not represent a limiting factor in iron uptake.

The uptake of non-Tf iron by rats and mouse RBCs and retics has been previously studied in vitro using radio-labeled iron. Under the experimental conditions used (e.g., high sucrose-containing medium), it was found that immature erythroid cells acquire non-Tf iron, most probably through their DMT1 transmembrane transport system. But, since physiologically all iron in the circulation is Tf-bound, DMT1 expressed at the plasma membrane has no substrate; it was assumed to function not as an external transporter but to mobilize iron intracellularly, for example, iron transport across the endosomal or the mitochondrial membranes [29].

The uptake of non-Tf iron by developing erythroid cells was studied in cultures derived from normal human erythroid progenitors. These cultures have been previously demonstrated to recapitulate erythropoiesis in vivo, including various aspects of iron metabolism [30]. Following culture in serum-containing medium, the cells were harvested, washed, loaded with CA, and resuspended in PBS or complete serum-containing culture medium. Iron entry was faster and to a larger extent in the absence of serum

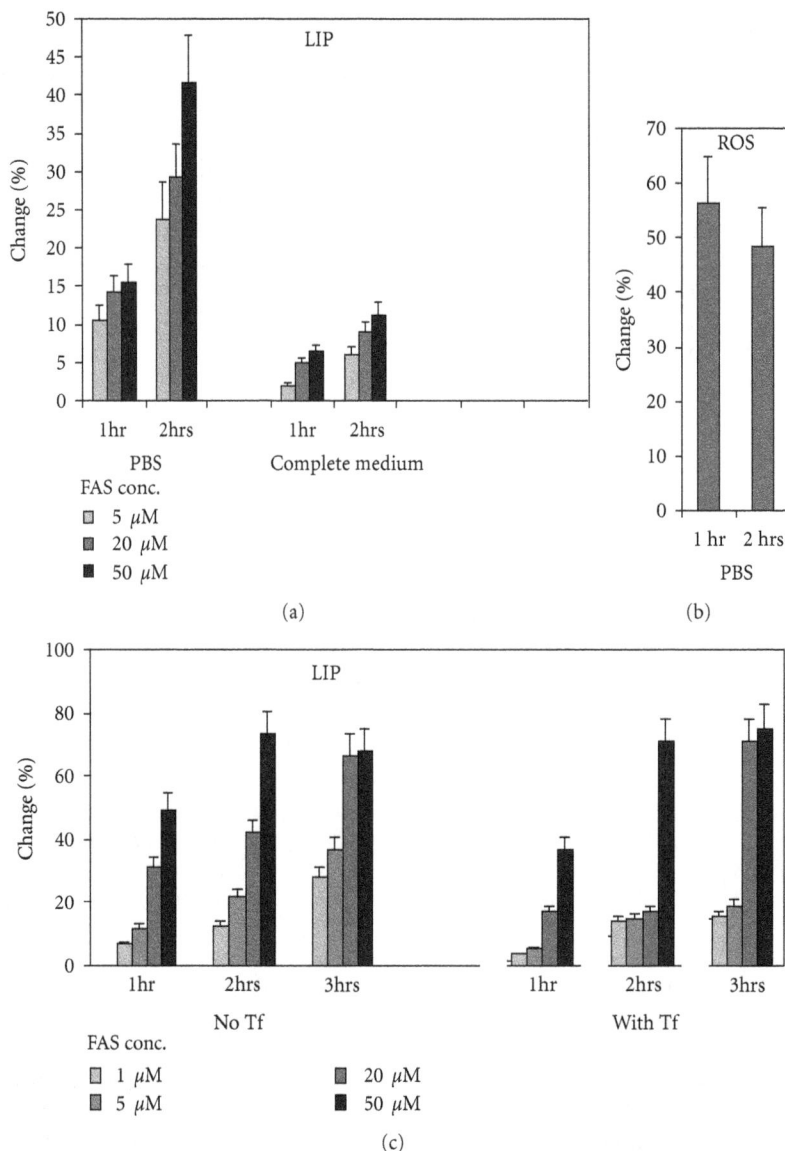

(a)

(b)

(c)

FIGURE 3: The effect of transferrin (Tf) on iron uptake and ROS by cultured erythroid precursors. Cultured human erythroid precursors were harvested on days 7-8 of phase II, washed and loaded with CA or DCF. (a) CA-loaded cells were washed and resuspended in PBS or in phase II medium (complete medium, containing 30% serum), and incubated for 1- or 2 hrs with the indicated concentrations of FAS. (b) DCF-loaded cells were washed and resuspended in PBS, and incubated for 1- or 2 hrs with the indicated concentrations of FAS. (c) CA-loaded cells were washed and resuspended in PBS supplemented with or without human holo-Tf (300 μg/mL) and incubated for 1–3 hrs with the indicated concentrations of FAS. The results indicated reduced iron uptake in the presence of Tf. The results are expressed as the percent (%) change (mean ± SD, $N = 4$) in the MFIs following incubation with and without Fe, calculated per the MFI−Fe.

indicating that Tf-independent iron uptake is operative in these cells too. We then studied the direct effect of Tf. The results indicated that iron uptake from Tf was much slower than that from FAS. When holo-Tf (90% saturated) was added together with FAS, iron uptake was retarded compared to FAS alone. It is interesting to note in this context that treating thalassemic mice with apo-Tf has been shown to reduce their iron load [31].

The results indicated that RBCs, retics as well as erythroid precursors at early stages of maturation take up iron through a Tf-independent pathway. It is unlikely that this pathway is operative normally, but only under pathological iron-overload situation when NTBI appears in the serum. Whether erythroid cells at various stages of maturation share the same mechanism of Tf-independent iron uptake is still an open question. Although the incoming non-Tf iron is found in the mitochondria of erythroid precursors, as determined by reducing the RPA fluorescence (Figure 4), it is not likely to participate in heme synthesis and Hb production. We have previously shown that, unlike Tf-iron and to some extent iron-ferritin and hemin, non-Tf iron cannot support the survival, proliferation, and hemoglobinization

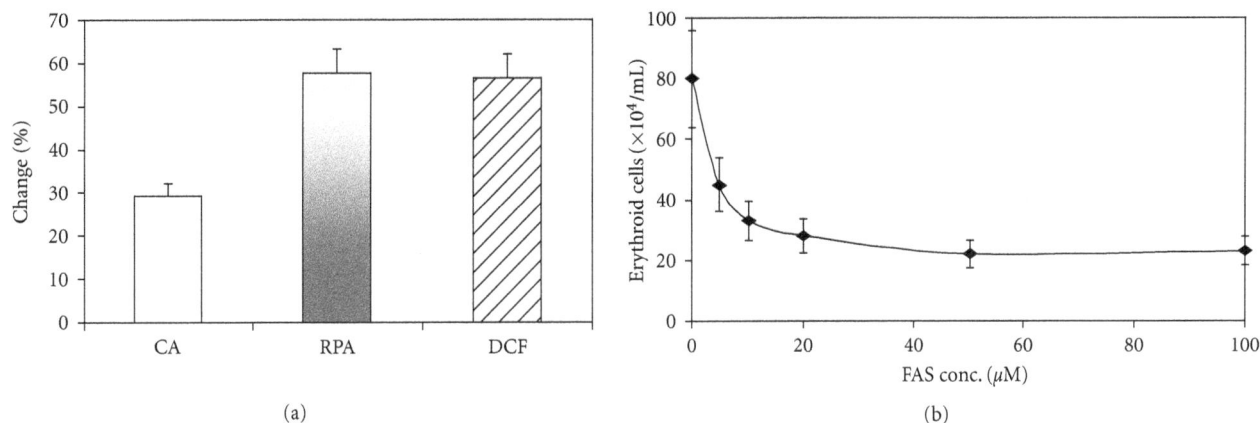

FIGURE 4: The effects of non-transferrin iron uptake on cytoplasmic and mitochondrial LIP and ROS generation by cultured erythroid precursors. Cultured human erythroid precursors were harvested on day 6 of phase II, incubated with or without 20 μM FAS for 1 hr, and stained with CA, RPA or DCF for measurement of cytoplasmic and mitochondrial LIPs and ROS generation, respectively. The results are expressed as the percent (%) change (mean ± SD, $N = 4$) in the MFIs following incubation with and without Fe, calculated per the MFI−Fe. (b) The indicated concentrations of FAS were added to day 6 cultures. Hb-containing cells were counted by benzidine staining on day 9. The results are expressed as the (mean ± SD, $N = 4$).

of erythroid precursors in vitro [32]. In contrast, non-Tf iron uptake involves in the induction of ROS generation and its cytopathological consequences, as demonstrated by a decrease in erythroid cell yield in cultures exposed to FAS (Figure 4).

Finally, our results suggest that flow cytometry analyses of LIP and ROS in RBCs might reflect "real-time" iron accumulation and as such might complement the measurements of serum ferritin—an acute phase reactant which is elevated in various inflammatory states, not necessarily related to iron overload [33]. The LIP assay does not reflect iron that has already accumulated in tissues and therefore cannot replace liver biopsy or MRI; however, since this assay is nonhazardous and much cheaper, when performed on multiple occasions, it might predict potential iron overload in tissues as well.

5. Conclusions

RBCs, retics, and developing erythroid precursors take up iron through a Tf-independent pathway. This pathway is operative under pathological iron-overload situation in the presence of non-Tf iron in the serum. The incoming non-Tf iron does not participate in heme synthesis and Hb production, but induces ROS generation, which results in cytotoxicity and a decrease in the erythroid cell yield. In addition, the flow cytometry methodology used in the present study may provide an analytical platform for practical and accurate measurements of LIP and ROS in RBCs for evaluating iron-overload and chelation therapy.

Authors Contribution

E. Prus performed the research, analyzed data and participated in writing the paper. E. Fibach designed the research, analyzed data and wrote the paper.

Conflict of Interests

The authors declare no competing financial interests.

Acknowledgment

The authors thank Mrs. Aliza Treves for her technical assistance.

References

[1] D. R. Richardson and P. Ponka, "The molecular mechanisms of the metabolism and transport of iron in normal and neoplastic cells," *Biochimica et Biophysica Acta*, vol. 1331, no. 1, pp. 1–40, 1997.

[2] M. D. Fleming, C. C. Trenor, M. A. Su et al., "Microcytic anaemia mice have a mutation in Nramp2, a candidate iron transporter gene," *Nature Genetics*, vol. 16, no. 4, pp. 383–386, 1997.

[3] Z. I. Cabantchik, OR. Kakhlon, S. Epsztejn, G. Zanninelli, and W. Breuer, "Intracellular and extracellular labile iron pools," *Advances in Experimental Medicine and Biology*, vol. 509, pp. 55–75, 2003.

[4] Z. I. Cabantchik, W. Breuer, G. Zanninelli, and P. Cianciulli, "LPI-labile plasma iron in iron overload," *Best Practice and Research: Clinical Haematology*, vol. 18, no. 2, pp. 277–287, 2005.

[5] A. Jacobs, "Low molecular weight intracellular iron transport compounds," *Blood*, vol. 50, no. 3, pp. 433–439, 1977.

[6] E. Fibach and E. Rachmilewitz, "The role of oxidative stress in hemolytic anemia," *Current Molecular Medicine*, vol. 8, no. 7, pp. 609–619, 2008.

[7] E. Prus and E. Fibach, "The labile iron pool in human erythroid cells," *British Journal of Haematology*, vol. 142, no. 2, pp. 301–307, 2008.

[8] E. H. Morgan, "Membrane transport of non-transferrin-bound iron by reticulocytes," *Biochimica et Biophysica Acta*, vol. 943, no. 3, pp. 428–439, 1988.

[9] A. Egyed, "Carrier mediated iron transport through erythroid cell membrane," *British Journal of Haematology*, vol. 68, no. 4, pp. 483–486, 1988.

[10] L. M. Garrick, K. G. Dolan, M. A. Romano, and M. D. Garrick, "Non-transferrin-bound iron uptake in Belgrade and normal rat erythroid cells," *Journal of Cellular Physiology*, vol. 178, no. 3, pp. 349–358, 1999.

[11] F. Canonne-Hergaux, AN. S. Zhang, P. Ponka, and P. Gros, "Characterization of the iron transporter DMT1 (NRAMP/DCT) in red blood cells of normal and anemic mk/mk mice," *Blood*, vol. 98, no. 13, pp. 3823–3830, 2001.

[12] E. Prus and E. Fibach, "Flow cytometry measurement of the labile iron pool in human hematopoietic cells," *Cytometry Part A*, vol. 73, no. 1, pp. 22–27, 2008.

[13] P. Ramos, L. Melchiori, S. Gardenghi et al., "Iron metabolism and ineffective erythropoiesis in β-thalassemia mouse models," *Annals of the New York Academy of Sciences*, vol. 1202, pp. 24–30, 2010.

[14] E. Fibach, D. Manor, A. Oppenheim, and E. A. Rachmilewitz, "Proliferation and maturation of human erythroid progenitors in liquid culture," *Blood*, vol. 73, no. 1, pp. 100–103, 1989.

[15] E. Fibach and E. Prus, "Differentiation of human erythroid cells in culture," in *Current Protocols in Immunology*, J. Coligan, B. Bierer, D. Margulies, E. Shevach, and W. Strober, Eds., vol. 2, supplement 69, pp. 22.F7.1–22.F7.10, John Wiley & Sons, Edison, NJ, USA, 2005.

[16] S. A. Weston and C. R. Parish, "New fluorescent dyes for lymphocyte migration studies: analysis by flow cytometry and fluorescence microscopy," *Journal of Immunological Methods*, vol. 133, no. 1, pp. 87–97, 1990.

[17] S. A. Weston and C. R. Parish, "Calcein: a novel marker for lymphocytes which enter lymph nodes," *Cytometry*, vol. 13, no. 7, pp. 739–749, 1992.

[18] W. Breuer, S. Epsztejn, and Z. I. Cabantchik, "Iron acquired from transferrin by K562 cells is delivered into a cytoplasmic pool of chelatable iron(II)," *Journal of Biological Chemistry*, vol. 270, no. 41, pp. 24209–24215, 1995.

[19] F. Petrat, D. Weisheit, M. Lensen, H. De Groot, R. Sustmann, and U. Rauen, "Selective determination of mitochondrial chelatable iron in viable cells with a new fluorescent sensor," *Biochemical Journal*, vol. 362, no. 1, pp. 137–147, 2002.

[20] J. Amer, A. Goldfarb, and E. Fibach, "Flow cytometric measurement of reactive oxygen species production by normal and thalassaemic red blood cells," *European Journal of Haematology*, vol. 70, no. 2, pp. 84–90, 2003.

[21] D. A. Bass, J. W. Parce, and L. R. Dechatelet, "Flow cytometric studies of oxidative product formation by neutrophils: a graded response to membrane stimulation," *Journal of Immunology*, vol. 130, no. 4, pp. 1910–1917, 1983.

[22] M. R. Loken, V. O. Shah, K. L. Dattilio, and C. I. Civin, "Flow cytometric analysis of human bone marrow: I. Normal erythroid development," *Blood*, vol. 69, no. 1, pp. 255–263, 1987.

[23] Y. Kohgo, K. Ikuta, T. Ohtake, Y. Torimoto, and J. Kato, "Body iron metabolism and pathophysiology of iron overload," *International Journal of Hematology*, vol. 88, no. 1, pp. 7–15, 2008.

[24] S. Rivella, "Ineffective erythropoiesis and thalassemias," *Current Opinion in Hematology*, vol. 16, no. 3, pp. 187–194, 2009.

[25] M. Kruszewski, "Labile iron pool: the main determinant of cellular response to oxidative stress," *Mutation Research*, vol. 531, no. 1-2, pp. 81–92, 2003.

[26] E. Prus and E. Fibach, "Effect of iron chelators on labile iron and oxidative status of thalassaemic erythroid cells," *Acta Haematologica*, vol. 123, no. 1, pp. 14–20, 2009.

[27] G. Rechavi and S. Rivella, "Regulation of iron absorption in hemoglobinopathies," *Current Molecular Medicine*, vol. 8, no. 7, pp. 646–662, 2008.

[28] E. Prus and E. Fibach, "Effect of iron chelators on labile iron and oxidative status of thalassaemic erythroid cells," *Acta Haematologica*, vol. 123, no. 1, pp. 14–20, 2009.

[29] A. S. Zhang, F. Canonne-Hergaux, S. Gruenheid, P. Gros, and P. Ponka, "Use of Nramp2-transfected Chinese hamster ovary cells and reticulocytes from mk/mk mice to study iron transport mechanisms," *Experimental Hematology*, vol. 36, no. 10, pp. 1227–1235, 2008.

[30] J. M. Leimberg, A. M. Konijn, and E. Fibach, "Developing human erythroid cells grown in transferrin-free medium utilize iron originating from extracellular ferritin," *American Journal of Hematology*, vol. 73, no. 3, pp. 211–212, 2003.

[31] H. Li, A. C. Rybicki, S. M. Suzuka et al., "Transferrin therapy ameliorates disease in β-thalassemic mice," *Nature Medicine*, vol. 16, no. 2, pp. 177–182, 2010.

[32] J. M. Leimberg, E. Prus, G. Link, E. Fibach, and A. M. Konijn, "Iron-chelator complexes as iron sources for early developing human erythroid precursors," *Translational Research*, vol. 151, no. 2, pp. 88–96, 2008.

[33] K. Kalantar-Zadeh, R. A. Rodriguez, and M. H. Humphreys, "Association between serum ferritin and measures of inflammation, nutrition and iron in haemodialysis patients," *Nephrology Dialysis Transplantation*, vol. 19, no. 1, pp. 141–149, 2004.

10

Iron Deficiency Anemia among Hospitalized Children in Konya, Turkey

Fatih Akin,[1] **Ece Selma Solak,**[1] **Cengizhan Kilicaslan,**[1] **Saltuk Bugra Boke,**[1] **and Sukru Arslan**[2]

[1] *Department of Pediatrics, Konya Training and Research Hospital, Meram, 42090 Konya, Turkey*
[2] *Department of Pediatric Nephrology, Konya Training and Research Hospital, 42090 Konya, Turkey*

Correspondence should be addressed to Fatih Akin; drfatihakin@gmail.com

Academic Editor: Aurelio Maggio

The aim of this study was to investigate the characteristics of our hospitalized patients with the diagnosis of iron deficiency anemia (IDA) and effects of the IDA prevention project of the Turkish Ministry of Health which was started in 2004. The recommended dose of prophylactic iron supplementation was 1-2 mg/kg/day. The files of 1519 patients who were hospitalized to Konya Education and Research Hospital Pediatrics Clinic were reviewed. A total of 50 patients consisting of 35 boys and 15 girls with the mean age of 16,59 ± 1,68 months were included into the study. The prevalence of IDA was 3.29% (boys: 4.23%, girls: 2.1%). Hgb and Hct of the patients >24 months were significantly higher than those of the patients with the age of 6–12 months. Iron supplementation receiving rates were very low. Of the 28 patients older than 12 months, only 44% of them had received a full course of iron supplementation for 8 months. In conclusion, although prophylactic iron supplementation lowered the prevalences of IDA, receiving rates of iron supplementation were not adequate. While IDA is still a public health problem, prophylactic approaches should be carried out more effectively.

1. Introduction

Iron deficiency is the most common and widespread nutritional disorder in the world [1]. It is the only nutrient deficiency which is also significantly prevalent in all industrialized nations. According to the data of the World Health Organisation (WHO), the prevalence of iron deficiency anaemia (IDA) in industrialized countries and in nonindustrialized countries is 10–20% and 50–60%, respectively [2]. Globally, the prevalence of IDA in preschool-age children (0.00–4.99 years) and school-age children is 47.4% and 25.4%, respectively [3].

Iron deficiency impairs the cognitive development of children from infancy through adolescence. It also damages immune mechanisms and is associated with increased morbidity rates. The importance of iron deficiency and anaemia as a public health problem has been increasingly recognized by health authorities and policy makers. Although efforts are targeted primarily to prevent iron deficiency, it is still the most common nutrient deficiency all over the world [2].

The Turkish Ministry of Health started a project in 2004, which aimed to give 1-2 mg/kg daily prophylactic iron supplementation to all children aged 4 months until 1 year. In 2009, it was reported that after starting this project the prevalence of IDA had decreased [4]. In this paper we aimed to investigate the effects of the project after 8 years and characteristics of our hospitalized patients with IDA.

2. Materials and Methods

The files of 1519 patients who were hospitalized in Konya Training and Research Hospital Pediatrics Clinic between July 2012 and December 2012 for an acute illness were reviewed retrospectively. 50 patients were found to have the diagnosis of IDA. If diagnosis of anaemia was noticed, further evaluations including the measurements of serum iron, total iron-binding capacity (TIBC), and ferritin were performed. When indicated, vitamin B12, folic acid levels, and haemoglobin (Hgb) electrophoresis we obtained to rule out other nutrient deficiencies and haemoglobinopathies that can cause anaemia.

The patients included into the study were divided into 3 groups according to age: Group 1: 6–12 months, Group 2: 12–24 months, and Group 3: >24 months. WHO Hgb thresholds were used to identify patients as anaemic (Hgb < 11 g/dL for patients 6–59 months old, Hgb < 11.5 for patients >59 month old). IDA was defined as Hgb values less than WHO thresholds with the presence of two or more of the following parameters; mean corpuscular volume (MCV) less than 70 fl, serum ferritin below 30 mcg/L, and transferrin saturation (TSAT) less than 16% [5, 6]. Patients having chronic illness, hematologic diseases, and thalassemia traits or receiving any chronic medication were not enrolled into the study. The variables examined in the study were Hgb, haematocrit (Hct), MCV, mean corpuscular haemoglobin (MCH), mean corpuscular haemoglobin concentration MCHC, red blood cell (RBC), red cell distribution width (RDW), white blood cell (WBC), platelet (Plt), iron, TIBC, TSAT, and ferritin levels of the patients.

2.1. Statistical Analysis. The statistical analysis was carried out using the SPSS 15.0 statistical software package for Windows. Descriptive statistics of continuous variables were expressed as mean ± standard deviation (sd). Independent samples *t*-test was used to compare the mean values of the groups. Mann Whitney-*U* test was used for nonnormally distributed variables (Iron and TSAT). When comparing the means of more than two groups, one-way ANOVA and Kruskal-Wallis test were conducted. If there was difference between groups, Tukeys test was performed to compare between the groups $P < 0.05$ was considered as significance level.

3. Results

A total of 50 patients were included into the study (35 boys and 15 girls). The age range of the patients was from 6 months to 80 months (mean age 16,59 ± 1,68 months). Mean age for boys and girls was 14,87 ± 1,41 and 20,56 ± 4,51 months, respectively.

Among a total of 1519 hospitalized patients, the prevalence of IDA was 3.29% (boys: 4.23%, girls: 2.1%). Mean values (mean ± sd) of Hgb, Hct, MCV, MCH, MCHC, RBC, RDW, WBC, Plt, iron, TIBC, ferritin, and TSAT according to sex are given in Table 1. There was no significant difference between girls and boys according to the variables except WBC. WBC levels of girls were significantly higher ($P < 0.05$).

RDW levels were significantly higher in patients aged between 13 and 24 months (17.66 ± 0.41) than the patients >24 months (15.61 ± 0.21).

With respect to age, the number of the subjects in Group 1, Group 2 and Group 3 was, 22, 21, and 7, respectively. Hgb levels were gradually increasing with age and this association was statistically significant (Table 2). Hgb and Hct of the patients >24 months old were significantly higher than those of the patients with the age of 6–12 months ($P < 0.05$). Additionally, when mean Hgb levels were compared with the

age-appropriate Hgb thresholds, the levels of Groups 1 and 2 were significantly lower than those of the thresholds.

Although prophylactic iron supplementation is recommended to be used from 4 months until 1 year, there were patients who never received or received only one bottle (a usage of nearly 1 month) of iron supplementation. Of the 28 patients older than 12 months, only 28% (8 patients; 6 boys, 2 girls) received full course of iron supplementation for 8 months, where 28% (8 patients; 7 boys 1 girl) of them receive it only for 1 month. The rest 44% did not receive iron supplementation despite the recommendations of their family physicians. Although rate of prophylactic iron supplementation use was significantly decreasing with age, there was no significant difference among variables according to receiving iron supplementation.

4. Discussion

Iron deficiency is the most widespread and common nutritional disorder in the world inspite of the efforts to decrease the frequency. The prevalence varies in different parts of the world with higher rates in the developing countries [5, 7]. The results of studies from different provinces of Turkey also showed that iron deficiency is the most important cause of anaemia. Koçak et al. reported that the prevalence of IDA was 17.2% with the highest prevalence in infants being 48% in southern Turkey [8]. Another study conducted in the western part of Turkey reported that the prevalence of IDA was 6.5% among adolescent age [9]. Kilinç et al. reported that the prevalence of IDA in the Southeastern Anatolia of Turkey was 15.5% among 2–5-year-old children [10]. Cetinkaya et al. investigated severe IDA among hospitalized children aged 7–24 months and reported that 61.6% of 3117 children had anaemia and 2.7% of them were severe IDA [11]. Comparing with these studies, the prevalence of IDA which is 3.29% is lower in our study. This may be due to the iron supplementation project of the health ministry started in 2004, as those studies were conducted before 2004.

WHO recommends prophylactic supplementation of iron at a dosage of 2 mg/kg/day to all children between 6 and 23 months of age, especially where the diet does not include fortified foods, or prevalence of anaemia in children approximately 1 year of age is severe [2]. The project of the Turkish Ministry of Health aimed to give iron supplementation to all children aged 4 months until 1 year. After 5 years in 2009, the ministry reported that prevalence of IDA had decreased to 7.8% from 15.2–62.5% prevalence rates, but IDA was still a public health problem in Turkey [4]. The low prevalence examined in our study may suggest that prophylactic iron supplementation has gradually increased. From the finding that the Hgb levels of patients aged 6–24 months were significantly lower than those of the age-appropriate thresholds, it can be considered that extension of prophylactic iron supplementation duration to 24 months might be more favorable.

Ferritin is an intracellular hollow protein shell composed of 24 subunits surrounding an iron core that may contain as many as 4000–4500 iron atoms. In the body, small amounts

TABLE 1: Laboratory characteristics of patients with IDA.

	Boys ($n = 35$)	Girls ($n = 15$)	P
Hgb (g/dL)	9.77 ± 0.14	9.69 ± 0.34	>0.05
Hct (%)	31.03 ± 0.48	31.37 ± 0.83	>0.05
MCV (fL)	6496 ± 0.87	64.13 ± 1.82	>0.05
MCH (pg)	20.50 ± 0.39	19.79 ± 0.73	>0.05
MCHC (gr/dL)	31.48 ± 0.25	30.79 ± 0.47	>0.05
RBC (M/mL)	4.81 ± 0.10	4.93 ± 0.18	>0.05
RDW (%)	16.75 ± 0.31	17.36 ± 0.57	>0.05
WBC (μL^{-1})	10.81 ± 0.63	13.75 ± 1.56	<0.05
PLT (μL^{-1})	384742.85 ± 22314.90	408000.00 ± 38686.28	>0.05
Iron (μg/dL)	29.17 ± 4.88	18.86 ± 2.71	>0.05
TIBC (μg/dL)	339.14 ± 18.48	345.73 ± 16.63	>0.05
Ferritin (μg/L)	29.43 ± 5.66	33.68 ± 7.87	>0.05
TSAT (%)	15.93 ± 6.65	5.40 ± 0.72	>0.05

TABLE 2: IDA parameters of the patients with respect to age.

Age	N	Hgb (g/dL)	MCV (fL)	Ferritin (μg/L)	TSAT (%)
6–12 months	22	9.40 ± 0.15	65.20 ± 1.17	25.44 ± 4.25	10.79 ± 3.20
12–24 months	21	9.81 ± 0.26	64.20 ± 1.17	29.94 ± 8.55	6.04 ± 0.67
>24 months	7	10.61 ± 0.22	64.72 ± 3.01	49.54 ± 14.83	39.19 ± 32.06

of ferritin are secreted into the plasma. The concentration of this plasma ferritin is positively correlated with the size of the total body iron stores in the absence of inflammation. Low serum ferritin values reflects depleted iron stores [12]. Ferritin levels, in contrast to Hgb, are not affected by residential elevation above sea level or smoking behaviour. However, ferritin is a positive acute phase response protein whereby concentrations increase during an inflammatory disease or subclinical infection. This makes the interpretation of normal or high serum ferritin values difficult in areas of widespread infection or inflammation [2]. The cutoff values of ferritin were revised in 1993 and it was reported that ferritin levels < 12 μg/L under 5 years of age, <15 μg/L above 5 years of age and <30 μg/L in the presence of infection reflect the depleted iron stores [12]. In the study of Phiri conducted on patients with severe anaemia in a high infection pressured area, they found mean ferritin levels to be 729.2 μg/L and suggested that it was necessary to change the cutoff limit of ferritin from 30 to 273 μg/L in order to improve its diagnostic efficiency [13]. The mean ferritin level of our patients was 30.71 ± 4.58 μg/L (min.: 2.4; max.: 179.4). 34% of our subjects had a ferritin level above 30 mcg/L with other parameters indicating IDA. All of these subjects had an accompanying inflammatory disease.

Anaemia is a late manifestation of iron deficiency, and iron deficiency without anaemia is even more widespread. If subtle effects of iron deficiency in infancy lay the ground for later problems in cognitive and behavioral functioning, then a large unrecognized population of children could be at risk due to perinatal iron deficiency, a nutritional problem that can be prevented or treated [14]. Consequences of IDA during childhood include growth retardation, reduced school achievement, impaired motor and cognitive development, and increased morbidity from infections including especially diarrhea and acute respiratory infections [2]. Specifically, iron deficiency can lead to deficits in memory and behavioural regulation as iron is required to make neurotransmitters such as dopamine, epinephrine, and serotonin while impaired myelination contributes to deficits in motor function [15–17]. Some of these impairments are thought to be irreversible if they occur at an early age and the consequences may continue even after treatment, reinforcing the importance of prevention [15, 18, 19].

5. Conclusions

In conclusion, although prophylactic iron supplementation lowered the prevalences of IDA, IDA is still a public health problem throughout the world. Iron deficiency impairs the cognitive development of children from infancy through adolescence. Therefore, prophylactic approaches should be carried out more effectively. It can be considered that extension of prophylactic iron supplementation duration to 24 months might be more favorable in our country. Because ferritin levels are increased during inflammatory processes, the cutoff levels should be reevaluated.

References

[1] E. DeMaeyer and M. Adiels-Tegman, "The prevalence of anaemia in the world," *World Health Statistics Quarterly*, vol. 38, no. 3, pp. 302–316, 1985.

[2] World Health Organisation, *Iron Deficiency Anaemia Assessment, Prevention, and Control*, A Guide for Programme Managers, WHO, 2001.

[3] World Health Organisation, *Worldwide Prevalence of Anaemia 1993–2005*, WHO Global Database on Anaemia, WHO, 2008.

[4] Turkish Ministry of Health, *The Report of the Study of Iron Usage among 12–23 Month-Old Children*, Turkish Ministry of Health, Ankara, Turkey, 2009.

[5] N. B. Lerner and R. Sills, "Iron deficiency anemia," in *Nelson Textbook of Pediatrics*, R. M. Kliegman, B. F. Stanton, J. St. Geme, N. Schor, and R. E. Behrman, Eds., pp. 1655–1658, Elsevier Saunders, Philadelphia, Pa, USA, 19th edition, 2011.

[6] C. Male, L. Å. Persson, V. Freeman, A. Guerra, M. A. Van't Hof, and F. Haschke, "Prevalence of iron deficiency in 12-mo-old infants from 11 European areas and influence of dietary factors on iron status (Euro-Growth study)," *Acta Paediatrica*, vol. 90, no. 5, pp. 492–498, 2001.

[7] World Health Organisation, *Preventing and Controlling Iron Deficiency Anaemia through Primary Health Care*, A Guide for Health Administrators and Programme Managers, WHO, Geneva, Switzerland, 1989.

[8] R. Koçak, Z. N. Alparslan, G. Ağridağ, F. Başlamisli, P. D. Aksungur, and S. Koltaş, "The frequency of anaemia, iron deficiency, hemoglobin S and beta thalassemia in the south of Turkey," *European Journal of Epidemiology*, vol. 11, no. 2, pp. 181–184, 1995.

[9] Y. Aydınok, Ş. Öztop, G. Nişli, K. Kavaklı, and N. Çetingül, "Percentile norms and curves for hematological values in Turkish adolescents," *Turkish Journal of Haematology*, vol. 15, pp. 169–173, 1998.

[10] M. Kilinç, G. T. Yüregir, and H. Ekerbiçer, "Anaemia and iron-deficiency anaemia in south-east Anatolia," *European Journal of Haematology*, vol. 69, no. 5-6, pp. 280–283, 2002.

[11] F. Cetinkaya, Y. Yildirmak, and G. Kutluk, "Severe iron-deficiency anemia among hospitalized young children in an urban hospital," *Pediatric Hematology and Oncology*, vol. 22, no. 1, pp. 77–81, 2005.

[12] World Health Organisation, *Serum Ferritin Concentrations for the Assessment of Iron Status and Iron Deficiency in Populations*, Vitamin and Mineral Nutrition Information System, WHO, Geneva, Switzerland, 2011.

[13] K. S. Phiri, J. C. J. Calis, A. Siyasiya, I. Bates, B. Brabin, and M. Boele van Hensbroek, "New cut-off values for ferritin and soluble transferrin receptor for the assessment of iron deficiency in children in a high infection pressure area," *Journal of Clinical Pathology*, vol. 62, no. 12, pp. 1103–1106, 2009.

[14] B. Lozoff, "Perinatal iron deficiency and the developing brain," *Pediatric Research*, vol. 48, no. 2, pp. 137–139, 2000.

[15] L. L. Iannotti, J. M. Tielsch, M. M. Black, and R. E. Black, "Iron supplementation in early childhood: health benefits and risks," *American Journal of Clinical Nutrition*, vol. 84, no. 6, pp. 1261–1276, 2006.

[16] R. J. D. Moy, "Prevalence, consequences and prevention of childhood nutritional iron deficiency: a child public health perspective," *Clinical and Laboratory Haematology*, vol. 28, no. 5, pp. 291–298, 2006.

[17] J. L. Beard, "Why iron deficiency is important in infant development," *Journal of Nutrition*, vol. 138, no. 12, pp. 2534–2536, 2008.

[18] B. Lozoff, "Iron deficiency and child development," *Food and Nutrition Bulletin*, vol. 28, no. 4, pp. S560–S571, 2007.

[19] I. A. Siddiqui, M. A. Rahman, and A. Jaleel, "Efficacy of daily vs. weekly supplementation of iron in schoolchildren with low iron status," *Journal of Tropical Pediatrics*, vol. 50, no. 5, pp. 276–278, 2004.

11

Safety and Efficacy of Intravenous Ferric Carboxymaltose (750 mg) in the Treatment of Iron Deficiency Anemia

Charles F. Barish,[1] Todd Koch,[2] Angelia Butcher,[2] David Morris,[3] and David B. Bregman[2,4]

[1] *Wake Gastroenterology and Wake Research Associates, Raleigh, NC 27612, USA*
[2] *Luitpold Pharmaceuticals, Inc., Norristown, PA 19403, USA*
[3] *WebbWrites, LLC, Durham, NC 27705, USA*
[4] *Department of Pathology, Albert Einstein College of Medicine, NY 10461, USA*

Correspondence should be addressed to Charles F. Barish, cfbgastro@aol.com

Academic Editor: Aurelio Maggio

Background. Iron deficiency anemia (IDA) is a common hematological complication with potentially serious clinical consequences that may require intravenous iron therapy. Ferric carboxymaltose (FCM) is a stable, nondextran iron formulation administered intravenously in large single doses to treat IDA. *Objective*. Two open-label, randomized, placebo-controlled trials evaluated safety of multiple or single 750 mg FCM doses compared to standard medical care (SMC) in IDA patients. Secondary endpoints were improvements in hemoglobin and iron indices. *Design and Patients*. Adults with hemoglobin ≤12 g/dL, ferritin ≤100 or ≤300 ng/mL with transferrin saturation ≤30% were randomized to receive single (n = 366) or weekly (n = 343) FCM or SMC (n = 360 and n = 366). *Results*. Significantly greater ($P \leq 0.001$) increases in hemoglobin and iron indices occurred in FCM groups versus SMC. In the multidose study, up to two infusions of FCM were needed to reach target iron levels versus 3–5 of intravenous iron comparators. FCM and SMC groups had similar incidences and types of adverse events and serious adverse events. Transient hypophosphatemia not associated with adverse events or clinical sequelae occurred in the FCM groups. *Conclusion*. Intravenous FCM is safe, well tolerated, and associated with improvements in hemoglobin and iron indices comparable to SMC when administered in single doses of up to 750 mg at a rate of 100 mg/min. Fewer FCM infusions were required to reach target iron levels compared to other intravenous iron preparations.

1. Introduction

Iron deficiency anemia (IDA) is a common hematological complication with a prevalence of 2% among adult men and 9–20% among adult women depending on race and ethnicity [1]. IDA occurs in several medical conditions including inflammatory bowel disease (IBD) and chronic kidney disease (CKD), in association with cancer and its treatment, and in cases of acute blood loss resulting from gastrointestinal (GI) bleeding, trauma, surgery, and obstetrics/gynecology conditions [2]. IDA contributes significantly to morbidity, disease burden, and decreased quality of life [3–5].

While oral iron is typically considered first-line treatment, high-dose intravenous (IV) iron therapy has a role in the treatment of varied clinical situations associated with IDA. IV iron is more effective in patients with IBD [6] and in oncology patients receiving erythropoietin-stimulating agents (ESAs) for chemotherapy-induced anemia [7]. IV iron is also preferred when iron requirements are too high to be corrected with oral iron therapy (e.g., gastrointestinal bleeding), when oral iron cannot be properly absorbed (e.g., after gastric bypass or in celiac disease), and when oral iron is not well tolerated because of gastrointestinal side effects. Approximately 10–20% of patients taking oral iron experience nausea, constipation, epigastric discomfort, and vomiting that may lead to noncompliance [8]. IV iron is recommended for hemodialysis-dependent CKD patients due to frequent blood losses on dialysis machines and difficulty utilizing oral iron [9, 10] and is also an option for treatment of predialysis CKD patients [9].

IV iron formulations available in the United States (US) vary in dosing regimens and indications and may be limited by the maximum dose that can be given in a single visit due to instability of the iron-carbohydrate moiety (e.g., iron sucrose and iron gluconate formulations) as well as by anaphylactic reactions due to dextran-containing iron formulations [11, 12]. Feraheme (ferumoxytol) is a recently approved IV iron product that can be administered as two injections of 510 mg [12]. Feraheme contains a modified dextran shell designed to reduce immunogenic potential, however anaphylaxis in the setting of previous hypersensitivity to iron dextran has been reported [13].

Ferric carboxymaltose (FCM) is a stable, non-dextran-containing iron formulation that permits the uptake of iron by the reticuloendothelial system with minimal release of free iron [14]. FCM was developed for rapid IV administration in high doses for the treatment of iron deficiency [15, 16] and the rapid infusion of up to 1000 mg of FCM over 15 min has been shown to be well tolerated. The FCM complex has a nearly neutral pH (5.0–7.0) with a physiologic osmolarity and no dextran cross-reactivity [17]. The iron-carbohydrate FCM complex is more stable than ferric gluconate or iron sucrose, permitting slow and controlled delivery of iron into target tissues.

Numerous clinical trials in over 2000 patients have shown that FCM improves hemoglobin levels and replenishes depleted iron stores [18]. FCM is effective and well tolerated in patients with IDA associated with a variety of medical conditions including IBD, CKD, heavy uterine bleeding, and postpartum anemia [19–23]. FCM treatment also improves symptoms, functional capacity, and quality of life in patients with chronic heart failure and iron deficiency with or without anemia [24]. FCM is approved in Europe for the treatment of iron deficiency when oral iron preparations are ineffective or cannot be used.

The primary objective of the present studies was to evaluate the safety of FCM at doses up to 750 mg compared to standard medical care (SMC) in patients with IDA.

2. Methods

Two phase 3, open-label, randomized, controlled, multicenter trials (NCT00703937 and NCT00704353) were conducted from July 2008 to July 2009 in 95 centers each. Study protocols (1VIT08019 and 21, Luitpold Pharmaceuticals) and informed consent forms were approved by institutional review boards of each center, and trials complied with the declaration of Helsinki. Enrolled subjects provided informed consent. Study 1VIT08019 was a FCM multidose study and Study 1VIT08021 was an FCM single-dose study. In both studies patients were randomized to either FCM or standard medical care (SMC). For patients in the SMC group, the treating physician could select approved oral or IV iron therapy thus permitting head-to-head comparisons to IV iron as well as oral iron.

2.1. Setting and Participants. Men and women 18 to 85 years of age with anemia attributable to iron deficiency were eligible if they were not dialysis dependent and had screening laboratory values for hemoglobin ≤11 (multidose study) or ≤12 g/dL (single-dose study), and ferritin ≤100 ng/mL or ≤300 ng/mL if transferrin saturation (TSAT) was ≤30%. Patients received study treatments on an outpatient basis.

Exclusion criteria included known hypersensitivity to any component of FCM, hemochromatosis or iron storage disorders, current treatment for asthma, recent treatment with IV iron, antibiotics or red blood cell transfusion, evidence of infection (including hepatitis B, hepatitis C, or HIV antibodies), concomitant severe cardiovascular diseases, pregnant or lactating women and women of child-bearing potential not using approved birth control methods, or any condition which, in the opinion of the investigator, made participation unacceptable.

2.2. Randomization and Interventions. Subjects underwent medical history and clinical evaluation during the screening phase and were randomized within 7 days to the treatment phase (Day 0) by a centralized interactive voice-response system if entry criteria were met. Randomization was stratified by baseline hemoglobin (≤8, 8.1 to 9.5, ≥9.6 g/dL), cardiovascular-disease risk (category 1 to 4 based on variables included in the Framingham risk model [25] including smoking status, prior history of cardiovascular disease, use of low-dose aspirin, and whether patients had diabetes, hypertension, or hyperlipidemia, where 1 is no known risk factor and 4 is a prior history of cardiovascular disease), use of immunosuppressive therapy, and past response to oral iron (poor/yes or poor/no). Subjects were randomized in a 1 : 1 ratio to receive FCM or SMC (including oral iron, IV iron, or no iron replacement) for treatment of IDA.

For the single-dose study, subjects received 750 mg FCM or 15 mg/kg, whichever was smaller, administered by IV push injection at 100 mg per minute on Day 0. For the multidose study, subjects received undiluted FCM 15 mg/kg up to a single dose of 750 mg at 100 mg per minute weekly until the calculated iron deficit dose had been administered (to a maximum cumulative dose of 2,250 mg). The FCM dose was determined by calculating the total iron requirement and dividing this total amount into one or more single dose(s) according to the Ganzoni formula: Total iron deficit (mg) = Body weight (kg) × (Target Hb − Actual Hb) (g/dL) × 2.4 + depot iron of 500 mg.

Subjects randomized to the SMC group received SMC from Day 0–30 for the single-dose study and Day 0–42 for the multidose study. Type of SMC was determined and documented by the investigator, and included approved oral or IV iron preparations. Feraheme [ferumoxytol] [12] is an IV iron formulation that was approved in June, 2009 (at about the time that these trials finished enrolling), and was therefore not included in the SMC options.

2.3. Outcomes and Followup. Clinical, laboratory, and safety data were collected at study visits on Days 0, 7 and 30/end-of-treatment visit for the single-dose study and

Days 0, 7, 14, 28, and 42/end-of-study visit for the multidose study. SMC subjects and subjects terminating early had a follow-up phone call 28–30 days after study-drug administration.

2.4. Statistical Analyses. The primary objective of both studies was to evaluate the safety of a maximum administered dose of 750 mg of FCM compared to SMC in the treatment of IDA. The safety population included all subjects administered study medication. Adverse events were reported from Day 0 to the completion of the study.

The multidose study included efficacy analyses that were based on a modified intent-to-treat (mITT) population consisting of all subjects from the safety population who had 2 baseline hemoglobin values (with less than a 1-gram difference between the 2) and at least 1 postbaseline hemoglobin assessment. Efficacy analyses were summarized for the following treatment groups:

(i) FCM.
(ii) Venofer (iron sucrose injection, USP) and Ferrlecit (sodium ferric gluconate).
(iii) Oral iron.
(iv) Other treatment.

Clinically meaningful hemoglobin increases were defined for the different patient populations: CKD $\geq$ 1 g/dL; heavy uterine bleeding or GI $\geq$ 2 g/dL; postpartum $\geq$ 3 g/dL; other $\geq$ 2 g/dL. The proportion of subjects in the mITT Population achieving a hemoglobin increase that was clinically meaningful for that population anytime between baseline and end of study or time of intervention was summarized for each therapy group. A 95% 2-sided confidence interval for the difference between FCM and each of the other therapy groups was based on the normal approximation for the binomial distribution, using the Wald continuity correction $[(1/n_1 + 1/n_2)/2]$. Logistic regression was used to provide a confidence interval for the comparison of FCM and each of the other therapy groups after adjusting for important baseline differences and potential baseline predictors of efficacy response.

No efficacy analyses were conducted in the single-dose study, although hemoglobin levels and other hematology indices were collected as part of the clinical chemistry and laboratory assessments.

A sample size of 500 subjects per group in each trial was estimated to provide approximately 80% power to detect a statistically significant difference with Fisher's exact test in the incidence of serious adverse events. However, by pooling the results of the two trials approximately 90% power could be achieved with a pooled sample size of approximately 700. Hence enrollment was stopped when 708 and 736 subjects were enrolled in the multidose and single-dose studies, respectively.

For baseline characteristics, treatment group differences for categorical characteristics (e.g., sex, race) were assessed with Fisher's exact test and quantitative characteristics (e.g., age, weight) were assessed using the *t*-test for independent groups. For safety assessments, comparison of incidence

rates was performed with the 2-sided Fisher's exact test. Comparisons of continuous endpoints, such as mean change in clinical laboratory findings were performed using the one-way analysis of variance (ANOVA) with a factor for randomized treatment group. The number of subjects with missing data was tabulated but excluded from Fisher's exact test. No formal statistical tests were performed for the incidence of abnormal laboratory values or vital signs.

3. Results

Seven hundred and thirty-eight patients were randomized in the single-dose study (366 in the FCM group, and 369 in the SMC group, 3 not treated) and 708 (343 in the FCM group and 360 in the SMC group, 5 not treated) in the multidose study. Disposition and reasons for not completing the studies are shown in Figure 1. The majority of subjects completed the studies. In the multidose study, the proportion of subjects completing the study in the FCM group was significantly greater than in the SMC group ($P = 0.03$).

No clinically significant differences were observed between the FCM and SMC groups for any demographic or baseline characteristic in either study (summarized in Table 1). Both studies were comprised primarily of women. Mean hemoglobin, TSAT, and ferritin values at screening were similar between the FCM and SMC groups. The majority of subjects were not currently using ESA, had received previous iron therapy, had no history of iron intolerance or drug allergy, had not used immunosuppressive therapy, and had a poor/no response to previous iron therapy. The cardiovascular disease risk for patients was primarily category 1 or 2, indicating the patient had no risk factors (category 1) or a single risk factor (category 2). The primary etiology of IDA included CKD, heavy uterine bleeding, gastrointestinal conditions, and postpartum causes. Just over half the subjects received oral iron. Among subjects receiving IV iron as SMC, Venofer and iron dextran were most commonly used.

The total doses of IV iron (mg) in either the FCM or the SMC groups are shown in Figure 2. In the single-dose study, the extent of iron exposure was similar in the FCM and SMC groups, although there was more variation in the SMC group. In the multidose study, the mean maximum single infusion in the FCM group was close to twice that of the SMC group (745.7 ± 45.1 mg versus 380.1 ± 407.2 mg). The number of infusions in the multidose study is also shown in Figure 2 (inset). In the FCM group, 1 or 2 infusions were needed over the course of the study to reach their target iron level, while in the SMC group, 3–5 infusions were needed.

3.1. Safety. Table 2 summarizes adverse event reporting in FCM and SMC groups. The overall incidences of treatment-emergent adverse events were similar across groups in both studies. In the single-dose study, the most common treatment-emergent events were nausea, vomiting constipation, diarrhea, urinary tract infection, and abdominal pain in the SMC group and nausea, headache, diarrhea, and fatigue in the FCM group. A statistically significantly greater proportion of subjects in the SMC group compared with the FCM

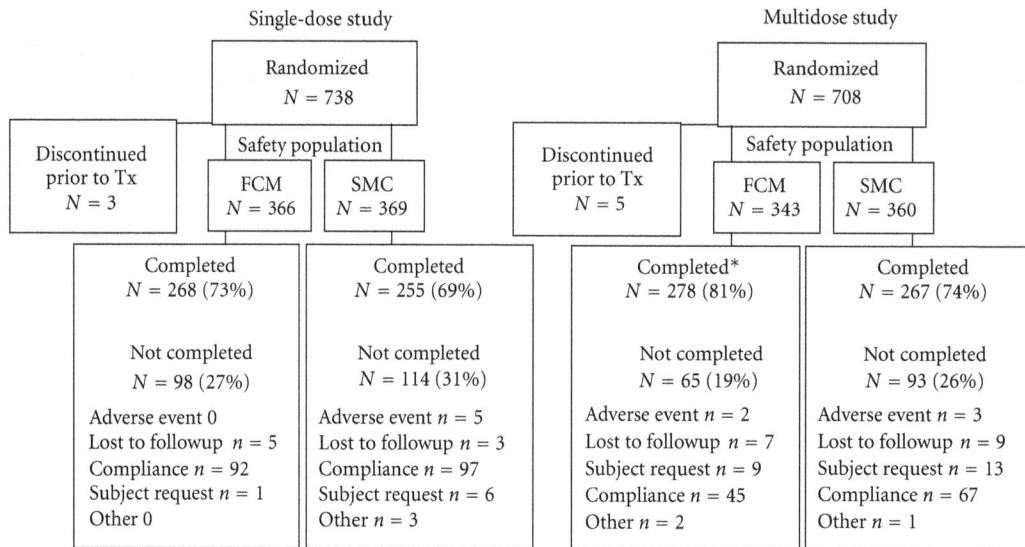

* Proportion of patients completing study was signicantly greater than in the SMC group, P = 0.03

FCM: ferric carboxymaltose
SMC: standard medical care

FIGURE 1: Disposition of subjects in the single-dose and multidose studies.

group experienced vomiting (4% versus 1%, $P = 0.029$) and urinary tract infection (2% versus 0.3%, $P = 0.038$).

In the multidose study, common ($\geq 5\%$) treatment-emergent adverse events in the SMC group were nausea, constipation, dizziness, and headache, and in the FCM group, headache. A statistically significantly greater proportion of subjects in the SMC group (7%) experienced constipation compared with those in the FCM group (4%), $P = 0.031$. A statistically significantly greater proportion in the FCM group compared to the SMC group experienced blood phosphorus decrease/hypophosphatemia (7% versus 0%, resp., $P < 0.001$) recorded by investigators as a result of clinical chemistry values below 2 mg/dL. None of the cases were considered serious or required action, and none resulted in discontinuation of a patient from the study.

The majority of treatment-emergent adverse events experienced during both studies were classified by the Investigator as Grade 1 or 2 in severity. In the single-dose study, 14 (4%) and 12 (3%) subjects in the FCM and SMC groups, respectively, experienced Grade 3 events, and 1 subject each in the SMC group experienced a Grade 4 and Grade 5 event. In the multidose study, 35 (10%) and 12 (3%) patients in the FCM and SMC groups, respectively, had Grade 3 treatment-emergent adverse events. Three subjects (0.9%) in the FCM group and 2 (0.6%) in the SMC group experienced events classified as Grade 4 severity.

In the single-dose study, there were no discontinuations in the FCM group and 6 (2%) in the SMC group due to an adverse events. In the multidose study, 17 (5%) subjects in the FCM group and 11 (3%) in the SMC group had at least 1 serious adverse events. One case in the FCM group (constipation) and 2 cases in the SMC group (renal infarct

and hypotension) were considered related to study medication. In the single dose study, 5 (1%) subjects in the FCM group and 9 (2%) in the SMC group experienced at least 1 serious adverse event, none of which were considered related to study medication. Two (2; 0.6%) and 3 (0.8%) subjects in the FCM and SMC groups, respectively, were discontinued from the multidose study due to an adverse event.

There were no deaths during the multidose study. In the single-dose study, one subject in the SMC group died from pneumonia.

The only significant differences in laboratory or clinical chemistry were the proportion of subjects in the FCM groups in both studies with phosphorus levels that dropped to less than 2 mg/dL from normal baseline in the range of 2.5–4.5 mg/dL. In the single dose study, 18% of subjects in the FCM group had decreases compared to 0.3% in the SMC group. In the multidose study, 47.9% of subjects in the FCM group showed a decline compared with 0.3% in the SMC group. These decreases were not associated with any clinical sequelae.

Evaluations of vital signs and physical examinations showed no clinically meaningful differences from baseline in either the FCM or SMC groups. In the single-dose study, 3 subjects in the FCM group and 1 in the SMC group experienced a nonserious hypersensitivity/allergic reaction, and in the multidose study, 1 (0.3%) and 3 (0.8%) subjects in the FCM and SMC groups, respectively, experienced hypersensitivity during the study. The events resolved after discontinuation of study drug (one FCM subject) or administration of antihistamines and/or glucocorticoids (3 subjects, 2 FCM, and 1 SMC). In the multidose study, 5 subjects in the FCM group and 1 in the SMC group who received

TABLE 1: Demographics and baseline characteristics of subjects (safety population).

	Multidose study		Single-dose study	
	FCM ($N = 343$)	SMC ($N = 360$)	FCM ($N = 366$)	SMC ($N = 369$)
Age (years)	49.3 ± 18.5	47.7 ± 17.6	49.2 ± 19.9	49.6 ± 19.9
Sex				
Female	292 (85.1)	318 (88.3)	322 (88.0)	315 (85.4)
Male	51 (14.9)	42 (11.7)	44 (12.0)	54 (14.6)
Race/Ethnicity				
Caucasian	185 (53.9)	180 (50.0)	171 (46.7)	205 (55.6)
African American	87 (25.4)	113 (31.4)	114 (31.1)	96 (26.0)
Hispanic	58 (16.9)	61 (16.9)	70 (19.1)	48 (13.0)
Asian	3 (0.9)	1 (0.3)	6 (1.6)	10 (2.7)
Other	10 (2.9)	5 (1.4)	5 (1.4)	10 (2.7)
Weight (kg)	82.2 ± 22.4	85.4 ± 22.0	83.2 ± 24.3	82.2 ± 22.9
IDA Etiology				
CKD	40 (11.7)	34 (9.4)	67 (18.3)	53 (14.4)
Uterine bleeding	77 (22.4)	103 (28.6)	61 (16.7)	79 (21.4)
GI related	69 (20.1)	66 (18.3)	49 (13.4)	47 (12.7)
Postpartum	35 (10.2)	36 (10.0)	56 (15.3)	49 (13.3)
Other/Unknown	122 (35.6)	121 (33.6)	133 (36.3)	141 (38.2)
Hb (g/dL)	9.6 ± 1.1	9.6 ± 1.1	10.8 ± 1.1	10.8 ± 1.0
Hb Category (g/dL)				
≤8.0	40 (11.7)	46 (12.8)	9 (2.5)	5 (1.4)
8.1–9.5	109 (31.8)	112 (31.1)	71 (19.4)	71 (19.2)
≥9.6	194 (56.6)	202 (56.1)	286 (78.1)	293 (79.4)
TSAT (%)	10.6 ± 7.9	10.5 ± 8.0	15.9 ± 9.2	15.0 ± 8.4
Ferritin (ng/mL)	25.6 ± 48.3	27.3 ± 66.4	38.1 ± 53.4	34.0 ± 51.1
No Current ESA use	337 (98.3)	356 (99.9)	347 (94.8)	351 (95.1)
No Iron Intolerance	283 (82.5)	302 (83.9)	333 (91.0)	318 (86.2)
Previous Iron Therapy	242 (70.6)	263 (73.1)	241 (65.8)	256 (69.4)
Response: Poor/No	208 (60.6)	217 (60.3)	246 (67.2)	248 (67.2)
No imm.supp. therapy	340 (99.1)	353 (98)	357 (97.5)	357 (96.7)
Cardiovascular risk				
≤2	201 (58.6)	222 (61.7)	217 (59.3)	230 (62.3)
>2	142 (41.4)	138 (38.3)	149 (40.7)	139 (37.7)
Type of SMC	NA		NA	
Oral Iron		187 (51.9)		210 (56.9)
IV Iron		154 (42.8)		128 (34.7)
Venofer		112 (31.1)		69 (18.7)
Iron Dextran		33 (9.2)		56 (15.2)
Ferrlecit		9 (2.5)		3 (0.8)
Other or no treatment		20 (5.6)		30 (4.6)

Values are expressed as mean ± standard deviation or number (percentage).
CKD: chronic kidney disease; ESA: erythropoiesis-stimulating agent; FCM: ferric carboxymaltose; Hb: hemoglobin; IDA: iron deficiency anemia; IV: intravenous; NA: not applicable; SMC: standard medical care; TSAT: transferring saturation.

Venofer had reported adverse events of hypotension (Grade 1 or 2) during the study. In the single-dose study, 3 subjects in the FCM group and none in the SMC group had low-blood-pressure readings recorded on the day of dosing in the absence of symptomatic hypotension.

3.2. *Efficacy.* In the single-dose study, statistically significantly greater ($P \leq 0.001$) mean increases from baseline to day 30 were observed in the FCM group compared with the SMC group for hemoglobin (1.15 ± 1.13 versus 0.78 ± 1.05 g/dL) and ferritin levels (146.4 ± 111.4 versus

TABLE 2: Incidence of treatment-emergent adverse events occurring in ≥2% of subjects.

| | Single-dose study | | |
| | FCM | SMC $N = 735$ | P value |
	$N = 366$	$N = 369$	
≥1 event	132 (36.0)	128 (34.6)	
Nausea	15 (4.1)	18 (4.9)	0.722
Headache	11 (3.0)	5 (1.4)	0.138
Diarrhea	10 (2.7)	8 (2.2)	0.642
Fatigue	10 (2.7)	7 (1.9)	0.474
Constipation	7 (1.9)	13 (3.5)	0.257
Vomiting	4 (1.1)	14 (3.8)	0.029*
Abdominal pain	2 (<1)	8 (2.2)	0.107
Urinary tract infection	1 (<1)	8 (2.2)	0.038*
	Multidose study $N = 703$		
	FCM $N = 343$	SMC $N = 360$	
≥1 event	185 (54.4)	198 (55.0)	
Decreased blood phosphorous	25 (7.3)	0	<0.001**
Headache	16 (4.7)	18 (5.0)	0.862
Nausea	14 (4.1)	27 (7.5)	0.055
Constipation	12 (3.5)	26 (7.2)	0.031*
Diarrhea	10 (2.9)	14 (3.9)	0.537
Dizziness	10 (2.9)	17 (4.7)	0.242
Upper respiratory tract infection	9 (2.6)	6 (1.7)	0.440
Arthralgia	8 (2.3)	8 (2.2)	1.000
Myalgia	8 (2.3)	2 (0.06)	0.058
Pain in extremity	9 (2.6)	4 (1.1)	0.167
Fatigue	9 (2.6)	5 (1.4)	0.287
Increased alanine aminotrasferase	7 (2.0)	5 (1/4)	0.570
Back pain	7 (2.0)	6 (1.7)	0.784
Nasopharyngitis	7 (2.0)	6 (1.7)	0.784
Urinary tract infection	7 (2.0)	6 (1.7)	0.784
Vomiting	6 (1.7)	13 (3.6)	0.164
Peripheral edema	3 (<1)	8 (2.2)	0.224
Cough	2 (<1)	8 (2.2)	0.108

Values are expressed as number of subjects (percentage).
FCM: ferric carboxymaltose; SMC: standard medical care.
*Statistically significant at 0.05 level.
**Statistically significant at 0.001 level.

67.1 ± 140.2 ng/mL), and hematocrit (3.4 ± 3.6 versus 2.4 ± 3.5%). Significantly greater mean increases from baseline to day 30 occurred in the FCM group compared with the SMC group in absolute reticulocyte count ($P = 0.016$), basophils, mean corpuscular hemoglobin, mean corpuscular volume, red-cell distribution width (all $P < 0.001$), and red-blood-cell counts ($P = 0.019$). A statistically significantly greater mean decrease from baseline to Day 30 was observed in the FCM group compared to the SMC group in platelets (i.e., decreases of 55 versus 35 thousand platelets per microliter from baselines of 312 and 315 thousand platelets per microliter, resp., $P < 0.001$). There were no significant differences between the two groups in the percent eosinophils,

lymphocytes, mean corpuscular hemoglobin concentration, monocytes, neutrophils, or white blood counts.

Mean changes from baseline in hemoglobin, ferritin, and TSAT are shown in Figure 3 for the mITT population in the multidose study. The mean increases from baseline to the highest value between baseline and the end of study or time of intervention in the FCM group were statistically significantly greater for hemoglobin, ferritin, and TSAT compared to subjects in the SMC group receiving Venofer or Ferrlecit, for hemoglobin and ferritin compared to the oral iron group, and for ferritin compared to other SMC treatment.

Table 3 shows the proportion of subjects in the multidose study mITT population achieving changes in hemoglobin

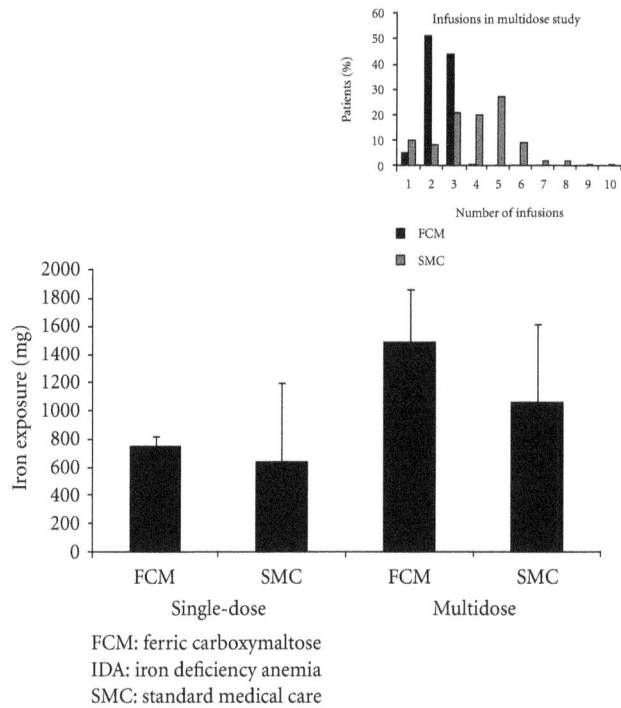

FIGURE 2: Extent of exposure to IV iron. Mean exposure with standard deviations for the FCM and SMC groups in the single-dose and multidose studies. The mean maximum single infusion in the multidose study was 745.7 ± 45.1 mg in the FCM group and 380.1 ± 407.2 mg in the SMC group. The insert shows the number of infusions administered in the multidose study.

FCM: ferric carboxymaltose
IDA: iron deficiency anemia
SMC: standard medical care

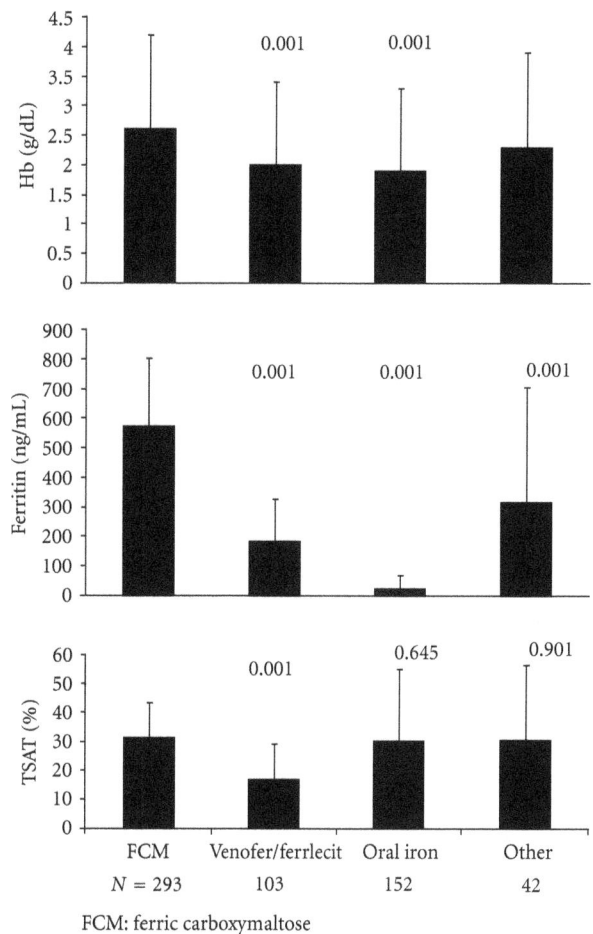

FCM: ferric carboxymaltose

FIGURE 3: Mean changes in hemoglobin, ferritin, and TSAT from baseline to the highest value between baseline and end of study or time of intervention for subjects in the multidose study (mITT population). P values for the differences between SMC groups versus FCM (determined by one-way ANOVA) are shown above the bars.

defined in the protocol as clinically meaningful for each population of patients (chronic kidney disease [CKD] ≥ 1 g/dL; heavy uterine bleeding or gastrointestinal (GI) ≥ 2 g/dL; postpartum ≥ 3 g/dL; other ≥ 2 g/dL) anytime between baseline (day 0) and end of treatment. These results are shown for the overall study population and stratified by IDA etiology for the FCM group and SMC subgroups. There were no statistically significant differences between the FCM group and SMC subgroups.

4. Discussion

The primary objective of these studies was to assess safety of FCM compared to SMC. FCM was well tolerated, and there were no clinically important differences in safety outcomes between the FCM and SMC group. The incidences of adverse events were similar overall, and the majority of adverse events were of grade 1 or 2 severity and were consistent with medical issues in these patient populations. Importantly, there were no deaths or anaphylactic reactions in the FCM groups in either study. FCM has been registered by the public health authorities in Europe since 2007 and has been used to treat iron deficiency in over 35 countries. FCM is in clinical development in the US.

The transient, asymptomatic hypophosphatemia observed in the FCM group in the present studies and as previously reported [20, 22, 23] is apparently not associated

with adverse events or clinical outcomes in patients with IDA. Selective decreased blood phosphate levels have been reported in acute hemolytic anemia, following hematopoietic reconstitution after allogeneic peripheral blood stem cell transplantation, and after iron administration [26–28]. Decreased levels may be a reflection of cellular uptake of extracellular phosphate associated with rapid expansion of erythropoiesis [22]. It may be associated with an increase in fibroblast growth factor 23, which plays a role in phosphate homeostasis [28]. A recent case study [29] described a renal transplant patient on long-term tacrolimus therapy who developed severe and symptomatic hypophosphatemia after IV FCM administration. While it remains unclear whether the tacrolimus therapy and resulting renal tubule toxicity contributed to the complication in this transplant recipient, in general, hypophosphatemia does not appear to alter the risk/benefit profile for use of FCM, and FCM is well tolerated in patients with IDA due to chronic kidney disease [30] or other causes.

TABLE 3: Proportion of subjects in the multidose study with a clinically meaningful increase in hemoglobin anytime between baseline and the end of study or time of intervention.

	FCM N = 293	Venofer or Ferrlecit N = 103	SMC subgroup Oral iron N = 152	Other treatment N = 42
			n (%)	
	187 (64)	59 (57)	68 (45)	22 (52)
Difference from FCM 95% CI		0.07 (−0.05, 0.18)	0.19 (0.09, 0.29)	0.11 (−0.06, 0.29)
			n/N (%)	
IDA Etiology				
CKD	15/34 (44)	8/16 (50)	2/11 (18)	1/4 (25)
Heavy uterine bleeding	55/71 (78)	16/25 (64)	25/52 (48)	8/11 (73)
IBD/GI related	41/61 (67)	19/25 (76)	4/15 (27)	7/15 (47)
Postpartum	16/24 (67)	0	8/18 (44)	1/1 (100)
Other/Unknown	60/103 (58)	16/37 (43)	29/56 (52)	5/11 (45)

FCM: ferric carboxymaltose; IDA: iron deficiency anemia; SMC: standard medical care.

The efficacy of FCM in treating IDA has been well documented in randomized clinical trials [19–23]. In the present studies, the mean increases from baseline to the highest value between baseline and the end of study or time of intervention for subjects in the FCM group were statistically significantly greater for hemoglobin, ferritin, and TSAT compared to subjects in the SMC group receiving Venofer or Ferrlecit, for hemoglobin and ferritin compared to the oral iron group, and for ferritin compared to other SMC treatment. Efficacy results were comparable across IDA associated with varied clinical conditions including gastrointestinal disorders, CKD, and obstetrics/gynecology conditions. The present studies did not show a statistically significant differences between FCM and SMC with respect to protocol-defined clinically meaningful increases in hemoglobin for each population (i.e., chronic kidney disease [CKD] ≥ 1 g/dL; heavy uterine bleeding or gastrointestinal (GI) ≥ 2 g/dL; postpartum ≥ 3 g/dL; other ≥ 2 g/dL) anytime between baseline (day 0) and end of treatment.

A single dose of 750 mg of FCM can be administered at a rate of 100 mg/min, thereby permitting use of FCM on an outpatient basis, and reducing clinic visits and venipunctures resulting in fewer disruptions to patients' lifestyles. Clinically, target hemoglobin levels may be achieved more rapidly, achieving stability earlier than when using multiple small doses. In the multidose study, the majority of patients (96%) in the FCM group required 1 or 2 doses to reach their target iron levels versus 3–5 doses required for the SMC treatments. Ferritin levels were also increased with 1 or 2 doses of FCM, and the increases were significantly greater than those occurring in the SMC groups. The reduced frequency of infusions with FCM may reduce health care visits, reduce the risk of infection, and preserve vein integrity. A further potential clinical benefit of high-dose intravenous iron is to overcome the inhibition of gastrointestinal iron absorption induced by hepcidin in patients with anemia of chronic disease or other inflammatory conditions (28, 29).

Strengths of the studies include the large sample sizes and the ability to confirm statistically and clinically significant improvements in hemoglobin indices even though several medical conditions contributing to IDA were represented in the trial. A potential weakness was the heterogeneity of the SMC comparators. Efficacy endpoints were compared to specific comparator agents (Venofer or Ferrlecit, oral iron) in some cases. Safety was compared to SMC although some adverse events would be expected to be different for oral versus intravenous comparators (e.g., constipation that is observed more prominently with oral iron).

In conclusion, FCM at single doses of up to 750 mg was safe and effective in patients with a broad range of IDA-associated medical conditions. Overall the FCM and SMC groups were similar in terms of incidences of adverse events and serious adverse events (including deaths). The transient hypophosphatemia observed in the FCM groups was not associated with adverse events or clinical sequelae. While improvements in hemoglobin and iron indices in patients treated with FCM were comparable to other IV iron formulations, fewer infusions of FCM were needed to reach target iron levels.

Authors' Contribution

C. Barish is an advisor/consultant to Salix, Synergy, Sucampo, and Abbott Pharmaceuticals. D. Bregman, T. Koch, and A. Butcher are employees of Luitpold Pharmaceuticals; D. Morris is a consultant to Luitpold Pharmaceuticals. All authors conceived and initiated the study and scrutinized eligible patients. All authors participated in writing, reviewing, and editing manuscript drafts and approved the final draft of the manuscript for submission.

Acknowledgments

Support for these studies was provided by Luitpold Pharmaceuticals, Inc. Medical writing support, funded by Luitpold Pharmaceuticals, Inc., was provided by Patrice C. Ferriola, PhD.

References

[1] S. Killip, J. M. Bennett, and M. D. Chambers, "Iron deficiency anemia," *American Family Physician*, vol. 75, no. 5, pp. 671–678, 2007.

[2] J. Umbreit, "Iron deficiency: a concise review," *American Journal of Hematology*, vol. 78, no. 3, pp. 225–231, 2005.

[3] J. P. Gisbert and F. Gomollón, "Common misconceptions in the diagnosis and management of anemia in inflammatory bowel disease," *American Journal of Gastroenterology*, vol. 103, no. 5, pp. 1299–1307, 2008.

[4] J. D. Haas and T. T. Brownlie, "Iron deficiency and reduced work capacity: a critical review of the research to determine a causal relationship," *Journal of Nutrition*, vol. 131, no. 2, pp. 676S–690S, 2001.

[5] S. Horton and C. Levin, "Commentary on 'evidence that iron deficiency anemia causes reduced work capacity'," *Journal of Nutrition*, vol. 131, no. 2, pp. 691S–696S, 2001.

[6] J. P. Gisbert, F. Bermejo, R. Pajares et al., "Oral and intravenous iron treatment in inflammatory bowel disease: hematological response and quality of life improvement," *Inflammatory Bowel Diseases*, vol. 15, no. 10, pp. 1485–1491, 2009.

[7] D. H. Henry, "The role of intravenous iron in cancer-related anemia," *Oncology*, vol. 20, no. 8, pp. 21–24, 2006.

[8] A. F. Goddard, M. W. James, A. S. McIntyre, and B. B. Scott, "Guidelines for the management of iron deficiency anaemia," *Gut*, vol. 60, pp. 309–1316, 2011.

[9] "KDOQI, National Kidney Foundation: II. Clinical practice guidelines and clinical practice recommendations for anemia in chronic kidney disease in adults," *American Journal of Kidney Diseases*, vol. 47, no. 5, supplement 3, pp. S16–S85, 2006.

[10] L. Gotloib, D. Silverberg, R. Fudin, and A. Shostak, "Iron deficiency is a common cause of anemia in chronic kidney disease and can often be corrected with intravenous iron," *Journal of Nephrology*, vol. 19, no. 2, pp. 161–167, 2006.

[11] W. Y. Qunibi, "The efficacy and safety of current intravenous iron preparations for the management of iron-deficiency anemia: a review," *Arzneimittel-Forschung*, vol. 60, no. 6 a, pp. 399–412, 2010.

[12] M. H. Rosner and M. Auerbach, "Ferumoxytol for the treatment of iron deficiency," *Expert Review of Hematology*, vol. 4, no. 4, pp. 399–406, 2011.

[13] S. Santosh, P. Podaralla, and B. Miller, "Anaphylaxis with elevated serum tryptase after administration of intravenous ferumoxytol," *NDT Plus*, vol. 3, no. 4, pp. 341–342, 2010.

[14] K. A. Lyseng-Williamson and G. M. Keating, "Ferric carboxymaltose: a review of its use in iron-deficiency anaemia," *Drugs*, vol. 69, no. 6, pp. 739–756, 2009.

[15] P. Geisser and J. Banké-Bochita, "Pharmacokinetics, safety and tolerability of intravenous ferric carboxymaltose: a dose-escalation study in volunteers with mild iron-deficiency anaemia," *Arzneimittel-Forschung*, vol. 60, no. 6 a, pp. 362–372, 2010.

[16] P. Geisser and V. Rumyantsev, "Pharmacodynamics and safety of ferric carboxymaltose: a multiple-dose study in patients with iron-deficiency anaemia secondary to a gastrointestinal disorder," *Arzneimittel-Forschung*, vol. 60, no. 6 a, pp. 373–385, 2010.

[17] F. Funk, P. Ryle, C. Canclini, S. Neiser, and P. Geisser, "The new generation of intravenous iron: chemistry, pharmacology, and toxicology of ferric carboxymaltose," *Arzneimittel-Forschung*, vol. 60, no. 6 a, pp. 345–353, 2010.

[18] R. A. Moore, H. Gaskell, P. Rose, and J. Allan4, "Meta-analysis of efficacy and safety of intravenous ferric carboxymaltose (Ferinject) from clinical trial reports and published trial data," *BMC Blood Disorders*, vol. 11, no. 1, article 4, 2011.

[19] S. Kulnigg, S. Stoinov, V. Simanenkov et al., "A novel intravenous iron formulation for treatment of anemia in inflammatory bowel disease: the ferric carboxymaltose (FERINJECT) randomized controlled trial," *American Journal of Gastroenterology*, vol. 103, no. 5, pp. 1182–1192, 2008.

[20] W. Y. Qunibi, C. Martinez, M. Smith, J. Benjamin, A. Mangione, and S. D. Roger, "A randomized controlled trial comparing intravenous ferric carboxymaltose with oral iron for treatment of iron deficiency anaemia of non-dialysis-dependent chronic kidney disease patients," *Nephrology Dialysis Transplantation*, vol. 26, no. 5, pp. 1599–1607, 2011.

[21] S. Tagboto, L. Cropper, J. Turner, and K. Pugh-Clarke, "The efficacy of a single dose of intravenous ferric carboxymaltose (Ferinject) on anaemia in a pre-dialysis population of chronic kidney disease patients," *Journal of Renal Care*, vol. 35, no. 1, pp. 18–23, 2009.

[22] D. B. Van Wyck, A. Mangione, J. Morrison, P. E. Hadley, J. A. Jehle, and L. T. Goodnough, "Large-dose intravenous ferric carboxymaltose injection for iron deficiency anemia in heavy uterine bleeding: a randomized, controlled trial," *Transfusion*, vol. 49, no. 12, pp. 2719–2728, 2009.

[23] D. B. Van Wyck, M. G. Martens, M. H. Seid, J. B. Baker, and A. Mangione, "Intravenous ferric carboxymaltose compared with oral iron in the treatment of postpartum anemia: a randomized controlled trial," *Obstetrics and Gynecology*, vol. 110, no. 2 I, pp. 267–278, 2007.

[24] S. D. Anker, J. C. Colet, G. Filippatos et al., "Ferric carboxymaltose in patients with heart failure and iron deficiency," *The New England Journal of Medicine*, vol. 361, no. 25, pp. 2436–2448, 2009.

[25] P. W. F. Wilson, R. B. D'Agostino, D. Levy, A. M. Belanger, H. Silbershatz, and W. B. Kannel, "Prediction of coronary heart disease using risk factor categories," *Circulation*, vol. 97, no. 18, pp. 1837–1847, 1998.

[26] A. C. Arroliga, K. K. Guntupalli, J. S. Beaver, W. Langholff, K. Marino, and K. Kelly, "Pharmacokinetics and pharmacodynamics of six epoetin alfa dosing regimens in anemic critically ill patients without acute blood loss," *Critical Care Medicine*, vol. 37, no. 4, pp. 1299–1307, 2009.

[27] Y. Shimizu, Y. Tada, M. Yamauchi et al., "Hypophosphatemia induced by intravenous administration of saccharated ferric oxide. Another form of FGF23-related hypophosphatemia," *Bone*, vol. 45, no. 4, pp. 814–816, 2009.

[28] B. J. Schouten, P. J. Hunt, J. H. Livesey, C. M. Frampton, and S. G. Soule, "FGF23 elevation and hypophosphatemia after intravenous iron polymaltose: a prospective study," *Journal of Clinical Endocrinology and Metabolism*, vol. 94, no. 7, pp. 2332–2337, 2009.

[29] L. Y. Mani, G. Nseir, J. P. Venetz, and M. Pascual, "Severe hypophosphatemia after intravenous administration of iron carboxymaltose in a stable renal transplant recipient," *Transplantation*, vol. 90, no. 7, pp. 804–805, 2010.

[30] A. C. Grimmelt, C. D. Cohen, T. Fehr, A. L. Serra, and R. P. Wüthrich, "Safety and tolerability of ferric carboxymaltose (FCM) for treatment of iron deficiency in patients with chronic kidney disease and in kidney transplant recipients," *Clinical Nephrology*, vol. 71, no. 2, pp. 125–129, 2009.

12

Rapid Assessment for Coexistence of Vitamin B12 and Iron Deficiency Anemia among Adolescent Males and Females in Northern Himalayan State of India

Ashok Bhardwaj,[1] Dinesh Kumar,[1] Sunil Kumar Raina,[1] Pardeep Bansal,[1] Satya Bhushan,[2] and Vishav Chander[1]

[1] Department of Community Medicine, Dr. Rajendra Prasad Government Medical College, Kangra, Himachal Pradesh 176001, India
[2] Department of Biochemistry, Dr. Rajendra Prasad Government Medical College, Kangra, Himachal Pradesh 176001, India

Correspondence should be addressed to Sunil Kumar Raina; ojasrainasunil@yahoo.co.in

Academic Editor: Bruno Annibale

Coexistence of folic acid and vitamin B12 deficiency has been observed among adolescents with iron deficiency anemia, but limited evidence is available from India. So, a rapid assessment was done to study the prevalence of iron, folic acid, and vitamin B12 deficiency among adolescent males and females in northern Himalayan state in India. *Methods.* Total 885 (female: 60.9%) adolescents (11 to 19 completed years) were surveyed from 30-cluster village from two community development blocks of Himachal Pradesh. Serum ferritin, folic acid, and vitamin B12 were estimated among randomly selected 100 male and 100 female adolescents. *Results.* Under-nutrition (BMI < 18.5 kg/m^2) was observed among 68.9% of adolescents (male: 67.1%; female: 70.7; $P = 0.29$). Anemia was observed to be prevalent among 87.2% males and 96.7% females ($P = 0.00$). Mild form of anemia was observed to be the most common (53.9%) form followed by moderate (29.7%) anemia. Strikingly, it was found that all the adolescents were deficient in vitamin B12 and none of the adolescents was observed to be deficient in folic acid. *Conclusion.* Among both male and female adolescents anemia with vitamin B12 deficiency was observed to be a significant public health problem. Folic acid deficiency was not observed as a problem among surveyed adolescents.

1. Introduction

Iron deficiency anemia is still a condition of a major public health concern for researchers and policy makers [1]. Period of adolescence is a significant phase of life as the physiologic growth spurt requires adequate nutrition in order to achieve healthy adulthood. Iron deficiency anemia reflects the state of undernutrition among adolescents. It results due to inadequate nutrition, blood loss, and inflammatory and infectious diseases. Iron deficiency anemia occurs because of poor intake and absorption is the most common form of anemia [2]. In India, the prevalence of iron deficiency anemia had been reported to be 55.8% among females and 30.2% among males in age group of 15–19 years [3]. Adolescent girls of 11–19 years across 16 districts observed the prevalence of anemia to be 90.0%, which was significantly more as compared to national level survey [4]. Iron requires haemglobin (Hb)

synthesis in red blood cells and low level of Hb clinically determines anemia. In addition to iron, the haematopoiesis requires sufficient amount of other nutrients, like folic acid and vitamin B12 require red blood cells production [5].

Folic acid is a water soluble vitamin involved in nucleic acid, blood cell, and nervous tissue synthesis. It is widely distributed in green leafy food items "foliage" and its deficiency will lead to megaloblastic anemia due to prolongation of synthesis phase of red blood cells and retarded maturation of germ cells in bone marrow. In addition to folic acid, vitamin B12 deficiency is the second common cause for megaloblastic anemia. Vitamin B12 is required for two important transmethylation reaction, one of which closely associated with folate in DNA synthesis and haematopoiesis. Not plants, but nonvegetarian food items are the source of vitamin B12 [6]. Low level of vitamin B12 has been considered to affect reproduction and can cause recurrent abortion, infertility, and preterm abortion among pregnant mothers [7]. Limited studies reported that there is coexistence of folic acid and vitamin B12 deficiency along with iron deficiency anemia [8, 9]. This coexistence was also observed among adolescent girls [10–13].

Iron, folic acid, and vitamin B12 deficiency is expected among adolescents with poor nutrition. Their deficiency is of concern in India, as undernutrition was observed among about 60.0% of female and 45.0% male adolescents [3]. Also, surveys have also observed significant prevalence of iron deficiency anemia among adolescents [3, 4]. Understanding their possible interrelationship and global concern due to their deficiency and limited evidence from country, a rapid assessment was done to study the prevalence of iron, folic acid, and vitamin B12 deficiency among adolescent males and females in northern Himalayan state in India. Majority of study population of the study area is consuming mainly vegetarian diet. Cereals, pulses, and rice are consumed daily by almost all the families of studied adolescents (both males and females).

2. Methods

It was a community based cross-sectional study done at Nichar block of district Kinnaur and Shahpur block of district Kangra, Himachal Pradesh, India. Nichar block has ranging altitude of 2,320 to 6,816 meters, and Shahpur has 427 to 6,401 meters above the sea level. A community-based survey was conducted in year 2010 by an independent trained field staff. During the survey total 885 adolescents (from 11 to 19 completed years) were surveyed and assessed for BMI and hemoglobin status. Serum ferritin, folates, and vitamin B12 were estimated among randomly selected 100 male and 100 female adolescents. Study participants were selected from study area using 30-cluster sampling technique, and the village was considered as a unit of cluster. From each cluster the estimated adolescents to be recruited were calculated by population proportion to size (PPS) method. Every cluster was hypothetically divided into four equal parts and study participants were recruited from each part for equal representation of cluster. Randomly, a house from each part was selected and adolescents were recruited till the sample size was met. Field staff administered a structured pretested interview-based questionnaire.

After the interview anthropometric assessment (height and weight) was done, and 5 mL venous blood sample was collected. For Hb estimation, blood (20 μL) was transferred to Whatman filter paper no. 1 and dried at room temperature. The paper was sealed in an envelope and transported to laboratory. The portion of filter paper with blood was placed in 5 mL Drabkin's solution and vortex for 5 minutes. After allowing solution to stand for 2 hours hemoglobin was assessed at 540 nm by spectrophotometer. For serum ferritin, folates, and vitamin B12 blood samples were centrifuged for separation of serum at the collection site and transported in cryocan (liquid nitrogen) to field laboratory for assessment. Ferritin, folates, and vitamin B12 were analyzed at IMMULITE 1000 (Chemiluminescent enzyme immunoassay) with control run. Kits of the same company (Siemens Health care diagnostics

Products limited) were used while performing the tests [14].

Standard diagnostic criteria were used for low hemoglobin (male: Hb < 13 g/dL; female: <12 g/dL), low ferritin (<12 ng/mL), vitamin B12 (<200 pg/mL), and folates (<2.7 ng/mL) levels [15]. Degree of deficiency was assessed for anemia as severe (male: Hb < 9.0 g/dL; female: <7.0 g/dL), mild (male: Hb 9–11.9 g/dL; female: 7.0–10.9 g/dL), and moderate (male: Hb 12.0–12.9 g/dL; female: 11.0–11.9 g/dL). As used in National family Health Survey (NFHS-3), the Body Mass Index (BMI) was categorized as moderate/severe thin (BMI < 17.0 kg/m^2), mild thin (BMI 17.0–18.4 kg/m^2), normal (BMI < 18.4–24.9 kg/m^2), overweight (BMI 25.0–29.9 kg/m^2), and obese (BMI > 30.0 kg/m^2) [3]. Ethical clearance was sought from institute ethics committee (IEC) before the data collection. Informed consent was also sought before interview and collection of blood sample. Statistical analysis was done by using Epiinfo 3.2.5 version (CDC), Chi square (χ^2), and unpaired student t-test was used to compare the proportions and means, respectively, [16]. As the study is rapid assessment that leads to differential distribution study participants subgroups (gender and age groups), the P value should be interpreted with caution.

3. Results

Total 885 (female: 60.9%) adolescents were surveyed. The mean age was found to be 14.0 (SD: ±2.5) and 14.8 (SD: ±2.5) year for males and females, respectively ($P = 0.00$). Participants were assessed for height and weight with an average BMI of 17.4 (SD: ±3.2) kg/m^2 for males and 17.2 (SD: ±2.9) kg/m^2 for females ($P = 0.33$). Assessment for anemia observed that the mean levels of Hb and ferritin among male (12.2 (SD: ±0.9) g/dL and 39.4 (SD: ±8.5) ng/mL) as compared to female adolescents (10.2 (SD: ±0.8) g/dL and 30.9 (SD: ±7.8) ng/mL) were significantly high ($P = 0.00$). On further assessment, it was found that among males the Hb level was 12.1 (SD: ±0.9) g/dL and 12.4 (SD: ±0.9) g/dL in age group of 11 to 15 and 16 to 19 years, respectively, and it was observed to be significant ($P = 0.00$). Whereas, in females the mean Hb was observed to be significantly ($P = 0.00$) low (9.9 (SD: ±0.8) g/dL) in age group of 16 to 19 years as compared to 11 to 15 years (10.9 (SD: ±0.9) g/dL). It was found that the average level of vitamin B12 ($P = 0.05$) and folate ($P = 0.08$) was low in age group of 16 to 19 as compared to 11 to 15 years. Among females of 16 to 19 year of age the average vitamin B12 was observed significantly higher ($P = 0.03$) (Table 1).

The mean vitamin B12 level was observed to be 34.7 (SD: ±11.5) and 33.5 (SD: ±11.0) pg/mL among both male and female adolescents, respectively ($P = 0.87$), which were very much low as per the required level of 200 pg/mL. Whereas, average folates level was observed to be within normal limits for both male (15.2 (SD: ±6.5) ng/mL) and female (14.1 (SD: ±6.1) ng/mL) adolescents ($P = 0.40$).

Undernutrition (BMI < 18.5 kg/m^2) was observed among 68.9% of adolescents (male: 67.1%; female: 70.7; $P = 0.29$), and the prevalence of moderate/severe level of thinness (BMI < 17.0 kg/m^2) was observed to be 49.8% and 47.7% among

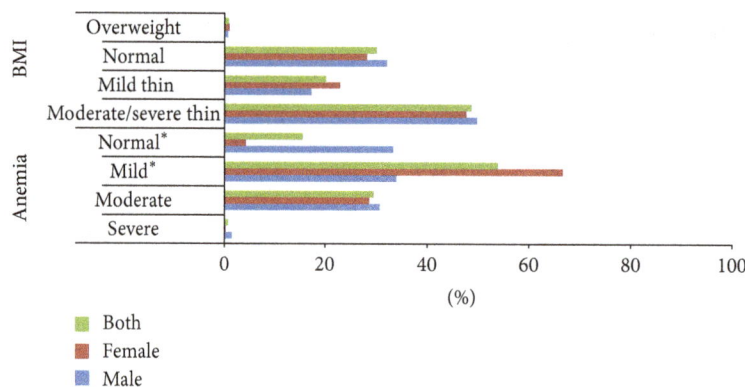

FIGURE 1: Prevalence of anemia and low BMI among studied adolescent males and females in Himalayan state of north India, 2010.

TABLE 1: Age and gender distribution of average Hb, ferritin, vitamin B12, and folate levels among studied adolescent males and females in Himalayan state of north India, 2010.

Variables Mean (±SD)	Gender	Age group (years)		t, P value
		11–15	16–19	
Hb	Male	12.1 (0.9)	12.4 (0.9)	3.3, 0.00
	Female	10.4 (0.8)	9.9 (0.8)	6.0, 0.00
	All	11.3 (1.2)	10.9 (1.4)	4.6, 0.00
Ferritin	Male	39.1 (11.2)	40.3 (11.5)	0.2, 0.83
	Female	27.5 (12.0)	34.3 (10.4)	1.9, 0.05
	All	39.4 (12.5)	36.0 (12.0)	0.8, 0.42
Vitamin B12	Male	36.0 (10.2)	30.3 (6.9)	0.4, 0.65
	Female	14.6 (7.5)	23.3 (3.5)	2.1, 0.03
	All	39.4 (21.0)	25.1 (4.2)	1.9, 0.05
Folate	Male	16.0 (6.4)	12.1 (3.7)	1.3, 0.18
	Female	14.6 (4.5)	13.5 (3.1)	0.9, 0.34
	All	15.0 (5.3)	13.1 (3.3)	1.7, 0.08

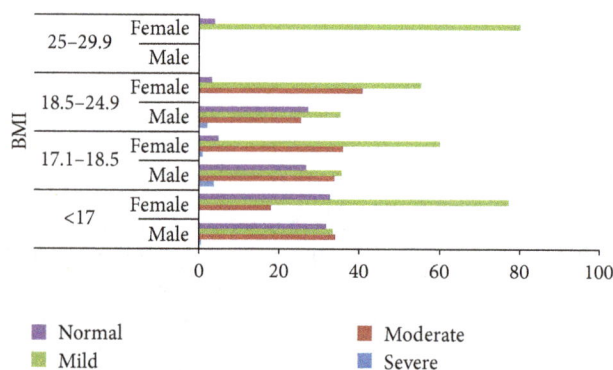

FIGURE 2: Prevalence of anemia as per different BMI categories among studied adolescents in Himalayan state of north India, 2010.

male and females, respectively (P = 0.63). Absolute 23.0% of female and 17.3% of male (P = 0.32) adolescent had mild level of thinness (BMI: 17.0–18.4 kg/m^2). Based upon standard cutoffs anemia was observed to be prevalent among 87.2% males and 96.7% females (P = 0.00). Mild form of anemia was observed to be most common (53.9%) form followed by moderate (29.7%) anemia. Severe anemia was observed to be very less (0.7%) among studied adolescents. Significantly (P = 0.00) more of female (66.6%), as compared to male (34.1%) adolescents, were exposed to mild anemia, whereas the prevalence of moderate anemia was observed to be 30.9% among male and 28.9% among female adolescents (P = 0.72) (Figure 1).

When assessed for prevalence of anemia among adolescents with their BMI, it was found that mild level of anemia was most common among all adolescents in all the categories of BMI. It was further observed that the prevalence of mild anemia was decreasing and moderate anemia was increasing among adolescents with moderate/severe thinness to normal appearance (Figure 2). Gender specific distribution

of type of anemia to different categories of BMI showed that significantly more of females were exposed to mild form of anemia in all categories of BMI. For adolescents with BMI of less than 17.0 kg/m^2, the prevalence of moderate anemia was 34.1% for males and 18.0% for females (P = 0.06) (Table 2).

The prevalence of low ferritin was also observed to be 15.0%, which was more among females (17.4%) than of males (12.2%) adolescents (P = 0.31). Strikingly, it was found that all the adolescents were deficient in vitamin B12 and none of adolescent was observed to be deficient in folic acid.

4. Discussion

Among adolescents, anemia remains a significant public health problem which reflects nutritional deficiency. It affects negatively on physical growth, morbidity, cognition, and reproduction [17]. It was further observed that, in addition to iron, folic, and vitamin B12 deficiency also predisposes the adolescent girls to preterm, low birth weight, and other congenital malformations in newborn during their period of pregnancy [5]. Very less studies were carried out among adolescent males, and the present study observed high prevalence of low Hb (male: 87.2% and females: 96.7%) in both genders, which was found to be similar as reported to be 90.0% among adolescent girls [4], whereas country wide survey did report

TABLE 2: Prevalence of anemia (g/dL) as per different BMI (kg/m^2) categories among studied adolescent males and females in Himalayan state of north India, 2010.

BMI	Severe			Moderate			Mild		
	Male	Female	χ^2, P value	Male	Female	χ^2, P value	Male	Female	χ^2, P value
	<9.0	<7.0		9.0–11.9	7.0–9.9		12.–12.9	10.–11.9	
<17.0	1 (0.5)	0 (0.0)	—	62 (34.1)	45 (18.0)	3.4, 0.06	61 (33.5)	193 (77.2)	41.0, 0.00
17.1–18.5	2 (3.6)	1 (0.8)	—	19 (33.9)	45 (36.0)	0.8, 0.35	20 (35.7)	75 (60.0)	3.9, 0.04
18.5–24.9	2 (2.0)	0 (0.0)	—	26 (25.5)	62 (40.8)	1.4, 0.23	36 (35.3)	84 (55.3)	3.5, 0.06
25.0–29.9	0 (0.0)	0 (0.0)	—	0 (0.0)	9 (20.0)	—	(0.0)	4 (80.0)	—

—: could not be calculated due less numbers.

that 55.8% of female and 30.2% of male adolescents but of 15–19 years had anemia [3], which was observed to be low as compared to present and earlier study [4].

Present study had showed that the mild anemia was of most common type, whereas, very less adolescents were observed with severe anemia. Mild anemia was observed among 53.9% of adolescents, whereas, it was 48.4% in country wide survey [3]. However, present study observed low prevalence of severe anemia (0.7%) as reported as 1.6% in national survey [3]. Moderate anemia was observed to be common (60.1%) and severe anemia among 13.1% studied adolescents girls in survey conducted in selected districts. But survey of a different selected district (different of present study area) but of the same state in which present study was carried out the prevalence of mild, moderate, and severe anemia was observed as 31.0%, 28.0%, and 2.0%, respectively, [4]. As compared to national survey, present study and survey in 16 different districts have observed the high prevalence of anemia, which could be attributed to different Hb estimation method in country wide survey (Hemocue) and in other studies (indirect cyanmethemoglobin) [18]. As the serum ferritin level determines the level of iron stores in the body, present study had observed the prevalence of low serum ferritin to be 12.2% among male and 17.4% among females. It was observed to be low when compared with study, which had reported the prevalence of low serum ferritin as 27.3% among adolescent girls with anemia [19]. Iron stores are expected to be low among anemic adolescents but can be further attributed to different poor dietary consumption and absorption of iron rich food items.

Folic acid and vitamin B12 deficiency impairs DNA and folate synthesis causing impaired and ineffective erythropoiesis [5]. Folic acid deficiency has been observed with iron deficiency, and the high prevalence was observed as 80.0% to 90.0% among studied adolescents in Venezuela [11, 12]. But about only 25.0% adolescent girls were observed to be deficient in folic acid in rural area of Bangladesh [13]. Strikingly, in the present study none of adolescent was observed to be deficient in folic acid and also the average level of folic acid was observed to be within normal limits.

It has been discussed that the vitamin B12 deficiency may also coexist with iron deficiency, and so far, with the existing background of evidences, there is an insignificant contribution of vitamin B12 deficiency, burden of anemia in the world [20]. However, sprouting evidence has shown that now the prevalence of vitamin B12 deficiency is becoming

a major type of nutritional deficient anemia. Its prevalence was observed to be around 20.0% among elderly population [12] and women of childbearing age [21]. A study among pregnant women of northern Indian state had revealed high prevalence (74.1%) of vitamin B12 deficiency [22]. Study among adolescents had shown that about 25.0% to 30.0% were deficient in vitamin B12 [11]. But the prevalence was only 7.0% for vitamin B12 deficiency that was observed among adolescent girls in rural area of Bangladesh [13]. A study found that that, among anemic adolescents, there was high prevalence of folic acid than that of vitamin B12 deficiency, whereas all the vitamin B12 deficient adolescents were anemic [12]. Present study showed that almost all of adolescents (about 90.0%) were anemic and all the studied adolescents were deficient in vitamin B12.

With the limited available evidence among adolescents, in the present study, a consistent finding for prevalence and type of anemia, but strikingly inconsistent observation like zero prevalence of folic acid deficiency and 100.0% prevalence of vitamin B12 deficiency was observed. Variation across the geographical regions for nutrient deficiencies like iron, folates, and vitamin B12 is associated with nutrition profile and prevalence of various inflammatory and infectious diseases in adolescents. Present study observed high prevalence of undernutrition among adolescents. Moderate/severe thinness was observed to be more common followed by mild thinness. In country wide survey—among adolescent of 15–19 years of age—the comparable prevalence of moderate/severe (male: 58.1%; female: 46.8%) and mild level of thinness (male: 28.8%; female: 25.9%) was observed [3]. So, observed 70.0% undernutrition prevalence, it is attributed to less consumption of recommended calorie intake and deficiency of other micro-nutrients. But present study observed no deficiency in folic acid, which could be associated with consumption of diet rich in folic acid, the iron folic acid supplementation (national program) in the study area. However, detailed dietary assessment and consumption of IFA tablets were not done in the present study and therefore cannot be attributed. Apart from them, the method of analysis and determined levels for nutrients use in various studies could also explain the variation.

Various surveys and studies across the country have shown anemia as an endemic public health problem. Country has initiated the distribution of IFA tablets among adolescents and pregnant women in order to reduce the anemia. In addition, various food supplementation programs for children, adolescents, and pregnant women have been in operation over the last three decades [23]. But, despite the significant efforts by the country the significant reduction in anemia is yet to be observed. A marked difference in IFA consumption due to considerable disparities in socioeconomic factors and health care delivery system was observed [24].

In present study, the iron deficiency anemia does not feel likely, as there was less prevalence of low serum ferritin and none of adolescent was observed to be deficient for folic acid. But inability to carry out the detailed hematological examination like total iron binding capacity, transferring receptor and peripheral blood smear should be considered as limitations of the study. Another limitation of study is that the estimation of Hb using dried filter paper could possibly lead to underestimation of Hb but could not be accounted as it was not validated. But considering the high prevalence of low hemoglobin and vitamin B12 deficiency among adolescents in present study would further require a carefully planned analytical study in order to establish the association of vitamin B12 deficiency and anemia. So, in addition to IFA supplementation, the role of other multivitamins in reducing anemia is becoming a major area of research.

References

[1] T. G. Sanghvi, P. W. J. Harvey, and E. Wainwright, "Maternal iron-folic acid supplementation programs: evidence of impact and implementation," *Food and Nutrition Bulletin*, vol. 31, no. 2, pp. S100–S107, 2010.

[2] G. S. Toteja and P. Singh, *Micronutrient Profile of Indian Population*, Indian Council of Medical Research, New Delhi, India, 2004.

[3] International Institute for Population Sciences (IIPS) and Macro International, *National Family Health Survey (NFHS-3), 2005-06*, vol. I, IIPS, Mumbai, India, 2007.

[4] G. S. Toteja, P. Singh, B. S. Dhillon et al., "Prevalence of anemia among pregnant women and adolescent girls in 16 districts of India," *Food and Nutrition Bulletin*, vol. 27, no. 4, pp. 311–315, 2006.

[5] S. M. Fishman, P. Christian, and J. West K.P., "The role of vitamins in the prevention and control anaemia," *Public Health Nutrition*, vol. 3, no. 2, pp. 125–150, 2000.

[6] E. Myhre, "Studies on megaloblasts in vitro," *Scandinavian Journal of Clinical & Laboratory Investigation*, vol. 16, p. 307, 1964.

[7] A. M. Molloy, P. N. Kirke, L. C. Brody, J. M. Scott, and J. L. Mills, "Effects of folate and vitamin B12 deficiencies during pregnancy on fetal, infant, and child development," *Food and Nutrition Bulletin*, vol. 29, no. 2, pp. S101–S111, 2008.

[8] U. Khanduri, A. Sharma, and A. Joshi, "Occult cobalamin and folate deficiency in Indians," *National Medical Journal of India*, vol. 18, no. 4, pp. 182–183, 2005.

[9] S. Arora, B. Singh, V. K. Gupta, and M. Venkatesan, "Burden of vitamin B12 deficiency in urban population in Delhi, India: a hospital based study," *International Journal of Pharma and Bio Sciences*, vol. 2, no. 1, pp. 521–528, 2011.

[10] P. Pathak, R. Saxena, S. K. Kapoor, S. N. Dwivedi, R. Singh, and U. Kapil, "Status of serum ferritin and folate levels amongst young women in a rural community of Haryana, India," *Nepal Medical College Journal*, vol. 6, no. 1, pp. 13–16, 2004.

[11] M. N. García-Casal, C. Osorio, M. Landaeta et al., "High prevalence of folic acid and vitamin B12 deficiencies in infants, children, adolescents and pregnant women in Venezuela," *European Journal of Clinical Nutrition*, vol. 59, no. 9, pp. 1064–1070, 2005.

[12] T. Suárez, M. Torrealba, N. Villegas, C. Osorio, and M. N. García-Casal, "Iron, folic acid and vitamin B12 deficiencies related to anemia in adolescents from a region with a high incidence of congenital malformations in Venezuela," *Archivos latinoamericanos de nutrición*, vol. 55, no. 2, pp. 118–123, 2005 (Spanish).

[13] F. Ahmed, M. R. Khan, C. P. Banu, M. R. Qazi, and M. Akhtaruz-zaman, "The coexistence of other micronutrient deficiencies in anaemic adolescent schoolgirls in rural Bangladesh," *European Journal of Clinical Nutrition*, vol. 62, no. 3, pp. 365–372, 2008.

[14] *Siemens Health Care Diagnostics*, Tarrytown, NY, USA.

[15] World Health Organization, "Nutritional anaemias. Report of a WHO scientific group," *World Health Organization Technical Report Series*, vol. 405, pp. 5–37, 1968.

[16] Centre for Disease Control, *Epiinfo: Release 3.2.5 TM*, Centre for Disease Control, Atlanta, Ga, USA, 2002.

[17] S. Seshadri, "Nutritional anaemia in South Asia," in *Malnutrition in South Asia: A Regional Profile*, S. K. Gillespie, Ed., pp. 75–124, UNICEF Regional Office for South Asia, 1997.

[18] M. Sari, S. De Pee, E. Martini et al., "Estimating the prevalence of anaemia: a comparison of three methods," *Bulletin of the World Health Organization*, vol. 79, no. 6, pp. 506–511, 2001.

[19] Y. A. Indriastuti Kurniawan, S. Muslimatun, E. L. Achadi, and S. Sastroamidjojo, "Anaemia and iron deficiency anaemia among young adolescent girls from peri urban coastal area of Indonesia," *Asia Pacific Journal of Clinical Nutrition*, vol. 15, no. 3, pp. 350–356, 2006.

[20] J. Metz, "A high prevalence of biochemical evidence of vitamin B12 or folate deficiency does not translate into a comparable prevalence of anemia," *Food and Nutrition Bulletin*, vol. 29, no. 2, pp. S74–S85, 2008.

[21] J. H. Zhu, D. J. Hu, L. Hao et al., "Iron, folate, and B12 deficiencies and their associations with anemia among women of childbearing age in a rural area in northern China," *International Journal for Vitamin and Nutrition Research*, vol. 80, no. 2, pp. 144–154, 2010.

[22] P. Pathak, U. Kapil, C. S. Yajnik, S. K. Kapoor, S. N. Dwivedi, and R. Singh, "Iron, folate, and vitamin B12 stores among pregnant women in a rural area of Haryana State, India," *Food and Nutrition Bulletin*, vol. 28, no. 4, pp. 435–438, 2007.

[23] Government of India, "Annual Report," Ministry of Health and Family Welfare, pp. 7–12, 2010.

[24] S.-R. Pasricha, B.-A. Biggs, N. Prashanth et al., "Factors influencing receipt of iron supplementation by young children and their mothers in rural India: local and national cross-sectional studies," *BMC Public Health*, vol. 11, article 617, 2011.

13

Erythrocyte and Reticulocyte Indices on the LH 750 as Potential Markers of Functional Iron Deficiency

Eloísa Urrechaga,[1] Luís Borque,[2] and Jesús F. Escanero[2]

[1] Hematology Laboratory, Hospital Galdakao—Usansolo, Galdakao, 48960 Vizcaya, Spain
[2] Department of Pharmacology and Physiology, Faculty of Medicine, University of Zaragoza, Zaragoza, Spain

Correspondence should be addressed to Eloísa Urrechaga, eloisa.urrechagaigartua@osakidetza.net

Academic Editor: Fernando Ferreira Costa

Reticulocyte hemoglobin content (CHr) and percentage of hypochromic cells (%Hypo) are restricted to the Siemens analysers. The aims of the study were to investigate the correlation of Red cells size factor (RSf) and low Hemoglobin density (LHD%), reported by Beckman-Coulter analysers, with CHr and %Hypo in the assessment of iron status in the presence of inflammation. 381 samples were run on both LH 750 (Beckman-Coulter) and Advia 2120 (Siemens) analysers. Correlation between parameters were calculated and the diagnostic performance of the new parameters was assessed. *Results.* Correlation between RSf and CHr, $r = 0.85$. ROC curve analysis for RSf in the diagnosis of iron restricted erythropoiesis defined as CHr < 28 pg: AUC 0.983; Cutoff 91.1%; Sensitivity 98.8%; Specificity 89.6% Correlation between LHD% and %Hypo, $r = 0.869$. ROC curve analysis for LHD% in the diagnosis of iron deficiency defined by %Hypo > 5%: AUC 0.954; Cut off 6.0%; Sensitivity 96.6%; Specificity 83.2% *Conclusions.* RSf and LHD% could be reliable parameters for the study of iron metabolism status.

1. Introduction

In iron deficiency anemia (IDA) iron supply depends on the quantity of iron storage in the body, while in functional iron deficiency (iron restricted erythropoiesis) supply depends on the rate of mobilization of iron from the stores. Functional iron deficiency is defined as an imbalance between the iron needs for erythropoiesis and the iron supply, with the latter not maintained at sufficient rate for adequate hemoglobinization of reticulocytes and mature erythrocytes [1].

The diagnosis of iron deficiency or functional iron deficiency is particularly challenging in patients with acute or chronic inflammatory conditions because most of the biochemical markers for iron metabolism are affected by acute phase reaction. This is the case of the anemia of chronic disease (ACD) and the anemia associated to chronic renal failure (CKD).

Serum ferritin, an indicator of iron storage but not of iron supply, is a positive acute phase reactant, while transferrin is a negative acute phase reactant, rendering the

calculation of transferrin saturation unreliable in this case [2–4].

For these reasons, an iron deficient erythropoiesis may occur despite that normal serum ferritin and transferrin saturation values and interest have been generated in the use of erythrocyte and reticulocyte parameters, available on the modern analysers based on flow cytometry technology.

Direct consequence of an imbalance between the erythroid marrow iron requirements and the actual supply is a reduction of red cell hemoglobin content, which causes hypochromic mature red cells and reticulocytes.

Reticulocyte hemoglobin content (CHr) and the percentage of hypochromic red blood cells (%Hypo) reflect iron availability and are reliable markers of functional iron deficiency [5, 6].

The measurement of CHr is a direct assessment of the incorporation of iron into erythrocyte hemoglobin (Hb) and thus an estimate of the recent functional availability of iron into the erythron; due to the life span of the reticulocytes, CHr is a sensitive indicator of iron deficient erythropoiesis [7–9].

The measurement of %Hypo (defined as the percentage of red blood cells with Hb concentration less than 280 g/L) is a sensitive method for quantifying the hemoglobinization of mature red cells. Because of the long circulating life span of mature erythrocytes %Hypo values are related to iron status in the last 2-3 months, and have been recognised as an indicator of iron deficiency [10, 11].

CHr and %Hypo have been used as a diagnostic tool, together with biochemical markers, to distinguish IDA from ACD, and are incorporated to National Kidney Foundation (NKF-K/DOQI) guidelines for the monitoring of recombinant human erythropoietin rHuEPO therapy [12–14].

To date, the measurement of CHr and %Hypo has been restricted to the analysers of a single manufacturer, Siemens (Siemens Medical Solutions Diagnostics, Tarrytown N.Y, USA). A second manufacturer has produced a comparable index, the so-called reticulocyte hemoglobin equivalent (Ret He) generated by the Sysmex XE 2100 analyser (Sysmex Corporation, Kobe, Japan).

Measurements of Ret He provides useful information in diagnosing anemia, iron restricted erythropoiesis, and functional iron deficiency and response to iron therapy during r-HuEPO. Twenty nine pg is the cutoff value that defines deficient erythropoiesis [15, 16]. Ret He correlates with CHr with the same clinical meaning [17]. The new Symex XE 5000 analyser reports the percentages of hypochromic red cells, but few data are already published about this parameter [18].

Beckman Coulter (Beckman Coulter Inc., Miami, Fl, USA) has recently introduced on the LH series analysers two new parameters

Red blood cell Size Factor (RSf) joins together the volume of mature red cells (MCV) and the volume of reticulocytes (MRV), both related to erythropoietic activity and hemoglobinization

$$RSf = \sqrt{MCV * MRV}. \qquad (1)$$

Compared to the mature erythrocyte population, reticulocytes have a mean volume 15–20 fL greater, they stay in the blood stream for 1–1.5 days, so the measurement of reticulocyte number and cellular characteristics, such as volume, provides real-time data regarding certain aspects of erythropoiesis that can influence the dimensions of red cells, such as iron availability. The examination of both precursors and mature cells provides an opportunity to detect and monitor acute and chronic changes in cellular hemoglobin status, related to cell volume [19].

Low hemoglobin density (LHD%) derives from the traditional mean cell hemoglobin concentration (MCHC), using the mathematical sigmoid transformation

$$LHD\% = 100 * \sqrt{1 - \left(\frac{1}{(1 + e^{1.8(30 - MCHC)})}\right)}. \qquad (2)$$

MCHC is an all-inclusive measure of both the availability of iron over the preceding 90–120 days, and of the proper introduction of iron into intracellular hemoglobin.

In the same way, LHD% is related to iron availability and the hemoglobinization of the mature red cells.

In this equation defining LHD%, in addition to the standard sigmoid function, a square root is applied to further enhance numerical resolution in the region corresponding to the lower end of %Hypo, to improve the differentiation between the normal and the abnormal among the blood samples having relatively low values of LHD% [20].

The aims of this study were

(i) to establish the reference range of RSf and LHD% and their values in different types of anemia;

(ii) to evaluate these recently introduced reticulocyte and erythrocyte parameters provided by the LH series analysers in terms of correlation with CHr and %Hypo as well as their diagnostic efficiency assuming CHr < 28.0 pg or %Hypo > 5% to detect iron restricted erythropoiesis and iron deficiency.

2. Materials and Methods

2.1. Criteria for Selecting the Groups of Patients. Samples from 120 healthy individuals, 72 iron deficiency anemia (IDA), 60 IDA with acute phase response (IDA APR), 71 chronic kidney disease (CKD), and 58 anemia of chronic disease (ACD) were randomly extracted from the routine workload and run sequentially on both LH 750 (Beckman Coulter Inc. Miami, Fl, USA) and Advia 2120 (Siemens Medical Solutions Diagnostics, Tarrytown N.Y., USA), analysers within 6 hours of collection.

Healthy group: 54 male and 66 female adult subjects, with no clinical symptoms of disease and with results of the complete blood count and biochemical iron metabolism markers within reference ranges.

A group of 132 IDA patients fulfilled traditional diagnostic criteria for iron deficiency anemia diagnosis, serum iron < 7.5 μmol/L, transferrin saturation < 20%, ferritin < 50 μg/L, and Hb < 110 g/L, were included before iron treatment.

This group was divided into a nonacute phase response group ($n = 72$, CRP < 5 mg/L) and acute phase response group ($n = 60$, CRP > 5 mg/L). Acute phase response included inflammation or infectious conditions, in addition to ferropenic status.

CKD patients were managed according to the recommendations of the NKF-K/DOQI guidelines [21]. All patients were treated with a variety of erythropoietin doses, the majority of them were treated with a maintenance dose of intravenous iron weekly, in order to maintain Hb at the recommended level 110–120 g/L.

ACD group included patients with a variety of diseases: chronic infections (tuberculosis); neoplasic disorders (Hodgkin's disease, breast carcinoma); noninfectious inflammatory diseases (rheumatoid arthritis, systemic lupus erythematosus).

ACD patients received treatment to maintain normal erythropoiesis and presented the traditional diagnostic criteria for "Functional iron-deficiency" diagnosis Transferrin saturation < 20%, Hb < 110 g/L, and serum ferritin values normal or over the reference range.

Table 1 shows the hematological and biochemical data of the different groups.

TABLE 1: Hematological and biochemical data of the healthy group ($n = 120$), iron deficiency anemia (IDA, $n = 72$), iron deficiency anemia and acute phase response (IDA APR, $n = 60$), anemia of chronic disease (ACD, $n = 58$), and chronic kidney disease (CKD, $n = 71$) patients.

	RBC 10^{12}/L	Hb g/L	MCV fL	MCH pg	MCHC g/L	Iron μmol/L	Transf g/L	Ferritin μg/L	Sat %
Healthy mean	4.9	154	91.1	31.3	343	16.5	2.53	75	31
(SD)	(0.27)	(6.4)	(2.55)	(1.53)	(5.2)	1(0.62)	(0.2)	(2.8)	(1.9)
IDA mean	4.6	95	70	22.5	320	4.8	3.31	14	6
(SD)	(0.61)	(14.2)	(10.3)	(4.23)	(17.3)	(2.15)	(0.53)	(9)	(3.6)
IDA APR mean	4.4	96	75.8	21.5	327	5.1	2.78	37	9
(SD)	(0.43)	(12.1)	(3.7)	(1.3)	(9.2)	(3.5)	(0.28)	(25)	(5.6)
ACD mean	3.5	101	93.2	31.9	343	10.0	2.68	522	15
(SD)	(0.48)	(11)	(6.0)	(2.23)	(10)	(6.8)	(0.66)	(704)	(5)
CKD mean	3.5	112	95.6	31.1	325	9.8	1.87	335	21
(SD)	(0.45)	(8.5)	(6.67)	(2.23)	(8)	(4.47)	(0.43)	(204)	(10)

RBC, red blood cells; Hb, hemoglobin; MCV, mean cell volume; MCH, mean cell hemoglobin; MCHC, mean cell hemoglobin concentration; Transf, transferrin; Sat, % transferrin saturation.

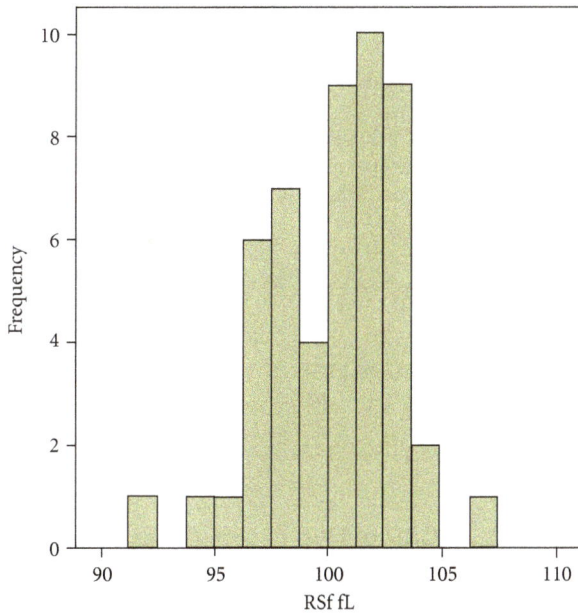

FIGURE 1: Red blood cell size factor (RSf) values in a population of 120 healthy adult subjects. The values showed Gaussian distribution (Kolmogorov-Smirnoff test, $P = .279$).

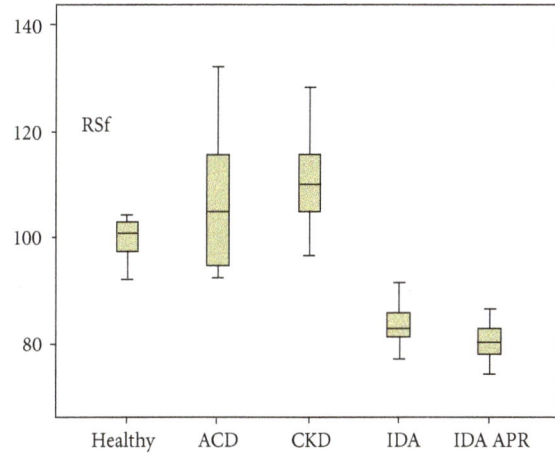

FIGURE 2: Comparison of red blood cell size factor (RSf) in the groups of anemic patients, anemia of chronic disease (ACD), chronic kidney disease (CKD), iron deficiency anemia (IDA) iron deficiency anemia and acute phase response (IDA APR), and in the healthy group.

2.2. *Statistical Evaluation of Analytical Results.* Statistical software package SPSS (SPSS; Chicago, IL, USA) version 17.0 for Windows was applied for statistical analysis of the results.

Reference ranges were calculated from the results obtained in the group of healthy subjects (95 central percentiles of the distribution). Kolmogorov—Smirnoff test was applied to verify the Gaussian distribution of RSf and LHD% values.

When the parameters under study presented a Gaussian distribution correlation, coefficients were calculated by Pearson method; independent samples t-test was performed in order to detect statistical deviations between the groups of patients; P values less than .05 were considered to be statistically significant.

When the parameters under study presented a non-Gaussian distribution correlation, coefficients were calcu-

lated by Spearman method; independent samples Mann-Whitney U-test was performed; P values less than .05 were considered to be statistically significant.

Receiver operating characteristic (ROC) curve analysis was utilized to illustrate the diagnostic performance of RSf and LHD% in the detection of iron deficiency status, defined by a CHr value 28 pg.

Cutoff values were established based on the optimal combination of sensitivity and specificity.

3. Results

The values of RSf were normally distributed ($P = .279$) (Figure 1). Reference range was 91.1–106.9 fL.

Figure 2 and Table 2 exhibit CHr and RSf mean values and standard deviation (SD) in the variety of anemia and healthy subjects included in the study.

The horizontal line in the center of the box shows the median value, the upper and lower limits of the box show the

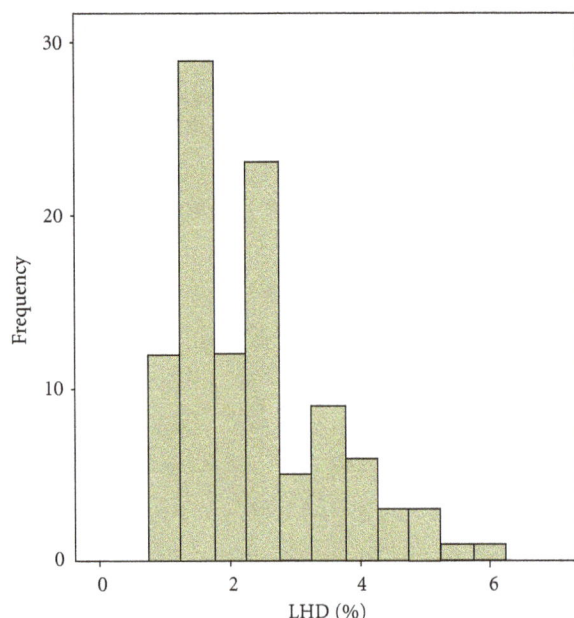

FIGURE 3: low hemoglobin density (LHD%) values in a population of 120 healthy adult subjects. The values showed a non-Gaussian distribution (Kolmogorov-Smirnoff test, P = .034).

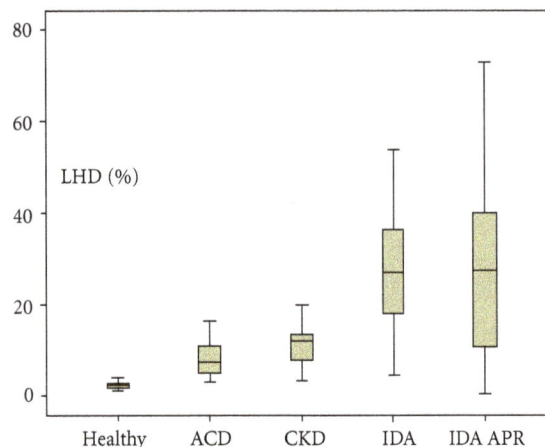

FIGURE 4: Comparison of low hemoglobin density (LHD%) in the groups of anemic patients, anemia of chronic disease (ACD), chronic kidney disease (CKD), iron deficiency anemia (IDA) iron deficiency anemia and acute phase response (IDA APR), and in the healthy group.

TABLE 2: Reticulocyte hemoglobin content (CHr) and red blood cell size factor (RSf) values, mean and standard deviation (SD), in the group of patients.

	CHr pgmean (SD)	RSf fLmean (SD)
Healthy	33.2 (1.6)	100.9 (5.3)
IDA	24.5 (4.4)	88.1 (7.8)
IDA APR	25.6 (2.5)	84.7 (4.1)
ACD	30.8 (5.1)	105.5 (10.9)
CKD	31.6 (3.5)	110.6 (8.7)

TABLE 3: Percentage of hypochromic red cells (% Hypo) values, mean and standard deviation (SD) and low hemoglobin density (LHD%) values, median (5th–95th interquartiles, IQ) in the group of patients.

	% Hypo Mean (SD)	LHD% Median (IQ)
Healthy	0.13 (0.15)	2.1 (0.9–4.1)
IDA	17.2 (17.4)	29.6 (7.5–76)
IDA APR	16.8 (15.5)	27.3 (8.3–71.2)
ACD	4.1 (4.4)	7.3 (5.1–30)
CKD	5.1 (6.7)	9.6 (5.6–27)

interquartile range, and the whiskers show the minimum and maximum values for each group.

The horizontal line in the center of the box shows the median value, the upper and lower limits of the box show the interquartile range, and the whiskers show the minimum and maximum values for each group.

Correlation between CHr and RSf values, Pearson regression coefficient 0.85, P < .001.

Independent samples t-test was performed in order to detect statistical deviations between the groups of patients.

Significant differences in RSf mean values (P < .001) were detected when groups with iron restricted erythropoiesis (IDA, mean 88.1 fL and IDA with APR, mean 84.7 fL) were compared with patients undergoing therapy (ACD, mean 108.9 fL and CKD, 110.6 fL) and the healthy subjects (mean 100.9 fL).

No statistic difference was found between IDA group and IDA patients with acute phase response (P = .481).

IDA and IDA with APR groups presented iron restricted erythropoiesis as is stated by CHr values (24.5 pg and 25.6 pg,

resp.) ACD and CKD patients receiving therapy maintained CHr levels higher than the cutoff value of 28 pg.

ROC curve analysis for RSf in the diagnosis of restricted erythropoiesis, defined by CHr < 28 pg, results were AUC 0.983, Cutoff 91.1 fL, sensitivity 98.8%, specificity 89.6%.

The values of LHD% were not normally distributed (P = .034) (Figure 3). Reference range was 0%–4.4%.

Figure 4 and Table 3 exhibit %Hypo values, mean and standard deviation (SD) and LHD% values, median and 5th–95th interquartiles, in the variety of anemias and healthy subjects included in the study.

The horizontal line in the center of the box shows the median value, the upper and lower limits of the box show the interquartile range, and the whiskers show the minimum and maximum values for each group.

Correlation between %Hypo and LHD% values, r = 0.869 (Spearman method) (P < .001). $y = 1.338x + 4.40$.

Independent samples U-test was performed in order to detect statistical deviations between the groups of patients.

Significant differences in LHD% values (P < .001) were detected when groups with iron deficiency (IDA, mean 29.6% and IDA with APR, mean 27.3%) were compared with patients undergoing therapy (ACD, mean 7.3%; CKD, mean 9.6%) and the healthy subjects (median 2.1%).

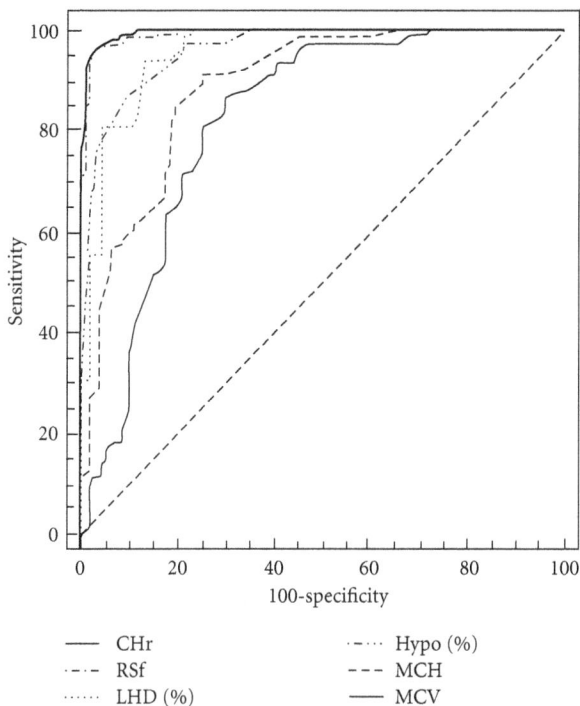

FIGURE 5: Receiver operating characteristic (ROC) curves for red blood cell size factor (RSf), low hemoglobin density (LHD%), reticulocyte hemoglobin content (CHr), percentage of hypochromic red cells (% Hypo), mean cell hemoglobin (MCH) and mean cell volume (MCV) in the diagnosis of iron deficiency, defined by CHr < 28 pg.

No statistic difference was found between IDA group and IDA patients with acute phase response ($P = .578$).

Receiver operating characteristic (ROC) curve analysis for LHD% in the diagnosis of iron deficiency, defined by %Hypo > 5% AUC 0.954, cutoff 6.0%, sensitivity 96.6%, specificity 83.3%.

Discriminant efficiency of biochemical parameters and classical erythrocyte indices:

mean cell hemoglobin (MCH), AUC 0.89; mean cell volume, (MCV), AUC 0.822; serum ferritin, AUC 0.722; serum iron, AUC 0.683 (Figure 5).

4. Discussion

Uncomplicated iron deficiency is not difficult to diagnose by means of the traditional laboratory tests. Biochemical markers are reliable parameters to diagnose iron deficiency in an uncomplicated clinical setting.

Serum ferritin, as a potent positive acute phase reactant is often increased in ACD and CKD patients [22]. Transferrin saturation is less than 15% to 20% in iron deficiency, but expression of serum transferrin is reported to be downregulated by inflammatory cytokines, so may not reliably reflect iron deficiency when anemia is complicated by inflammation [23].

Efforts have been made to evaluate some readily available and relatively inexpensive laboratory parameters as indirect markers of iron restricted erythropoiesis and iron availability

in a clinical context influenced by inflammation and acute phase reaction.

The best combination of hematological indices for iron deficiency is an increased percentage of hypochromic erythrocytes and a reduced hemoglobin content of reticulocytes [24].

Measurements of reticulocyte hemoglobin content (CHr) have been shown to provide useful information in diagnosing functional iron deficiency during r-HuEPO therapy [25, 26] and response to iron therapy [27, 28].

Recent studies confirm the clinical reliability of mature erythrocyte parameters, such as hypochromic red cells (Hypo %), as markers of iron deficiency in hemodialysis patients [29, 30].

Beckman Coulter (Beckman Coulter Inc. Miami, Fl, USA) applies the Volume Conductivity Scatter technology to this field and new parameters are now available on the LH series analysers.

The main purpose of the present study was to determine the diagnostic performance of RSf and LHD% and to assess whether the new parameters correlate with the existing diagnostic tests CHr and %Hypo for restricted erythropoiesis and functional iron deficiency diagnosis.

This study shows a reasonable level of agreement between RSf and CHr.

Despite the fact that CHr is a measurement of the reticulocyte hemoglobin content and RSf is a measurement of both mature red cells and reticulocyte size, a high concordance between these parameters has been observed and values of both parameters showed the same trend in the different groups.

In patients with iron restricted erythropoiesis, (IDA and IDA APR) RSf values were lower than the reference range 91.1 fL.

ACD and CKD patients were receiving therapy, they suffered a mild anemia but maintained bone marrow activity, as the CHr values state (30.8 and 31.6 pg, resp.). RSf values in these patients were in the reference range of RSf, but the macrocytosis associated to CKD and hemodialysis treatment causes that 15% of the patients in this group had RSf values slightly over the reference range, 106.6 fL.

Diagnostic sensitivity, specificity, and efficiency of RSf were good when compared to a 28 pg value of CHr. In particular, a cutoff value of 91.1 fL for RSf showed the best diagnostic efficiency, with a sensitivity of 98.8% and a specificity of 89.6%.

This study shows a reasonable agreement between % Hypo and LHD% and their values showed the same trend in the different groups.

%Hypo values in patients undergoing therapy were near the threshold of iron deficient erythropoiesis 5% (ACD 4.1%, CKD 5.1%).

The LHD% values obtained in these groups of patients were statistically lower (ACD 7.3%, CKD 9.6%) than the iron deficient ones (29.6%, 27.3%) but, as all of them had a mild anemia, LHD% values in these patients were above the reference range 4.4%.

The optimal cutoff point for LHD% was 6.0%, which provided sensitivity 96.6%, specificity 83.2%, and area under curve 0.954, for iron deficiency detection, defined by %Hypo > 5%.

In this study, it has been stated that RSf and LHD% could be reliable parameters for the study of iron status and the amount of the supply available for erythropoiesis.

Iron metabolism is a dynamic process which cannot be defined by one test parameter only. The analysis of these new parameters can be performed simultaneously in the course of routine blood counts, with no incremental costs and no additional needs of more blood sampling. In conjunction with standard blood cell counts and iron, parameters could enable the diagnosis to be made rapidly and accurately.

The new parameters derived from Beckman-Coulter technology seem to be an acceptable alternative to CHr and %Hypo in the routine practice, with the same clinical meaning, but more prospective and longitudinal studies are needed in order to verify the results obtained, to determine their reliability for clinical purposes or whether the additional information provided could be used in managing the iron requirements of patients.

References

[1] I. Cavill and I. C. Macdougall, "Functional iron deficiency," *Blood*, vol. 82, no. 4, p. 137, 1993.

[2] S. Fishbane, L. J. Imbriano, E. A. Kowalski, and J. K. Maesaka, "The evaluation of iron status in patients receiving recombinant human erythropoietin," *Journal of the American Society of Nephrology*, vol. 7, pp. 654–657, 1996.

[3] A. Mast, "The clinical utility of peripheral blood tests in the diagnosis of iron deficiency anemia," *Bloodline*, vol. 1, pp. 7–9, 2001.

[4] D. Coyne, "Iron indices: what do they really mean?" *Kidney International*, vol. 69, no. 101, supplement, pp. S4–S8, 2006.

[5] I. C. Macdougall, I. Cavill, B. Hulme, et al., "Detection of functional iron deficiency during erythropoietin treatment: a new approach," *British Medical Journal*, vol. 304, no. 6821, pp. 225–226, 1992.

[6] J. F. Navarro and M. L. Macia, "Hypochromic red cells as an indicator of iron deficiency," *The Journal of Rheumatology*, vol. 24, no. 4, pp. 804–805, 1997.

[7] S. Fishbane, C. Galgano, R. C. Langley Jr., W. Canfield, and J. K. Maesaka, "Reticulocyte hemoglobin content in the evaluation of iron status of hemodialysis patients," *Kidney International*, vol. 52, no. 1, pp. 217–222, 1997.

[8] A. E. Mast, M. A. Blinder, Q. Lu, S. Flax, and D. J. Dietzen, "Clinical utility of the reticulocyte hemoglobin content in the diagnosis of iron deficiency," *Blood*, vol. 99, no. 4, pp. 1489–1491, 2002.

[9] C. Brugnara, "Iron deficiency and erythropoiesis: new diagnostic approaches," *Clinical Chemistry*, vol. 49, no. 10, pp. 1573–1578, 2003.

[10] I. C. Macdougall, "Merits of percentage hypochromic red cells as a marker of functional iron deficiency," *Nephrology Dialysis Transplantation*, vol. 13, no. 4, pp. 847–849, 1998.

[11] C. Bovy, A. Gothot, J.-M. Krzesinski, and Y. Beguin, "Mature erythrocyte indices: new markers of iron availability," *Haematologica*, vol. 90, no. 4, pp. 549–551, 2005.

[12] I. C. Macdougall, W. H. Horl, C. Jacobs, et al., "European best practice guidelines 6–8: assessing and optimizing iron stores," *Nephrology Dialysis Transplantation*, vol. 15, no. 4, pp. 20–32, 2000.

[13] S. Kotisaari, J. Romppanen, I. Penttila, and K. Punnonen, "The Advia 120 red blood cell and reticulocyte indices are useful in diagnosis of iron-deficiency anemia," *European Journal of Haematology*, vol. 68, no. 3, pp. 150–156, 2002.

[14] F. Locateli, P. Aljama, P. Barany, et al., "Revised European best practice guidelines for the management of anaemia in patients with chronic renal failure," *Nephrology Dialysis Transplantation*, vol. 19, supplement 2, pp. 1–47, 2004.

[15] M. Buttarello, V. Temporin, R. Ceravolo, G. Farina, and P. Burian, "The new reticulocyte parameter RET Y of the Sysmex XE 2100. Its use in the diagnosis and monitoring of post treatment sideropenic anemia," *American Journal of Clinical Pathology*, vol. 121, pp. 489–495, 2004.

[16] L. Thomas, S. Franck, M. Messinger, J. Linssen, M. Thome, and C. Thomas, "Reticulocyte hemoglobin measurement—comparison of two methods in the diagnosis of iron-restricted erythropoiesis," *Clinical Chemistry and Laboratory Medicine*, vol. 43, no. 11, pp. 1193–1202, 2005.

[17] A. E. Mast, M. A. Blinder, and D. J. Dietzen, "Reticulocyte hemoglobin content," *American Journal of Hematology*, vol. 83, no. 4, pp. 307–310, 2008.

[18] E. Urrechaga, L. Borque, and J. F. Escanero, "Potential utility of the new sysmex XE 5000 red blood cell extended parameters in the study of disorders of iron metabolism," *Clinical Chemistry and Laboratory Medicine*, vol. 47, no. 11, pp. 1411–1416, 2009.

[19] E. Urrechaga, "Clinical utility of the new beckman-coulter parameter red blood cell size factor in the study of erithropoiesis," *International Journal of Laboratory Hematology*, vol. 31, no. 6, pp. 623–629, 2009.

[20] E. Urrechaga, "The new mature red cell parameter, low haemoglobin density of the Beckman-Coulter LH750: clinical utility in the diagnosis of iron deficiency," *International Journal of Laboratory Hematology*, vol. 32, no. 1, part 1, pp. e144–e150, 2010.

[21] "NKF-K/DOQI clinical practice guidelines and clinical practice recommendations for anemia in chronic kidney disease in adults," *American Journal of Kidney Diseases*, vol. 47, no. 5, supplement 3, pp. S11–S145, 2006.

[22] S. Fishbane, W. Shapiro, P. Dutka, O. F. Valenzuela, and J. Faubert, "A randomized trial of iron deficiency testing strategies in hemodialysis patients," *Kidney International*, vol. 60, no. 6, pp. 2406–2411, 2001.

[23] A. Besarab, "Evaluating iron sufficiency: a clearer view," *Kidney International*, vol. 60, no. 6, pp. 2412–2414, 2001.

[24] C. Brugnara, "A hematologic "gold standard" for iron-deficient states?" *Clinical Chemistry*, vol. 48, no. 7, pp. 981–982, 2002.

[25] C. Brugnara, M. R. Laufer, A. J. Friedman, K. Bridges, and O. Platt, "Reticulocyte hemoglobin content (CHr): early indicator of iron deficiency and response to therapy," *Blood*, vol. 83, no. 10, pp. 3100–3101, 1994.

[26] F. Valderrabano, W. H. Horl, C. Jacobs, et al., "European best practice guidelines 1–4: evaluating anaemia and initiating treatment," *Nephrology Dialysis Transplantation*, vol. 15, no. 4, pp. 8–14, 2000.

[27] C. Brugnara, M. R. Laufer, A. J. Friedman, and O. Platt, "Reticulocyte hemoglobin content (CHr): early indicator of iron deficiency and response to therapy," *Blood*, vol. 82, A93, 1993.

[28] C. Thomas and L. Thomas, "Biochemical markers and hematologic indices in the diagnosis of functional iron deficiency," *Clinical Chemistry*, vol. 48, no. 7, pp. 1066–1076, 2002.

[29] U. Arndt, J. P. Kaltwasser, R. Gottschalk, D. Hoelzer, and B. Möller, "Correction of iron-deficient erythropoiesis in the treatment of anemia of chronic disease with recombinant human erythropoietin," *Annals of Hematology*, vol. 84, no. 3, pp. 159–166, 2005.

[30] C. Bovy, A. Gothot, P. Delanaye, X. Warling, J.-M. Krzesinski, and Y. Beguin, "Mature erythrocyte parameters as new markers of functional iron deficiency in haemodialysis: sensitivity and specificity," *Nephrology Dialysis Transplantation*, vol. 22, no. 4, pp. 1156–1162, 2007.

14

Iron Deficiency Anemia: Focus on Infectious Diseases in Lesser Developed Countries

Julia G. Shaw[1, 2] and Jennifer F. Friedman[2, 3]

[1] Public Health Program, Division of Biology and Medicine, Brown University, Providence, RI 02912, USA
[2] Lifespan Hospital Center for International Health Research, 55 Claverick Street, Suite 100, Providence, RI 02903, USA
[3] Warren Alpert School of Medicine, Brown University, Providence, RI 02912, USA

Correspondence should be addressed to Jennifer F. Friedman, jennifer_friedman@brown.edu

Academic Editor: Ajit C. Gorakshakar

Iron deficiency anemia is thought to affect the health of more than one billion people worldwide, with the greatest burden of disease experienced in lesser developed countries, particularly women of reproductive age and children. This greater disease burden is due to both nutritional and infectious etiologies. Individuals in lesser developed countries have diets that are much lower in iron, less access to multivitamins for young children and pregnant women, and increased rates of fertility which increase demands for iron through the life course. Infectious diseases, particularly parasitic diseases, also lead to both extracorporeal iron loss and anemia of inflammation, which decreases bioavailability of iron to host tissues. This paper will address the unique etiologies and consequences of both iron deficiency anemia and the alterations in iron absorption and distribution seen in the context of anemia of inflammation. Implications for diagnosis and treatment in this unique context will also be discussed.

1. Introduction

Anemia is a worldwide public health problem, with global prevalence estimated at 24.8% (95% CI: 22.9–26.7). The majority of the global disease burden of anemia is shouldered by the developing world, with prevalence in Africa and South East Asia as high as two thirds among children under five, and nearly half among women [1]. The World Health Organization (WHO) has classified anemia as a severe public health problem (prevalence $\geq 40\%$) for children under five in 69 countries, and for pregnant women in 68 countries [1]. The causes of anemia in the developing world are multifactorial and include nutritional deficiencies, extra-corporal blood loss, higher prevalence of hemoglobinopathies, and inflammation. These etiologies often coexist and are difficult to distinguish due to limited diagnostic capabilities in resource-poor settings. High fertility rates also contribute to the burden of anemia among pregnant women and infants, with short interbirth intervals placing women at higher risk for iron deficiency anemia with concomitant increased risk of iron deficiency for the newborn [2–4]. This papaer will focus primarily on the etiology of iron deficiency anemia in the context of infectious diseases endemic in lesser developed countries.

The WHO notes that anemia is often used as an inappropriate proxy for iron deficiency, given the coexistence of many etiologies [5]. Recent studies demonstrate that the role of anemia of inflammation in the pathogenesis of anemia in the developing world is underestimated [6], as it plays a central role in the context of infectious diseases prevalent in these regions [7–14]. Though both iron deficiency anemia and anemia of inflammation ultimately lead to host tissue iron insufficiency, it is likely that health outcomes related to each differ. Improved diagnostic tools to define etiology, including multiple concurrent etiologies, are an important first step to understanding how different causes of anemia adversely impact health outcomes. Due to recent advances in our understanding of the etiology of anemia of inflammation, and specifically the role of hepcidin in altering iron metabolism, improvements in diagnostic tools to distinguish iron deficiency anemia and anemia of inflammation will be increasingly possible.

2. Iron Deficiency in the Developing World

Iron deficiency is thought to affect the health of more than one billion people worldwide [15]. The WHO/World Bank has ranked iron deficiency anemia as the third leading cause of Disability Adjusted Life Years (DALY's) lost for females of childbearing age [16], and among the top 10 disease burdens for men in this age group (15–44 years) [16]. Among infants, iron deficiency is the most common micronutrient deficiency and cause of anemia worldwide [17, 18]. Young children and women in lesser-developed countries (LDCs) are most significantly affected by iron deficiency anemia [15], which has numerous causes specific to the developing world including blood loss due to poor dietary iron intake, high fertility rates, and fecal iron loss in the context of parasitic infections such as hookworm, schistosomiasis, and trichuriasis.

Iron deficiency occurs at a higher prevalence among women than among their male counterparts due to menstrual iron losses and the extreme iron demands of pregnancy (approximately two times those of a nonpregnant state). The growing fetus requires a large supply of iron, which is taken up from maternal blood via transferrin-receptor mediated endocytosis [19]. Once maternal iron stores are depleted, she becomes anemic and transfer of iron to the developing fetus may be compromised [2, 20]. In utero acquisition of iron determines newborn iron stores [21] and remains associated with iron status at 9 [22] and 24 months of age [23]. Thus, infants who are born with insufficient iron stores are unlikely to reacquire adequate iron supplies, particularly in LDCs where maternal breast milk may contain inadequate iron and weaning foods are notoriously iron poor. This risk persists, and even increases, for young children in LDCs where diets are often poor in bio-available iron, particularly in areas where iron fortification programs are not in effect. Young children remain a particularly vulnerable group due to the increased iron requirements during periods of rapid growth, which are almost 10 times higher per kilogram of body weight than that of an adult male.

One of the major consequences of iron deficiency for infant health is cognitive impairment, as infancy is a key period for brain growth and development, and iron uptake into the brain is maximal during this period [24]. Iron is required for several important brain functions including myelination of nerve fibers, energy metabolism, and acting as a cofactor for a number of enzymes involved in neurotransmitter synthesis [21, 25]. Many well-designed studies conducted in LDCs among infants and young children have demonstrated that iron supplementation leads to improvements in specific domains of cognition [26, 27]. Domains that are more amenable to iron therapy include language and motor development [26]. Of note, some studies have found that the effect of treatment is modified by baseline characteristics, such that children with poorer nutritional or hemoglobin status at baseline are more likely to benefit [28]. Further, many studies have demonstrated impairment of development even at mild or moderate degrees of iron deficiency anemia [26, 27, 29, 30]. It should be noted, however, that a number of randomized controlled trials have demonstrated no benefit of iron therapy on cognitive performance. This may be due to short periods of followup, capture of domains of cognition that may not be as sensitive to iron insufficiency, or examination of domains of cognition that may be related to iron insufficiency, but are no longer "plastic" or amenable to treatment [31].

Iron deficiency is also thought to cause decreased work capacity [32]. This has more significant implications for LDCs, where a greater proportion of a nation's gross national product is related to manual labor. In a study based in China, migrant schoolchildren with severe iron deficiency were found to have decreased aerobic capacity and habitual physical activity [33]. In addition, studies have been conducted examining the relationship between treatment for helminth infections and physical work capacity. Studies have demonstrated increased work capacity following treatment for both schistosomiasis and hookworm [34, 35]. Though much of this benefit is likely due to improvements in iron status with treatment, it should be noted that improved work capacity in these contexts might also be due to improved nutritional status and reduction in parasite-related symptomatology.

3. Infectious Diseases and Iron Deficiency

3.1. Hookworm. Hookworm infection is one of the most important parasitic diseases in humans in terms of Disability Adjusted Life Years (DALYs) lost, outranking schistosomiasis, African trypanosomiasis, Chagas disease, and leprosy [36, 37]. Much of the burden of hookworm is due to extra-corporeal iron loss [38], and interventions to treat hookworm infection have demonstrated significant improvements in hemoglobin [39]. Iron-deficiency anemia resulting from chronic intestinal blood loss due to hookworm infection often causes long-term morbidity [40, 41]. Blood loss is caused predominantly by parasite release of coagulases, causing ongoing blood loss in the stool, rather than actual blood consumption by the parasite. For example, *A. duodenale* is estimated to cause up to 0.25 mL of blood loss per worm per day [41]. A hookworm burden of 40–160 worms (depending on the iron status of the host) is associated with iron deficiency anemia [42]. Women of childbearing age, pregnant women, and young children are at greatest risk for hookworm-associated iron deficiency anemia due to low iron stores resulting from diets insufficient to meet demands.

The development of hookworm-related iron deficiency anemia depends on the level of an individual's iron stores, the intensity of infection, and the infecting species as *A. duodenale* causes a greater blood loss than *N. americanus*. A study conducted in Tanzania examined 525 school-age children, comparing the degree of anemia and iron deficiency among children infected with each species. It was found that among children with *N. americanus*, anemia was prevalent in 60.5% and iron deficiency anemia in 33.1%. Among children infected with *A. duodenale*, prevalence was 80.55% and 58.9%, respectively, suggesting that *A. duodenale* is associated with a greater burden of iron deficiency [40].

Hookworm is unique among helminths in that infection intensities tend to peak in adulthood [43]. Rather than peaking in childhood and adolescence and then declining as is the case of many other parasitic infections, the intensity of hookworm infection follows a steady rise during childhood and does not reach a peak or plateau until adulthood [42]. A study conducted in Hainan Province, China, which examined risk factors associated with *N. americanus* in people 50 years of age and older, found that age still accounted for 27% of the variation in the intensity of hookworm infection [44]. This is likely due to the fact that neither age- nor exposure-related immunity develops in the majority of hookworm-infected people [45]. This further supports the concern that hookworm infection may continue to affect work capacity among the most productive members of society.

The association between hookworm infection intensity and increasing age has serious implications for women of reproductive age who are already at risk for anemia due to low iron stores related to poor dietary intake, menstrual blood loss, and pregnancy. Hookworm is likely a major contributor to the adverse birth outcomes associated with iron deficiency anemia, most notably low birth weight [46]. In a randomized, double blind placebo controlled trial among pregnant women in Sri Lanka, the proportions of stillbirths and perinatal deaths were significantly lower in the group treated with mebendazole compared to the control group (1.9 versus 3.3%, 0.55 (95% CI 0.4–0.77)), as was the proportion of low-birthweight babies (1.1 versus 2.3%, 0.47 (95% CI 0.32–0.71)). Of note, the authors found a slight increase in the odds for major congenital defects among the women who received mebendazole, "contrary to medical advice," during the first trimester only (odds ratio 1.66 (0.1–3.56), $P = .23$). In a separate study conducted in Uganda, where the prevalence of maternal anemia was 40% at enrollment, investigators found no overall effect of albendazole on maternal anemia or birthweight, but a suggestion of benefit for anemia among women with moderate to heavy intensities of hookworm infection at baseline (OR 0.45; 95% CI, 0.21–0.98; $P = .15$ for interaction).

There has been significant debate regarding the role of soil-transmitted helminths (STH), which include hookworm, ascaris, and trichuris, in cognitive impairment. Though other mechanisms have been discussed [47], iron deficiency is consistently proposed as a primary mechanism leading to cognitive impairment. Many factors have contributed to conflicting results. Of note, early cross-sectional studies that demonstrated relationships between soil-transmitted helminths (STH) and cognitive function have been criticized for lack of control for important confounders such as SES [47]. While some cross-sectional studies that have adjusted for potential confounders have found a relationship between cognitive performance and STH infection [48], other studies have not. Further, randomized controlled trials examining the effects of treatment for STH have had differing results [28, 49]. A recent meta-analysis addressing the topic of treatment for STH and cognitive outcomes concluded that a relationship between antihelmintic treatment and improved cognitive performance could not be determined [50]. This papaer noted that the quality of even the randomized controlled trials was generally poor. This meta-analysis was highly controversial, with many ensuing published and unpublished differences of opinion [51–54]. One major critique was that baseline infection status of the children was not determined in the majority of trials included, such that both infected and uninfected children were randomized and treated. This "mass treatment" approach leads to an underestimation of the effect of treatment among those who are infected with STHs. In fact, one critique noted that among the studies that were able to stratify analyses by baseline infection status, a treatment effect was seen [49]. In addition, studies were conducted in parts of the world with varying intensities of each STH and with drugs that have varying effect on each STH. In addition, short follow-up periods in the context of randomized controlled trials may have also obscured the ability to capture improvements, as children likely need to recover iron stores before significant gains can be appreciated. Finally, children with long-standing helminth infections may develop deficits in the actual ability to learn and process new information, which may take long periods of time to develop or reacquire. Conclusions from this meta-analysis are thus limited to the impact of a mass treatment approach, which may not lead to significant improvements in cognitive performance in a target population with varying intensities of infection. It is likely, however, that among children who are infected, particarly at higher intensities of infection, treatment does lead to improvement in specific areas of cognitive function [49]. Despite these controversies, expected improvements in cognitive and school performance have been among the key reasons cited in recent initiatives for widespread, regular antihelmintic treatment of school children in endemic areas [42, 55].

4. Schistosomiasis: Iron Deficiency Anemia and Anemia of Inflammation

A number of cross-sectional studies have examined the relationship between the three most prevalent human schistosomes and anemia [8, 56–62]. However, due to the numerous nutritional deficiencies and infectious diseases that co-exist with schistosome infections, which are also related to increased risk for anemia, careful control for confounding variables or use of an experimental design is necessary to quantify this association. Recent cross-sectional studies have better adjusted for potential confounders, allowing for an improved estimation of the true relationship between schistosomiasis and anemia [59–61]. These recent studies have observed an inverse relationship between *S. japonicum* intensity of infection [60, 61] and hemoglobin, and *S. haematobium* infection and risk of anemia among young children and adolescents [59].

Many randomized controlled trials have found that therapy with praziquantel and albendazole [63–65] or metrifonate [66, 67], which is efficacious against schistosome and hookworm infections, leads to improvements in hemoglobin. The use of combination therapy makes inferences regarding the schistosomiasis-attributable benefit of treatment for anemia difficult, though most authors suggest that a portion of observed improvement in hemoglobin was likely due to reduced schistosome burden.

Only two randomized controlled trials have been conducted utilizing monotherapy with a drug efficacious predominantly against schistosomes [68, 69]. One study conducted in an *S. japonicum* endemic village in Leyte, the Philippines demonstrated significant differences in hemoglobin six months after therapy between children in the intervention and control arms. The magnitude of effect was approximately 1.1 g/dL. Of note, males experienced a greater increase in hemoglobin with treatment than did females. The experimental design of this study and the "isolation" of schistosomiasis support a role for *S. japonicum* in the etiology of anemia in regions of the developing world where it is endemic. Another randomized controlled trial examined praziquantel treatment alone for *S. haematobium*, and found no effect of treatment on hemoglobin [68]. This is unlikely to be due to lack of statistical power ($N = 104$ in placebo and 105 in praziquantel), low prevalence of anemia (70%), or inadequate followup (eight months). However, it is possible that this null finding was due to the exclusion of children with high intensity infections.

4.1. Anemia of Inflammation.

Anemia of inflammation must be mentioned in the context of iron status in LDCs, as this process leads to both decreased iron absorption and sequestration of iron into storage forms, rendering it less available to host tissues. Further, the etiology of anemia (iron deficiency anemia or anemia of inflammation, or both) is difficult to determine in the developing world context where assays to determine biomarkers of iron status are not available. Anemia of inflammation is characterized by decreased red blood cell production through a series of mechanisms, mediated in part by proinflammatory cytokines, particularly TNF-alpha and IL-6. These mechanisms include suppression of the normal response of bone marrow to erythropoietin, decreased synthesis of erythropoietin, dyserythropoiesis (disturbances of bone marrow cellular division), and alterations in iron metabolism such that iron is sequestered into storage forms, such as ferritin, making it less bio-available [70].

Recently, major advances have been made in our understanding of anemia of inflammation [71]. In response to inflammation, in particular IL-6, hepcidin is synthesized [72]. This protein has pleiotropic effects on iron metabolism. Hepcidin causes sequestration of iron from bio-available forms to storage forms, as well as decreased intestinal absorption of iron [73, 74]. Both processes are due to the binding of hepcidin to ferroportin, the only iron egress protein in humans. Hepcidin-ferroportin binding causes the internalization and degradation of ferroportin [75], thus trapping iron inside cells. This results in the inability to absorb iron from the gut and to mobilize iron from reticuloendothelial macrophages [73, 76, 77]. In the proximal small intestine, iron is trapped in intestinal epithelial cells and lost during normal cell turnover [74, 78]. Decreased absorption and iron sequestration leads to decreased iron bio-availability to meet needs such as erythropoeisis. This is of great public health

importance given that anemia of inflammation contributes to, or is the primary cause of, anemia in the context of many common infectious diseases in LDCs including malaria, HIV, schistosomiasis, tuberculosis, and others [7, 14, 62, 79, 80].

4.2. HIV.

While HIV is not a significant cause of iron deficiency anemia, its role as a major cause of anemia in LDCs warrants special mention due to the "functional" iron deficiency caused by HIV-related anemia of inflammation. Anemia is highly prevalent among people with HIV-infection, and has been identified as a marker for disease progression and associated with decreased survival [3, 81–83]. There is significant evidence to support anemia of inflammation as the primary cause of anemia in the context of HIV infection [3]. A study conducted among infants in Uganda found the prevalence of IDA (Hb < 11.0 g/dL and ferritin < 12 g/L) to be approximately equal among HIV-infected and uninfected infants, with prevalence of any anemia significantly higher in the HIV-infected group than the uninfected group (90.9% and 76.9%, resp.). The authors attribute the excess anemia among HIV-infected infants to anemia of inflammation [3, 84]. Another study conducted among antiretroviral-naïve HIV-infected children in South Africa found that prevalence of anemia increased with HIV disease stage from 42% for children with no evidence of immunosuppression to 85% for children with severe immunosuppression. Iron deficiency anemia was present in only 17% of the children, further supporting the primary role of anemia of inflammation in the pathogenesis anemia in the context of HIV infection [3, 85].

5. Trichuris

The prevalence of infection with *T. trichiura* in the developing world is high, approaching 95% in areas of endemicity and affecting an estimated 1049 million people [86]. Although low-intensity infections with *T. trichiura* appear to be asymptomatic, high-intensity infections and Trichuris Dysentery Syndrome (TDS) are associated with growth stunting and anemia [87, 88]. Potential mechanisms of trichuris-related anemia include worm consumption of blood in the context of heavy infections, colonic lesions with associated bleeding, or chronic reduction in food and micronutrient intake due to the anorexia inducing effects of TNF-alpha released in response to infection [86, 89]. Of note, one study assessing occult blood loss with *T. trichiura* found that trichuriasis does not lead to significant occult gastrointestinal bleeding in the absence of TDS [90].

6. Bacterial Dysentery Syndromes

Occult blood loss due to Shigellosis or Enteroinvasive *Escherichia coli* dysentery may contribute to iron deficiency anemia among infants and children in areas of the developing world where these pathogens cause frequent childhood illness. Absolute blood loss due to dysentery or its contribution to IDA have not been well quantified.

7. *Helicobacter pylori*

The greatest prevalence of *H. pylori* is in LDCs, where the majority of infections are acquired during early childhood [91, 92]. *H. pylori* neutralizes and decreases secretion of gastric acid resulting in hypochlorhydria, and causes chronic inflammation of the gastrointestinal tract. Studies conducted among both adults and children have implicated *H. pylori* as a cause of iron deficiency anemia [92–97]. It is hypothesized that *H. pylori*-associated iron deficiency anemia is caused by both compromised absorption of bioavailable iron in the context of hypochlorhydria, and the competing iron demands of *H. pylori* and the host [92, 98, 99].

8. Malaria

Malaria is a major contributor to anemia in the developing world. Though the primary cause of anemia in the context of malaria is hemolytic, studies have demonstrated that anemia of inflammation plays an important role as well by inducing changes in iron absorption and distribution [14, 100]. Both clinical and asymptomatic malaria have been associated with anemia of inflammation. In a study in Indonesia, de Mast et al. found that asymptomatic children with *P. falciparum* or *P. vivax* parasitemia had significantly lower hemoglobin concentrations than aparasitemic controls (12.6 and 12.2 g/dL versus 14.4 g/dL; $P < .01$), as well as significantly higher serum hepcidin concentrations (5.2 and 5.6 nM versus 3.1 nM; $P < .05$) [100]. These results support the concept that prolonged sequestration of iron into storage forms due to inflammation caused by malaria parasitemia is likely a major cause of anemia in the developing world.

Exceptionally high rates of maternal morbidity and mortality are a major concern in the developing world, particularly in sub-Saharan Africa [101]. Much of this excess morbidity and mortality is attributable to malaria [102, 103]. Risk of malarial infection is especially high in HIV-infected individuals [104]. Studies have shown that HIV infection contributes to the burden of malarial anemia by increasing risk for parasitemia, severe anemia, and treatment failure [3]. Women are more susceptible to *P. falciparum* malaria during pregnancy, and the risk of disease and death is high for both the mother and her fetus. In areas of stable malaria transmission, an estimated one in four women has evidence of malarial infection at the time of delivery [105]. This underestimates the burden throughout gestation as it is ascertained only at delivery and does not take into account effects of infections preceding delivery [103]. In stable transmission areas, severe maternal anemia and low birth weight are frequent sequelae and account for an enormous loss of life [106, 107]. To address this, WHO recommends provision of intermittent prophylactic treatment in pregnancy (IPTp) to reduce the risk of pregnancy malaria and related in malaria-endemic regions. IPTp entails provision of sulfadoxine-pyrimethamine (SP) during the second and third trimester [107]. Early studies found that SP-IPTp significantly reduced the frequency of both placental and peripheral parasitemia [108–110], increased maternal hemoglobin levels, and reduced the prevalence of moderate to severe anemia [108, 111]. Approximately one in four cases of severe maternal anemia may be prevented with adequate prevention of malaria during pregnancy [112]. There is growing concern, however, with respect to malaria resistance to SP and the efficacy of this regimen [113]. New studies are underway to evaluate the safety and efficacy of newer antimalarial drugs in pregnancy.

Treatment for malaria and anemia in LDCs is further complicated by concerns that provision of iron in malaria endemic regions may increase the risk for malaria-related morbidity and mortality [114–116]. Studies in Tanzania found that pregnant women who were iron-replete versus iron-deficient at delivery were three times more likely to have placental parasitemia [114, 117]. In addition, among iron-replete mothers, placental malaria led to an increased risk of anemia among newborns [117]. The deleterious interaction between iron and malaria has also been demonstrated among children. Iron plus folate supplementation given during a recent randomized, placebo-controlled trial in a high *P. falciparum* transmission area of Zanzibar resulted in a 15% increase in all cause mortality [116]. Enhanced malarial morbidity was concentrated in children who were iron-replete at baseline. Children receiving iron and folate suffered 16% ($P = .02$) greater risk of clinical malaria and a 70% greater risk ($P = .02$) of cerebral malaria. In a separate study in Kenya, clinical malaria was significantly less frequent among iron-deficient children [118]. In Papua New Guinea, iron supplementation increased the prevalence of parasitemia and splenomegaly among infants [119]. Iron supplementation did not, however, increase the risk of malaria among children under intensive health surveillance in Kenya [120]. Taken together, these findings suggest that routine supplementation with iron may place populations in malaria endemic settings at increased risk for malaria-specific morbidity and mortality [116]. Effects of baseline iron status, acquired immunity, or intensity of health surveillance could explain some of the variability in results. Further studies are warranted and underway to more clearly evaluate the balance of risks and benefits and potential effect modifiers of this risk for specific populations.

9. Iron Supplementation in Pregnancy

Despite WHO recommendations to provide prenatal vitamins with iron [121], studies do not support an association between iron interventions and birth outcomes [122, 123]. A recent Cochrane review of this topic reaffirmed this conclusion [124], and a separate earlier review concluded that "the currently available evidence from studies with designs appropriate to establish a causal relationship is insufficient to support or reject the practice (prenatal iron supplementation) for the specific purposes of raising birth weight or lowering the rate of preterm birth" [122]. This is further supported by animal data including a primate study of iron supplementation during pregnancy [125]. In that study using Rhesus monkeys, neonatal neurobehavioral test scores, number of stillbirths, birth weight, and maternal weight gain were not significantly different between dams fed a diet containing iron (100 μg Fe/g) and those monkeys deprived of iron ($<10\,\mu$g Fe/g). Further, maternal monkeys receiving the iron-replete diet did differ significantly in hematocrit, MCV, transferrin saturation, serum ferritin, and serum iron compared to those receiving an iron-deplete diet. However, newborn monkeys did have higher hemoglobin values with maternal supplementation.

Ongoing discrepancies across studies with respect to benefits of iron supplementation during pregnancy are likely due to the underrecognized role of anemia of inflammation in the developing world. This is highlighted by a recent study that examined a wide range of nutritional and nonnutritional causes of anemia in pregnancy in Malawi, including bone marrow aspiration [6]. Investigators found that CRP concentrations were elevated in 54% of anemic pregnant women with *no nutritional deficiencies* and in 73.5% of the anemic women who were iron-replete by bone marrow assessment. This study demonstrates the important role played by anemia of inflammation in the pathogenesis of anemia in pregnancy. In the context of anemia of inflammation, the absorption of prenatal iron supplements will be limited and absorbed iron will be shunted from bio-available forms to storage forms, limiting maternal use and potentially inhibiting delivery of iron to the fetus. The possible exacerbation of malaria-related morbidity in pregnancy associated with provision of prenatal iron may also explain disparate findings, if iron provision in this context is increasing malarial anemia [114, 117].

Other benefits of prenatal iron supplementation have been identified, however. In particular, many studies have demonstrated improvements in maternal hemoglobin with prenatal iron supplementation [123]. This may be of greater significance in the developing world where there is a higher prevalence of moderate to severe iron deficiency anemia with consequent greater risk of perinatal mortality related to postpartum hemorrhage. Prenatal iron supplementation may also have beneficial effects for the newborn. Preziozi et al. found that newborn iron status is dependent on maternal iron status during pregnancy and that children born to iron-treated mothers have higher serum ferritin, greater body length, and increased Apgar scores in comparison to those treated with placebo [126]. Other studies conducted in LDCs have shown that concentrations of hemoglobin, iron, and ferritin are significantly lower in the cord blood newborns of anemic mothers, with linear relationships demonstrated with maternal hemoglobin and ferritin levels [2].

9.1. Diagnosis and Treatment. Despite the enormous global burden of disease due to anemia and the multiple causes of anemia in LDCs, diagnostic tests to distinguish primary etiologies are limited, particulary in these cost-constrained settings. Given iron deficiency anemia (due to dietary insufficiency and infectious diseases) and anemia of inflammation are the two leading causes of anemia in LDCs, and interventions to address these differ, diagnostic tools to differentiate the two are of paramount importance.

Until recently, there has been a lack of valid biomarkers to distinguish the causes of anemia. Hemoglobin and ferritin have proven to be poor diagnostic tools [127], largely due to the fact that ferritin is decreased in the context of iron deficiency, but increased in the context of anemia of inflammation as iron is sequestered in storage forms. The emergence of hepcidin as a biomarker for anemia of inflammation may help to fill this diagnostic gap, and assist in effectively selecting individuals who will benefit most from iron therapy [100]. Treatment of anemia of inflammation requires diagnosis and treatment of the underlying causes of inflammation, highlighting the importance of treatment programs for HIV, helminth infections and malaria (both clinical and subclinical) in curbing anemia in the LDCs.

References

[1] World Health Organization, *Worldwide Prevalence of Anaemia 1993–2005*, World Health Organization, Geneva, Switzerland, 2008.

[2] A. Kumar, A. K. Rai, S. Basu, D. Dash, and J. S. Singh, "Cord blood and breast milk iron status in maternal anemia," *Pediatrics*, vol. 121, no. 3, pp. e673–e677, 2008.

[3] K. Tolentino and J. F. Friedman, "An update on anemia in less developed countries," *American Journal of Tropical Medicine and Hygiene*, vol. 77, no. 1, pp. 44–51, 2007.

[4] T. Hokama, S. Takenaka, K. Hirayama et al., "Iron status of newborns born to iron deficient anaemic mothers," *Journal of Tropical Pediatrics*, vol. 42, no. 2, pp. 75–77, 1996.

[5] WHO, UNICEF, and University U, *Iron Deficiency Anaemia Assessment, Prevention and Control: A Guide for Programme Managers*, World Health Organization, Geneva, Switzerland, 2001.

[6] N. R. Van Den Broek and E. A. Letsky, "Etiology of anemia in pregnancy in south Malawi," *American Journal of Clinical Nutrition*, vol. 72, no. 1, pp. 247S–256S, 2000.

[7] J. F. Friedman, P. Mital, H. K. Kanzaria, G. R. Olds, and J. D. Kurtis, "Schistosomiasis and pregnancy," *Trends in Parasitology*, vol. 23, no. 4, pp. 159–164, 2007.

[8] T. Leenstra, L. P. Acosta, G. C. Langdon et al., "Schistosomiasis japonica, anemia, and iron status in children, adolescents, and young adults in Leyte, Philippines," *American Journal of Clinical Nutrition*, vol. 83, no. 2, pp. 371–379, 2006.

[9] T. Leenstra, H. M. Coutinho, L. P. Acosta et al., "Schistosoma japonicum reinfection after praziquantel treatment causes anemia associated with inflammation," *Infection and Immunity*, vol. 74, no. 11, pp. 6398–6407, 2006.

[10] A. L. Richards, "Tumour necrosis factor and associated cytokines in the host's response to malaria," *International Journal for Parasitology*, vol. 27, no. 10, pp. 1251–1263, 1997.

[11] P. Kern, C. J. Hemmer, H. Gallati et al., "Soluble tumor necrosis factor receptors correlate with parasitemia and disease severity in human malaria," *Journal of Infectious Diseases*, vol. 166, no. 4, pp. 930–934, 1992.

[12] N. Meda, B. Dao, and A. Ouangré, "HIV, maternal anemia and perinatal intervention using zidovudine," *International Journal of Gynecology and Obstetrics*, vol. 61, no. 1, pp. 65–66, 1998.

[13] R. Ramon, D. Sawadogo, F. S. Koko et al., "Haematological characteristics and HIV status of pregnant women in Abidjan, Cote d'Ivoire, 1995-96," *Transactions of the Royal Society of Tropical Medicine and Hygiene*, vol. 93, no. 4, pp. 419–422, 1999.

[14] C. Menendez, A. F. Fleming, and P. L. Alonso, "Malaria-related anaemia," *Parasitology Today*, vol. 16, no. 11, pp. 469–476, 2000.

[15] F. Trowbridge and R. Martorell, "Forging effective strategies to combat iron deficiency. Summary and recommendations," *Journal of Nutrition*, vol. 132, no. 4, pp. 875S–879S, 2002.

[16] R. Yip, "Prevention and control of iron deficiency: policy and strategy issues," *Journal of Nutrition*, vol. 132, no. 4, pp. 802S–805S, 2002.

[17] S. J. Fomon, S. E. Nelson, and E. E. Ziegler, "Retention of iron by infants," *Annual Review of Nutrition*, vol. 20, pp. 273–290, 2000.

[18] N. Kretchmer, J. L. Beard, and S. Carlson, "The role of nutrition in the development of normal cognition," *American Journal of Clinical Nutrition*, vol. 63, no. 6, pp. 997S–1001S, 1996.

[19] J. E. Levy, O. Jin, Y. Fujiwara, F. Kuo, and N. C. Andrews, "Transferrin receptor is necessary for development of erythrocytes and the nervous system," *Nature Genetics*, vol. 21, no. 4, pp. 396–399, 1999.

[20] L. Gambling, R. Danzeisen, C. Fosset et al., "Iron and copper interactions in development and the effect on pregnancy outcome," *Journal of Nutrition*, vol. 133, no. 5, pp. 1554S–1556S, 2003.

[21] R. Rao and M. K. Georgieff, "Neonatal iron nutrition," *Seminars in Neonatology*, vol. 6, no. 5, pp. 425–435, 2001.

[22] M. K. Georgieff, S. W. Wewerka, C. A. Nelson, and R. A. DeRegnier, "Iron status at 9 months of infants with low iron stores at birth," *Journal of Pediatrics*, vol. 141, no. 3, pp. 405–409, 2002.

[23] G. Hay, B. Sandstad, A. Whitelaw, and B. Borch-Iohnsen, "Iron status in a group of Norwegian children aged 6-24 months," *Acta Paediatrica, International Journal of Paediatrics*, vol. 93, no. 5, pp. 592–598, 2004.

[24] E. M. Taylor and E. H. Morgan, "Developmental changes in transferrin and iron uptake by the brain in the rat," *Developmental Brain Research*, vol. 55, no. 1, pp. 35–42, 1990.

[25] J. L. Beard, "Iron biology in immune function, muscle metabolism and neuronal functioning," *Journal of Nutrition*, vol. 131, no. 2, pp. 568S–580S, 2001.

[26] B. Lozoff, I. De Andraca, M. Castillo, J. B. Smith, T. Walter, and P. Pino, "Behavioral and developmental effects of preventing iron-deficiency anemia in healthy full-term infants," *Pediatrics*, vol. 112, no. 4, pp. 846–854, 2003.

[27] M. E. K. Moffatt, S. Longstaffe, J. Besant, and C. Dureski, "Prevention of iron deficiency and psychomotor decline in high-risk infants through use of iron-fortified infant formula: a randomized clinical trial," *Journal of Pediatrics*, vol. 125, no. 4, pp. 527–534, 1994.

[28] R. J. Stoltzfus, J. D. Kvalsvig, H. M. Chwaya et al., "Effects of iron supplementation and anthelmintic treatment on motor and language development of preschool children in Zanzibar: double blind, placebo controlled study," *BMJ*, vol. 323, no. 7326, pp. 1389–1393, 2001.

[29] T. Lind, BO. Lönnerdal, H. Stenlund et al., "A community-based randomized controlled trial of iron and zinc supplementation in Indonesian infants: effects on growth and development," *American Journal of Clinical Nutrition*, vol. 80, no. 3, pp. 729–736, 2004.

[30] J. Williams, A. Wolff, A. Daly, A. MacDonald, A. Aukett, and I. W. Booth, "Iron supplemented formula milk related to reduction in psychomotor decline in infants from inner city areas: randomised study," *BMJ*, vol. 318, no. 7185, pp. 693–698, 1999.

[31] S. Grantham-McGregor and C. Ani, "A review of studies on the effect of iron deficiency on cognitive development in children," *Journal of Nutrition*, vol. 131, no. 2, pp. 649S–668S, 2001.

[32] J. D. Haas and T. Brownlie IV, "Iron deficiency and reduced work capacity: a critical review of the research to determine a causal relationship," *Journal of Nutrition*, vol. 131, no. 2, pp. 676S–690S, 2001.

[33] J. Wang, J. S. Huo, J. Sun, and Z. X. Ning, "Physical performance of migrant schoolchildren with marginal and severe iron deficiency in the suburbs of Beijing," *Biomedical and Environmental Sciences*, vol. 22, no. 4, pp. 333–339, 2009.

[34] J. Ndamba, N. Makaza, M. Munjoma, E. Gomo, and K. C. Kaondera, "The physical fitness and work performance of agricultural workers infected with Schistosoma mansoni in Zimbabwe," *Annals of Tropical Medicine and Parasitology*, vol. 87, no. 6, pp. 553–561, 1993.

[35] L. S. Stephenson, "Helminth parasites, a major factor in malnutrition," *World Health Forum*, vol. 15, no. 2, pp. 169–172, 1994.

[36] N. R. De Silva, S. Brooker, P. J. Hotez, A. Montresor, D. Engels, and L. Savioli, "Soil-transmitted helminth infections: updating the global picture," *Trends in Parasitology*, vol. 19, no. 12, pp. 547–551, 2003.

[37] A. Loukas, S. L. Constant, and J. M. Bethony, "Immunobiology of hookworm infection," *FEMS Immunology and Medical Microbiology*, vol. 43, no. 2, pp. 115–124, 2005.

[38] R. J. Stoltzfus, H. M. Chwaya, J. M. Tielsch, K. J. Schulze, M. Albonico, and L. Savioli, "Epidemiology of iron deficiency anemia in Zanzibari schoolchildren: the importance of hookworms," *American Journal of Clinical Nutrition*, vol. 65, no. 1, pp. 153–159, 1997.

[39] R. J. Stoltzfus, H. M. Chway, A. Montresor et al., "Low dose daily iron supplementation improves iron status and appetite but not anemia, whereas quarterly anthelminthic treatment improves growth, appetite and anemia in Zanzibari preschool children," *Journal of Nutrition*, vol. 134, no. 2, pp. 348–356, 2004.

[40] M. Albonico, R. J. Stoltzfus, L. Savioli et al., "Epidemiological evidence for a differential effect of hookworm species, Ancylostoma duodenale or Necator americanus, on iron status of children," *International Journal of Epidemiology*, vol. 27, no. 3, pp. 530–537, 1998.

[41] R. W. Steketee, "Pregnancy, nutrition and parasitic diseases," *Journal of Nutrition*, vol. 133, no. 5, pp. 1661S–1667S, 2003.

[42] P. J. Hotez, S. Brooker, J. M. Bethony, M. E. Bottazzi, A. Loukas, and S. Xiao, "Hookworm infection," *New England Journal of Medicine*, vol. 351, no. 8, pp. 799–841, 2004.

[43] J. Bethony, S. Brooker, M. Albonico et al., "Soil-transmitted helminth infections: ascariasis, trichuriasis, and hookworm," *Lancet*, vol. 367, no. 9521, pp. 1521–1532, 2006.

[44] J. Bethony, J. Chen, S. Lin et al., "Emerging patterns of hookworm infection: Influence of aging on the intensity of Necator infection in Hainan Province, People's Republic of China," *Clinical Infectious Diseases*, vol. 35, no. 11, pp. 1336–1344, 2002.

[45] S. M. Geiger, C. L. Massara, J. Bethony, P. T. Soboslay, and R. Corrêa-Oliveira, "Cellular responses and cytokine production in post-treatment hookworm patients from an endemic area in Brazil," *Clinical and Experimental Immunology*, vol. 136, no. 2, pp. 334–340, 2004.

[46] D. W. T. Crompton, "The public health importance of hookworm disease," *Parasitology*, vol. 121, pp. S39–S50, 2000.

[47] A. E. Ezeamama, J. F. Friedman, L. P. Acosta et al., "Helminth infection and cognitive impairment among Filipino children," *American Journal of Tropical Medicine and Hygiene*, vol. 72, no. 5, pp. 540–548, 2005.

[48] H. Sakti, C. Nokes, W. S. Hertanto et al., "Evidence for an association between hookworm infection and cognitive function in Indonesian school children," *Tropical Medicine and International Health*, vol. 4, no. 5, pp. 322–334, 1999.

[49] D. T. Simeon, S. M. Grantham-McGregor, J. E. Callender, and M. S. Wong, "Treatment of Trichuris trichiura infections improves growth, spelling scores and school attendance in some children," *Journal of Nutrition*, vol. 125, no. 7, pp. 1875–1883, 1995.

[50] R. Dickson, S. Awasthi, P. Williamson, C. Demellweek, and P. Garner, "Effects of treatment for intestinal helminth infection on growth and cognitive performance in children: systematic review of randomised trials," *BMJ*, vol. 320, no. 7251, pp. 1697–1701, 2000.

[51] A. Bhargava, "Treatment for intestinal helminth infection. Conclusions should have been based on broader considerations," *BMJ*, vol. 321, no. 7270, p. 1224, 2000.

[52] E. Cooper, "Treatment for intestinal helminth infection. Message does not follow from systematic review's findings," *BMJ*, vol. 321, no. 7270, pp. 1225–1226, 2000.

[53] E. Michael, A. Bhargava, D. Bundy et al., "Treatment for intestinal helminth infection," *BMJ*, vol. 321, no. 7270, pp. 1224–1227, 2000.

[54] L. Savioli, M. Neira, M. Albonico et al., "Treatment for intestinal helminth infection. Review needed to take account of all relevant evidence, not only effects on growth and cognitive performance," *BMJ*, vol. 321, no. 7270, pp. 1226–1227, 2000.

[55] B. Lozoff, E. Jimenez, J. Hagen, E. Mollen, and A. W. Wolf, "Poorer behavioral and developmental outcome more than 10 years after treatment for iron deficiency in infancy," *Pediatrics*, vol. 105, no. 4, p. E51, 2000.

[56] A. Prual, H. Daouda, M. Develoux, B. Sellin, P. Galan, and S. Hercberg, "Consequences of Schistosoma haematobium infection on the iron status of schoolchildren in Niger," *American Journal of Tropical Medicine and Hygiene*, vol. 47, no. 3, pp. 291–297, 1992.

[57] M. M. Mansour, W. M. Francis, and Z. Farid, "Prevalence of latent iron deficiency in patients with chronic S. mansoni infection," *Tropical and Geographical Medicine*, vol. 37, no. 2, pp. 124–128, 1985.

[58] L. Yuesgeng, Y. Dongbao, L. Yi, X. Yang, and X. Meng, "Morbidity and Health impact of schistosomiasis japonica in Dongting Lake area. A final report," in *WHO Collaborating Centre for Research and Control on Schistosomiasisis in Lake Region*, WHO, Geneva, Switzerland, 1992.

[59] S. Tatala, U. Svanberg, and B. Mduma, "Low dietary iron availability is a major cause of anemia: a nutrition survey in the Lindi District of Tanzania," *American Journal of Clinical Nutrition*, vol. 68, no. 1, pp. 171–178, 1998.

[60] J. F. Friedman, H. K. Kanzaria, L. P. Acosta et al., "Relationship between Schistosoma Japonicum and nutritional status among children and young adults in Leyte, the Philippines," *American Journal of Tropical Medicine and Hygiene*, vol. 72, no. 5, pp. 527–533, 2005.

[61] H. K. Kanzaria, L. P. Acosta, G. C. Langdon et al., "Schistosoma japonicum and occult blood loss in endemic villages in Leyte, The Philippines," *American Journal of Tropical Medicine and Hygiene*, vol. 72, no. 2, pp. 115–118, 2005.

[62] J. F. Friedman, H. K. Kanzaria, and S. T. McGarvey, "Human schistosomiasis and anemia: the relationship and potential mechanisms," *Trends in Parasitology*, vol. 21, no. 8, pp. 386–392, 2005.

[63] H. Friis, D. Mwaniki, B. Omondi et al., "Effects on haemoglobin of multi-micronutrient supplementation and multi-helminth chemotherapy: a randomized, controlled trial in Kenyan school children," *European Journal of Clinical Nutrition*, vol. 57, no. 4, pp. 573–579, 2003.

[64] G. R. Olds, C. King, J. Hewlett et al., "Double-blind placebo-controlled study of concurrent administration of albendazole and praziquantel in schoolchildren with schistosomiasis and geohelminths," *Journal of Infectious Diseases*, vol. 179, no. 4, pp. 996–1003, 1999.

[65] M. Taylor, C. C. Jinabhai, I. Couper, I. Kleinschmidt, and V. B. Jogessar, "The effect of different anthelmintic treatment regimens combined with iron supplementation on the nutritional status of schoolchildren in KwaZulu-Natal, South Africa: a randomized controlled trial," *Transactions of the Royal Society of Tropical Medicine and Hygiene*, vol. 95, no. 2, pp. 211–216, 2001.

[66] N. M. R. Beasley, A. M. Tomkins, A. Hall et al., "The impact of population level deworming on the haemoglobin levels of schoolchildren in Tanga, Tanzania," *Tropical Medicine and International Health*, vol. 4, no. 11, pp. 744–750, 1999.

[67] L. S. Stephenson, M. C. Latham, S. N. Kinoti, and M. L. Oduori, "Regression of splenomegaly and hepatomegaly in children treated for Schistosoma haematobium infection," *American Journal of Tropical Medicine and Hygiene*, vol. 34, no. 1, pp. 119–123, 1985.

[68] L. S. Stephenson, S. N. Kinoti, M. C. Latham, K. M. Kurz, and J. Kyobe, "Single dose metrifonate or praziquantel treatment in Kenyan children. I. Effects on Schistosoma haematobium, hookworm, hemoglobin levels, splenomegaly, and hepatomegaly," *American Journal of Tropical Medicine and Hygiene*, vol. 41, no. 4, pp. 436–444, 1989.

[69] S. T. McGarvey, G. Aligui, K. K. Graham, P. Peters, G. Richard Olds, and R. Olveda, "Schistosomiasis japonica and childhood nutritional status in northeastern Leyte, the Philippines: a randomized trial of praziquantel versus placebo," *American Journal of Tropical Medicine and Hygiene*, vol. 54, no. 5, pp. 498–502, 1996.

[70] R. T. Means Jr., "The anaemia of infection," *Bailliere's Best Practice and Research in Clinical Haematology*, vol. 13, no. 2, pp. 151–162, 2000.

[71] N. C. Andrews, "Forging a field: the golden age of iron biology," *Blood*, vol. 112, no. 2, pp. 219–230, 2008.

[72] E. Nemeth, S. Rivera, V. Gabayan et al., "IL-6 mediates hypoferremia of inflammation by inducing the synthesis of the iron regulatory hormone hepcidin," *Journal of Clinical Investigation*, vol. 113, no. 9, pp. 1271–1276, 2004.

[73] G. Nicolas, C. Chauvet, L. Viatte et al., "The gene encoding the iron regulatory peptide hepcidin is regulated by anemia, hypoxia, and inflammation," *Journal of Clinical Investigation*, vol. 110, no. 7, pp. 1037–1044, 2002.

[74] T. Ganz, "Hepcidin, a key regulator of iron metabolism and mediator of anemia of inflammation," *Blood*, vol. 102, no. 3, pp. 783–788, 2003.

[75] T. Ganz, "Hepcidin and its role in regulating systemic iron metabolism," *Hematology / American Society of Hematology. Education Program*, pp. 29–507, 2006.

[76] Y. Beguin, H. A. Huebers, G. Weber, M. Eng, and C. A. Finch, "Hepatocyte iron release in rats," *Journal of Laboratory and Clinical Medicine*, vol. 113, no. 3, pp. 346–354, 1989.

[77] C. Hershko, J. D. Cook, and C. A. Finch, "Storage iron kinetics. VI. The effect of inflammation on iron exchange in the rat," *British Journal of Haematology*, vol. 28, no. 1, pp. 67–75, 1974.

[78] G. Nicolas, M. Bennoun, A. Porteu et al., "Severe iron deficiency anemia in transgenic mice expressing liver hepcidin," *Proceedings of the National Academy of Sciences of the United States of America*, vol. 99, no. 7, pp. 4596–4601, 2002.

[79] G. Antelman, G. I. Msamanga, D. Spiegelman et al., "Nutritional factors, and infectious, disease contribute to anemia among pregnant women with human immunodeficiency virus in Tanzania," *Journal of Nutrition*, vol. 130, no. 8, pp. 1950–1957, 2000.

[80] U. Devi, C. M. Rao, V. K. Srivastava, P. K. Rath, and B. S. Das, "Effect of iron supplementation on mild to moderate anaemia in pulmonary tuberculosis," *British Journal of Nutrition*, vol. 90, no. 3, pp. 541–550, 2003.

[81] P. S. Sullivan, D. L. Hanson, S. Y. Chu, J. L. Jones, and J. W. Ward, "Epidemiology of anemia in human immunodeficiency virus (HIV)-infected persons: results from the multistate adult and adolescent spectrum of HIV disease surveillance project," *Blood*, vol. 91, no. 1, pp. 301–308, 1998.

[82] A. Mocroft, O. Kirk, S. E. Barton et al., "Anaemia is an independent predictive marker for clinical prognosis in HIV-infected patients from across Europe," *AIDS*, vol. 13, no. 8, pp. 943–950, 1999.

[83] R. D. Moore, J. C. Keruly, and R. E. Chaisson, "Anemia and survival in HIV infection," *Journal of Acquired Immune Deficiency Syndromes and Human Retrovirology*, vol. 19, no. 1, pp. 29–33, 1998.

[84] D. Totin, C. Ndugwa, F. Mmiro, R. T. Perry, J. Brooks Jackson, and R. D. Semba, "Iron deficiency anemia is highly prevalent among human immunodeficiency virus-infected and uninfected infants in Uganda," *Journal of Nutrition*, vol. 132, no. 3, pp. 423–429, 2002.

[85] B. S. Eley, A. A. Sive, M. Shuttleworth, and G. D. Hussey, "A prospective, cross-sectional study of anaemia and peripheral iron status in antiretroviral naïve, HIV-1 infected children in Cape Town, South Africa," *BMC Infectious Diseases*, vol. 2, article no. 3, 2002.

[86] L. S. Stephenson, C. V. Holland, and E. S. Cooper, "The public health significance of Trichuris trichiura," *Parasitology*, vol. 121, pp. S73–S95, 2000.

[87] D. D. Ramdath, D. T. Simeon, M. S. Wong, and S. M. Grantham-McGregor, "Iron status of schoolchildren with varying intensities of Trichuris trichiura infection," *Parasitology*, vol. 110, no. 3, pp. 347–351, 1995.

[88] L. J. Robertson, D. W. T. Crompton, D. Sanjur, and M. C. Nesheim, "Haemoglobin concentrations and concomitant infections of hookworm and Trichuris trichiura in Panamanian primary schoolchildren," *Transactions of the Royal Society of Tropical Medicine and Hygiene*, vol. 86, no. 6, pp. 654–656, 1992.

[89] E. M. Duff, N. M. Anderson, and E. S. Cooper, "Plasma insulin-like growth factor-1, type 1 procollagen, and serum tumor necrosis factor alpha in children recovering from Trichuris dysentery syndrome," *Pediatrics*, vol. 103, no. 5, article e69, 1999.

[90] S. M. Raj, "Fecal occult blood testing of Trichuris-infected primary school children in northeastern peninsular Malaysia," *American Journal of Tropical Medicine and Hygiene*, vol. 60, no. 1, pp. 165–166, 1999.

[91] L. M. Brown, "*Helicobacter pylori*: epidemiology and routes of transmission," *Epidemiologic Reviews*, vol. 22, no. 2, pp. 283–297, 2000.

[92] H. J. Windle, D. Kelleher, and J. E. Crabtree, "Childhood *Helicobacter pylori* infection and growth impairment in developing countries: a vicious cycle?" *Pediatrics*, vol. 119, no. 3, pp. e754–e759, 2007.

[93] J. Yakoob, W. Jafri, and S. Abid, "*Helicobacter pylori* infection and micronutrient deficiencies," *World Journal of Gastroenterology*, vol. 9, no. 10, pp. 2137–2139, 2003.

[94] V. M. Cardenas, Z. D. Mulla, M. Ortiz, and D. Y. Graham, "Iron deficiency and *Helicobacter pylori* infection in the United States," *American Journal of Epidemiology*, vol. 163, no. 2, pp. 127–134, 2006.

[95] S. DuBois and D. J. Kearney, "Iron-deficiency anemia and *Helicobacter pylori* infection: a review of the evidence," *American Journal of Gastroenterology*, vol. 100, no. 2, pp. 453–459, 2005.

[96] N. Milman, S. Rosenstock, L. Andersen, T. Jorgensen, and O. Bonnevie, "Serum ferritin, hemoglobin, and *Helicobacter pylori* infection: a seroepidemiologic survey comprising 2794 Danish adults," *Gastroenterology*, vol. 115, no. 2, pp. 268–274, 1998.

[97] A. J. Parkinson, B. D. Gold, L. Bulkow et al., "High prevalence of *Helicobacter pylori* in the Alaska Native population and association with low serum ferritin levels in young adults," *Clinical and Diagnostic Laboratory Immunology*, vol. 7, no. 6, pp. 885–888, 2000.

[98] B. Annibale, G. Capurso, E. Lahner et al., "Concomitant alterations in intragastric pH and ascorbic acid concentration in patients with *Helicobacter pylori* gastritis and associated iron deficiency anaemia," *Gut*, vol. 52, no. 4, pp. 496–501, 2003.

[99] C. Ratledge and L. G. Dover, "Iron metabolism in pathogenic bacteria," *Annual Review of Microbiology*, vol. 54, pp. 881–941, 2000.

[100] Q. de Mast, D. Syafruddin, S. Keijmel et al., "Increased serum hepcidin and alterations in blood iron parameters associated with asymptomatic P. falciparum and P. vivax malaria," *Haematologica*, vol. 95, no. 7, pp. 1068–1074, 2010.

[101] WHO, UNICEF, and UNFPA, *Maternal Mortality in 2005: estimates developed by WHO, UNICEF, UNFPA, and the World Bank*, World Health Organization, Geneva, Switzerland, 2007.

[102] S. Dellicour, A. J. Tatem, C. A. Guerra, R. W. Snow, and F. O. Ter Kuile, "Quantifying the number of pregnancies at risk of malaria in 2007: a demographic study," *PLoS Medicine*, vol. 7, no. 1, Article ID e1000221, 2010.

[103] M. Desai, F. O. ter Kuile, F. Nosten et al., "Epidemiology and burden of malaria in pregnancy," *Lancet Infectious Diseases*, vol. 7, no. 2, pp. 93–104, 2007.

[104] P. Patnaik, C. S. Jere, W. C. Miller et al., "Effects of HIV-1 serostatus, HIV-1 RNA concentration, and CD4 cell count on the incidence of malaria infection in a cohort of adults in rural Malawi," *Journal of Infectious Diseases*, vol. 192, no. 6, pp. 984–991, 2005.

[105] H. L. Guyatt and R. W. Snow, "Impact of malaria during pregnancy on low birth weight in sub-Saharan Africa," *Clinical Microbiology Reviews*, vol. 17, no. 4, pp. 760–769, 2004.

[106] P. E. Duffy and M. Fried, "Malaria in the pregnant woman," *Current Topics in Microbiology and Immunology*, vol. 295, pp. 169–200, 2005.

[107] WHO, *Technical Expert Group meeting on intermittent preventive treatment in pregnancy (IPTp)*, WH. Organization, Ed., World Health Organization, Geneva, Switzerland, 2007.

[108] K. Kayentao, M. Kodio, R. D. Newman et al., "Comparison of intermittent preventive treatment with chemoprophylaxis for the prevention of malaria during pregnancy in Mali," *Journal of Infectious Diseases*, vol. 191, no. 1, pp. 109–116, 2005.

[109] M. E. Parise, J. G. Ayisi, B. L. Nahlen et al., "Efficacy of sulfadoxine-pyrimethamine for prevention of placental malaria in an area of Kenya with a high prevalence of malaria and human immunodeficiency virus infection," *American Journal of Tropical Medicine and Hygiene*, vol. 59, no. 5, pp. 813–822, 1998.

[110] A. M. Van Eijk, J. G. Ayisi, F. O. Ter Kuile et al., "Effectiveness of intermittent preventive treatment with sulphadoxine-pyrimethamine for control of malaria in pregnancy in western Kenya: a hospital-based study," *Tropical Medicine and International Health*, vol. 9, no. 3, pp. 351–360, 2004.

[111] C. E. Shulman, "Intermittent sulphadoxine-pyrimethamine to prevent severe anaemia secondary to malaria in pregnancy: a randomised placebo-controlled trial," *Lancet*, vol. 353, no. 9153, pp. 632–636, 1999.

[112] H. L. Guyatt and R. W. Snow, "The epidemiology and burden of Plasmodium Falciparum-related anemia among pregnant women in sub-Saharan Africa," *American Journal of Tropical Medicine and Hygiene*, vol. 64, no. 1-2, pp. 36–44, 2001.

[113] W. E. Harrington, T. K. Mutabingwa, A. Muehlenbachs et al., "Competitive facilitation of drug-resistant Plasmodium falciparum malaria parasites in pregnant women who receive preventive treatment," *Proceedings of the National Academy of Sciences of the United States of America*, vol. 106, no. 22, pp. 9027–9032, 2009.

[114] E. R. Kabyemela, M. Fried, J. D. Kurtis, T. K. Mutabingwa, and P. E. Duffy, "Decreased susceptibility to Plasmodium falciparum infection in pregnant women with iron deficiency," *Journal of Infectious Diseases*, vol. 198, no. 2, pp. 163–166, 2008.

[115] S. J. Oppenheimer, S. B. J. Macfarlane, J. B. Moody, and C. Harrison, "Total dose iron infusion, malaria and pregnancy in Papua New Guinea," *Transactions of the Royal Society of Tropical Medicine and Hygiene*, vol. 80, no. 5, pp. 818–822, 1986.

[116] S. Sazawal, R. E. Black, M. Ramsan et al., "Effects of routine prophylactic supplementation with iron and folic acid on admission to hospital and mortality in preschool children in a high malaria transmission setting: community-based, randomised, placebo-controlled trial," *Lancet*, vol. 367, no. 9505, pp. 133–143, 2006.

[117] J. F. Friedman, J. D. Kurtis, E. R. Kabyemela, M. Fried, and P. E. Duffy, "The iron trap: iron, malaria and anemia at the mother-child interface," *Microbes and Infection*, vol. 11, no. 4, pp. 460–466, 2009.

[118] A. M. Nyakeriga, M. Troye-Blomberg, J. R. Dorfman et al., "Iron deficiency and malaria among children living on the coast of Kenya," *Journal of Infectious Diseases*, vol. 190, no. 3, pp. 439–447, 2004.

[119] S. J. Oppenheimer, F. D. Gibson, S. B. Macfarlane et al., "Iron supplementation increases prevalence and effects of malaria: report on clinical studies in Papua New Guinea," *Transactions of the Royal Society of Tropical Medicine and Hygiene*, vol. 80, no. 4, pp. 603–612, 1986.

[120] H. Verhoef, C. E. West, S. M. Nzyuko et al., "Intermittent administration of iron and sulfadoxine-pyrimethamine to control anaemia in Kenyan children: a randomised controlled trial," *Lancet*, vol. 360, no. 9337, pp. 908–914, 2002.

[121] World Health Organization, *Iron Deficiency Anemia: Assessment, Prevention, and Control*, World Health Organization and United Nations Children's Fund, Geneva, Switzerland, 2001.

[122] K. M. Rasmussen, "Is there a causal relationship between iron deficiency or iron-deficiency anemia and weight at birth, length of gestation and perinatal mortality?" *Journal of Nutrition*, vol. 131, no. 2, pp. 590S–603S, 2001.

[123] L. Reveiz, G. M. L. Gyte, and L. G. Cuervo, "Treatments for iron-deficiency anaemia in pregnancy," *Cochrane Database of Systematic Reviews*, no. 2, Article ID CD003094, 2007.

[124] J. P. Peña-Rosas and F. E. Viteri, "Effects and safety of preventive oral iron or iron+folic acid supplementation for women during pregnancy," *Cochrane Database of Systematic Reviews*, no. 4, Article ID CD004736, 2009.

[125] M. S. Golub, C. E. Hogrefe, A. F. Tarantal et al., "Diet-induced iron deficiency anemia and pregnancy outcome in rhesus monkeys," *American Journal of Clinical Nutrition*, vol. 83, no. 3, pp. 647–656, 2006.

[126] P. Preziosi, A. Prual, P. Galan, H. Daouda, H. Boureima, and S. Hercberg, "Effect of iron supplementation on the iron status of pregnant women: consequences for newborns," *American Journal of Clinical Nutrition*, vol. 66, no. 5, pp. 1178–1182, 1997.

[127] C. M. Chaparro, "Setting the stage for child health and development: prevention of iron deficiency in early infancy," *Journal of Nutrition*, vol. 138, no. 12, pp. 2529–2533, 2008.

15

Effect of Maternal Iron Deficiency Anemia on the Iron Store of Newborns in Ethiopia

Betelihem Terefe,[1] Asaye Birhanu,[2] Paulos Nigussie,[3] and Aster Tsegaye[2]

[1]*Department of Hematology and Immunohematology, University of Gondar, Gondar, Ethiopia*
[2]*School of Medical Laboratory Science, Addis Ababa University, Addis Ababa, Ethiopia*
[3]*Ethiopian Health and Nutrition Research Institute (EHNRI), Addis Ababa, Ethiopia*

Correspondence should be addressed to Betelihem Terefe; betch.nym@gmail.com

Academic Editor: Aurelio Maggio

Iron deficiency anemia among pregnant women is a widespread problem in developing countries including Ethiopia, though its influence on neonatal iron status was inconsistently reported in literature. This cross-sectional study was conducted to compare hematologic profiles and iron status of newborns from mothers with different anemia status and determine correlation between maternal and neonatal hematologic profiles and iron status in Ethiopian context. We included 89 mothers and their respective newborns and performed complete blood count and assessed serum ferritin and C-reactive protein levels from blood samples collected from study participants. Maternal median hemoglobin and serum ferritin levels were 12.2 g/dL and 47.0 ng/mL, respectively. The median hemoglobin and serum ferritin levels for the newborns were 16.2 g/dL and 187.6 ng/mL, respectively. The mothers were classified into two groups based on hemoglobin and serum ferritin levels as iron deficient anemic (IDA) and nonanemic (NA) and newborns of IDA mothers had significantly lower levels of serum ferritin ($P = 0.017$) and hemoglobin concentration ($P = 0.024$). Besides, newborns' ferritin and hemoglobin levels showed significant correlation with maternal hemoglobin ($P = 0.018$; $P = 0.039$) and ferritin ($P = 0.000$; $P = 0.008$) levels. We concluded that maternal IDA may have an effect on the iron stores of newborns.

1. Background

Iron deficiency (ID) is the most important cause of nutritional anemia and is the most common micronutrient deficiency worldwide, especially in developing countries [1]. Pregnant women are particularly vulnerable to ID because of the increased metabolic demands imposed by pregnancy involving a growing placenta, fetus, and maternal tissues, coupled with associated dietary risks [2].

In developing countries including Ethiopia, pregnant women commonly begin gestation with depleted or low body iron stores which might make them prone to developing iron deficiency anemia (IDA) [3]. Frequently, the anemia is severe in degree and it coexists with maternal malnutrition [3]. Under these situations, the competing demands of mother and fetus may disturb the normal maternal-fetal iron homeostasis [3–5]. This may have a resultant effect both on

the mother and on the fetus, such as premature delivery, intrauterine growth retardation, and neonatal and perinatal death [6]. As the main source of iron for infants until the age of 6 months is the iron endowed from maternal circulation [7], it is logical to question the extension of the effect of maternal IDA on the fetus during and beyond its stay in the womb.

In spite of many researches conducted on this specific issue, consistent findings were not evident. Some have reported the negative impact of maternal IDA on iron stores of newborns [3, 5, 8–11], while others could not find any relationship in between [12–14]. Most of the studies have used serum ferritin as a measurement of iron store, but this serum ferritin has one known drawback as it is an acute phase reactant (APR); it increases during infection, including sub-clinical infections [15]. Therefore in this study, we incorporated another APR that is C-reactive protein

(CRP) test to minimize the bias that can be caused due to infection and tried to determine the effect of IDA on the iron store of term newborns.

2. Methods

This study was conducted from December 2011 to February 2012 in Obstetrics and Gynecology Department of St. Paul's hospital, Addis Ababa, Ethiopia. Mothers who had bleeding during pregnancy, preterm delivery (<37 weeks), multiple pregnancy, eclampsia, diabetes mellitus, heart, kidney, lung disease, and hematologic disease were excluded.

A total of 101 mothers and their respective newborns were included first. However, 12 of them were withdrawn from the study because they had anemia other than IDA. Therefore, the final sample comprised 89 mothers and their respective newborns.

Sociodemographic characteristics of study participants were collected using pretested questionnaires and blood samples were collected at the median cubital vein of the mothers during the process of labor and at the placental end of the umbilical cord. Pairs of samples were collected from each mother and cord using K_3EDTA test tubes (for complete blood counting, CBC) and test tubes with serum gel separator (for ferritin determination and CRP measurement).

CBC and ferritin concentrations were analyzed using Cell-dyn 1800 (Abbott Laboratories, Abbott Park, Illinois) and fully automated Cobas e 411 (Roche Diagnostics GmbH, D-68298 Mannheim, Germany), respectively. CRP was determined by a qualitative slide agglutination test using Cromatest (Linear Chemicals SL, Barcelona, Spain). The instruments were calibrated before the beginning of analyses. Precision test was carried out to assure reproducibility of results provided by the Cell-dyn 1800 analyzer and it was within the acceptable limit stated by the manufacturer. In addition, commercial quality control samples were included in every session of analyses for both CBC enumeration and serum ferritin level determination. Three levels of whole blood controls (high, medium, and low), two levels of plasma control (low, normal), and serum control (positive and negative) were used for CBC ferritin and CRP determinations, respectively. Levy-Jennine (LJ) charts were plotted and the controls were within the 2SD limits with no shifts or drifts detected.

We entered the data from the analyzers and questionnaire into Microsoft Excel and analyzed it using MedCalc Software Version 12.1.4. D'Agostino-Pearson test was used to check the normality of data distribution. Since all of the analytes studied were not normally distributed, nonparametric tests were applied. Frequencies, percentages, medians, and interquartile ranges (IQR) were computed to summarize the data. In order to compare quantitative and qualitative variables between the groups, Mann-Whitney and Chi-square tests were applied, respectively. Association of maternal and newborns parameters were assessed by spearman's correlation. P value of <0.05 was considered as statistically significant in all analyses.

The study protocol was approved by the Research Ethics Review Committees of Addis Ababa University and St. Paul's Hospital. In addition, informed verbal consents were collected from the mothers.

3. Result

3.1. Description of the Sociodemographic and Obstetric Data of Study Participants. We included 89 mothers with their respective newborns. The median age of the mothers was 23 years (IQR = 21–27 years). As clearly presented in Table 1, about one-third of the mothers (34.8%; n = 31) had educational level above secondary school, while 29.2% (n = 26) of the mothers were illiterates. Housewives were dominant and accounted for 75.3% (n = 67) of the participants.

The majority of mothers were primiparous (64.0%; n = 57), and also were attending antenatal care (ANC) during their pregnancy. Those mothers who have been taking iron during their pregnancy accounted for 58.4% (n = 52) (Table 1).

Most of the babies were delivered through vaginal delivery (78.7%; n = 70) and the proportion of male (49.4%; n = 44) and female (50.6%; n = 45) newborns were almost equal. The babies had median weight of 3100 g (IQR = 2800–3400 g) and a few (12.4%; n = 11) had low birth weight (Table 1).

3.2. Hematological and Ferritin Status of Mothers and Their Newborns. The median hemoglobin and serum ferritin levels for the mothers were 12.2 g/dL (IQR = 11.3–12.9 g/dL) and 45.5 ng/mL (IQR = 26.8–80.34 ng/mL), respectively (Table 2). The median hemoglobin and serum ferritin levels for the newborns were 16.2 g/dL (IQR = 15.0–17.2 g/dL) and 191.5 ng/mL (IQR = 140.5–264.8 ng/mL), respectively (Table 2). Table 2 also summarizes the median and the IQRs of other studied CBC parameters among mothers and their newborns.

3.3. Grouping Study Participants. The mothers were grouped into two categories, NA and IDA based on hemoglobin and serum ferritin concentrations. We used 11 g/dL as cutoff value for maternal hemoglobin concentration after altitude corrections as per World Health Organization (WHO) recommendation [16]. Similarly, the cutoff value for maternal ferritin level was set at 15 ng/mL for those mothers who were not reactive to CRP test and 30 ng/mL for those mothers who were reactive to CRP test in order to balance the effect of infection as recommended by the WHO [15].

Then, mothers showing low hemoglobin concentration (<11 g/dL) and low ferritin level (<15 ng/mL or <30 ng/mL as per their CRP reaction status) were grouped under IDA. Mothers with normal hemoglobin concentration (≥11 g/dL) were classified as NA. Accordingly, 21 mothers (23.6%) were grouped under IDA category while the rest 68 mothers (76.4%) were grouped under NA category. Prevalence of anemia, median differences in hemoglobin, and ferritin levels among newborns of mothers in the two categories were computed and presented in Table 3.

3.4. Correlations between Mothers and Newborns Laboratory Parameters. The newborns ferritin level has significant correlation with hemoglobin (r_s = 0.25, P = 0.018) and ferritin (r_s = 0.38, P < 0.001) levels of their mothers (Table 4). In addition, the newborns hemoglobin had significant correlation with hemoglobin (r_s = 0.22, P = 0.039) and ferritin

TABLE 1: Summary of sociodemographic and obstetric characteristics of mothers and their newborns gender and weight attending at St. Paul's Hospital, Addis Ababa.

Characteristics	Total ($n = 89$) frequency (%)	IDA ($n = 21$) frequency (%)	NA ($n = 68$) frequency (%)	P value[*]
Maternal age				
≤24 yrs	52 (58.4%)	11 (52.4%)	41 (60.3%)	0.700
>24 yrs	37 (41.6%)	10 (47.6%)	27 (39.7%)	
Maternal education level				
No education	26 (29.2%)	6 (28.6%)	20 (29.4%)	
Primary school	19 (21.4%)	6 (28.6%)	13 (19.1%)	0.805
Secondary school	13 (14.6%)	3 (14.2%)	10 (14.7%)	
Above secondary school	31 (34.8%)	6 (28.6%)	25 (36.8%)	
Maternal occupation				
Housewives	67 (75.3%)	16 (76.2%)	51 (75.0%)	0.858
Employed	22 (24.7%)	5 (23.8%)	17 (25.0%)	
Parity				
Primiparous	57 (64.0%)	12 (57.1%)	45 (66.2%)	0.621
Multiparous	32 (36.0%)	9 (42.9%)	23 (33.8%)	
Delivery				
Vaginal	70 (78.7%)	17 (81.0%)	53 (77.9%)	0.992
Cesarean section	19 (21.3%)	4 (19.0%)	15 (22.1%)	
ANC followup				
Yes	79 (88.8%)	17 (81.0%)	62 (91.2%)	0.367
No	10 (11.2%)	4 (19.0%)	6 (8.8%)	
Iron intake during pregnancy				
Yes	52 (58.4%)	10 (47.6%)	42 (61.8%)	0.370
No	37 (41.6%)	11 (52.4%)	26 (38.2%)	
Newborns' gender				
Female	45 (50.6%)	10 (47.6%)	35 (51.5%)	0.953
Male	44 (49.4%)	11 (52.4%)	33 (48.5%)	
Weight of newborns				
Normal birth weight	78 (87.6%)	19 (90.5%)	59 (86.8%)	0.942
Low birth weight	11 (12.4%)	2 (9.5%)	9 (13.2%)	

IDA = iron deficient anemic; NA = nonanemic. [*]Data are from the Chi-square test.

($r_s = 0.28$, $P = 0.008$) levels of their mothers (Table 4); additionally the newborns hemoglobin showed significant correlation with mothers mean corpuscular hemoglobin (MCH) and mean corpuscular hemoglobin concentration (MCHC) values (Table 4).

4. Discussion

In our study, we determined that maternal IDA may have an effect on the iron stores of newborns as hemoglobin ($P = 0.025$) and ferritin concentrations ($P = 0.027$) were significantly lower in newborns delivered from IDA mothers than newborns delivered from NA mothers (Table 3 and Figure 1). These findings were in accordance with previous reports elsewhere [3, 8, 17, 18]. However, there are also findings in contrary to the present study which showed that iron accretion in the fetus was independent of maternal iron status [12–14].

The disagreements might be raised due to differences in cutoff value for serum ferritin (<10 ng/mL, which has low sensitivity), failure to incorporate tests that rule out infection (which may mask the actual ferritin status) [13], and differences in condition of study participants including mothers who were taking iron supplementation during pregnancy, which may have masked the relationship of maternal and newborns iron status [14].

It is well established that serum ferritin is an indicator of the level of body iron sores [19]. Thus, the significantly lower level of ferritin in newborns delivered from IDA mothers compared to NA mothers suggests reduced iron stores in these newborns. Additionally, the newborns delivered from IDA mothers had a significantly lower concentration of hemoglobin than newborns from NA mothers that might contribute for a decreased amount of recycled heme iron resultantly decreasing its contribution for the iron pool. Here, we were not surprised to see no statistically significant

TABLE 2: Hematological profile and ferritin status of mothers and their newborns at St. Paul's Hospital, Addis Ababa ($n = 89$).

Parameters	Median (IQR)[a]		P value[*]
	Mothers	Newborns	
Hemoglobin (g/dL)	12.2 (11.2–12.9)	16.2 (15.0–17.2)	<0.001
Mean cell volume (fL)	90.0 (88.1–93.5)	105.5 (102.7–109.7)	<0.001
Mean cell hemoglobin (pg)	30.7 (30.2–31.8)	37.3 (36.2–38.2)	<0.001
Mean cell hemoglobin concentration (%)	34.2 (33.9–34.8)	35.0 (34.3–35.8)	<0.001
Red cell distribution width (%)	14.1 (13.5–14.9)	16.3 (15.6–17.1)	<0.001
Serum ferritin (ng/mL)	47.0 (26.5–79.7)	187.6 (140.0–264.7)	<0.001

IDA = iron deficient anemic; NA = nonanemic. [a]IQR, 25th to 75th quartiles, [*]data are from Mann-Whitney test.

TABLE 3: Hematological profile and ferritin status of newborns by anemia and iron status of their mothers[a] at St. Paul's Hospital, Addis Ababa ($n = 89$).

Parameters	Group median (IQR)[b]		P value
	IDA ($n = 21$)	NA ($n = 68$)	
Hgb (g/dL)	15.6 (14.8–16.4)	16.7 (15.5–17.6)	**0.024**[*]
MCV (fL)	105.1 (101.6–108.4)	105.9 (103.0–109.9)	0.588[*]
MCH (pg)	37.0 (35.9–38.1)	37.5 (36.4–38.3)	0.344[*]
MCHC (%)	35.0 (33.9–35.4)	35.1 (34.3–35.9)	0.227[*]
RDW (%)	16.0 (15.5–16.5)	16.4 (15.7–17.3)	0.080[*]
Ferritin (ng/mL)	138.9 (105.0–211.7)	200.7 (151.4–265.3)	**0.017**[*]
Frequency (%) of anemia	3 (14.3%)	5 (7.9%)	0.593[**]

Hgb = hemoglobin; MCV = mean cell volume; MCH = mean cell hemoglobin; MCHC = mean cell hemoglobin concentration; RDW = red cell distribution width. [a]IDA = iron deficient anemic; NA = nonanemic. [b]IQR, 25th to 75th quartiles. [*]Data are from Mann-Whitney test. [**]Data are from the Chi-square test.

TABLE 4: Spearman's correlation coefficients (r) comparing hematological profile and ferritin status of mothers and their respective newborns at St. Paul's Hospital, Addis Ababa ($n = 89$).

Newborns parameters	Mother's parameters r_s (P value)					
	Hgb	MCV	MCH	MCHC	RDW	Ferritin
Hgb	0.22[a]	0.09	0.23[a]	0.35[c]	−0.00	0.28[b]
MCV	0.06	−0.03	−0.03	−0.05	−0.08	0.12
MCH	0.15	0.02	0.09	0.14	−0.06	0.10
MCHC	0.16	0.24[a]	0.31[b]	0.39[c]	−0.02	0.04
RDW	−0.01	−0.19	−0.16	0.04	0.03	0.01
Ferritin	0.25[a]	0.10	0.13	0.11	−0.21	0.38[c]

Hgb = hemoglobin; MCV = mean cell volume; MCH = mean cell hemoglobin; MCHC = mean cell hemoglobin concentration; RDW = red cell distribution width. [a]P value < 0.05, [b]P value < 0.01, and [c]P value < 0.001.

difference in prevalence of anemia among newborns of the two groups of mothers ($P = 0.593$). This is because visible difference that can be evidenced in the form of anemia is not expected at such an early stage in life [7]. However, later in life, anemia prevalence could be different among newborns from the two groups of mothers since newborns are highly dependent on the stored iron acquired from the mother during pregnancy till the age of 6 months [20, 21]. Therefore, the significantly lower ferritin level and hemoglobin concentration in newborns delivered from IDA mothers compared to NA mothers may make them prone to iron deficiency and

anemia in early infancy. This may have serious consequences on cognitive development and cellular immunity [22].

The evidence presented in this study also denotes that all the hematological and ferritin parameters studied were markedly higher in newborns than in their mothers. Similar findings were also documented in previous studies [3, 5, 8–11]. The higher ferritin levels in newborns can be explained by the existence of active transfer of iron across placenta from mother to the fetus [23]. Also, it can be due to the upregulation of transferrin receptor synthesis in the case of iron deficiency, which enables placenta to compete more effectively for circulating transferrin iron with erythroid marrow of the pregnant mothers intending adequate iron supply of the growing fetus [7, 11, 24].

In this study, newborns ferritin level has significant correlation with hemoglobin and ferritin levels of mothers. In addition, the newborns hemoglobin had significant correlation with hemoglobin and ferritin levels of mothers. Several investigators have determined the correlation between hemoglobin and ferritin parameters of newborns and their mothers; however, the results vary from study to study. Kumar et al., for example, have showed that maternal ferritin levels had significant correlations with Hgb levels ($r_s = +0.488$; $P < 0.001$) and ferritin ($r_s = +0.440$; $P < 0.001$) in cord blood [3]. Singla et al. have also found that maternal serum ferritin was significantly correlated with cord blood Hgb ($r_s = +0.390$, $P < 0.01$) and cord serum ferritin ($r_s = +0.523$; $P < 0.001$) [8]. The relatively lower correlation observed in this study compared to the two studies may be due to the absence of any severe anemia cases in our study, while there were severe anemia cases in the two studies.

In this study, we determined that the deleterious effect of maternal IDA may extend beyond pregnancy, in an Ethiopian context. This suggests the need for strengthening strategy to improve the maternal iron status. Improving the nutritional status of pregnant women could have a positive impact on improving the iron status of the mothers and also their newborns. The other option might be delayed clamping of the umbilical cord after birth for improving the iron status of young infants [25].

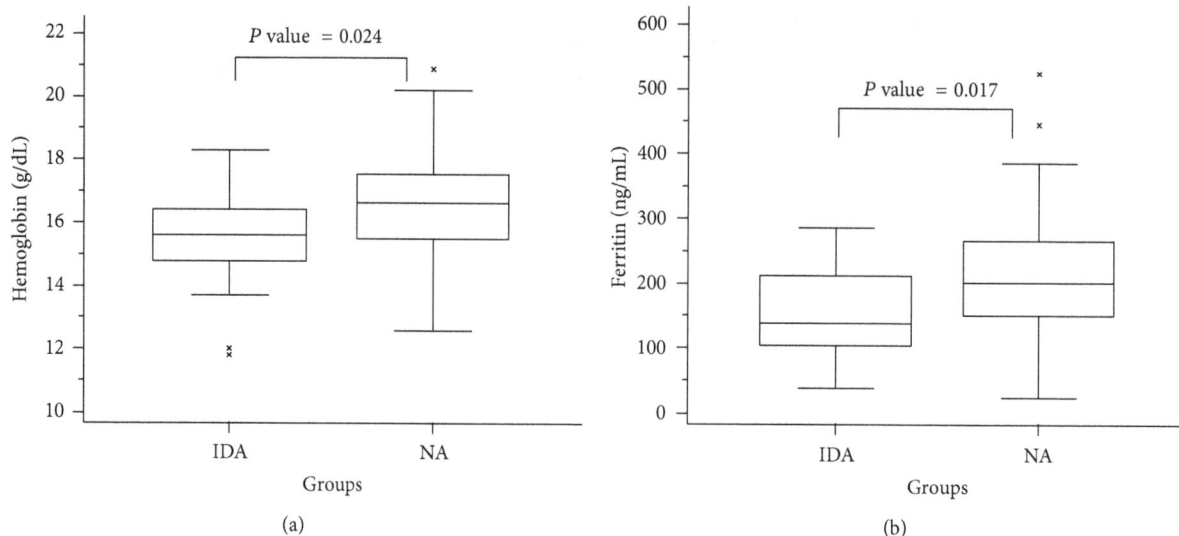

FIGURE 1: Box plots of hematological profile and ferritin parameters in newborns according to anemia and iron status of the mothers. IDA = iron deficient anemic; NA = nonanemic. P values are from the Mann-Whitney test.

5. Conclusion

Median hemoglobin and ferritin concentrations were significantly lower in newborns delivered from IDA mothers compared to NA mothers. Additionally newborns hemoglobin and ferritin concentration had a significant correlation with hemoglobin and ferritin concentration of the mothers. Based on these findings we can conclude that maternal IDA may have an effect on the iron stores of newborns.

Conflict of Interests

The authors declare that they have no competing interests.

Authors' Contribution

Betelihem Terefe, Asaye Birhanu, and Aster Tsegaye have participated in the conception and design of the study. Betelihem Terefe and Paulos Nigussie have participated in the selection of study participants. Betelihem Terefe and Paulos Nigussie have participated in the laboratory analysis and acquisition of data. All authors have participated in preparing and critically reviewing the draft paper. All authors also have read and approved the final paper.

Acknowledgments

The authors would like to thank Addis Ababa University for the financial support and Paul's Hospital Laboratory for their Cell-dyn 1800 reagent supply. The authors thank the study participants for their kind collaboration.

References

[1] A. Krafft, R. Huch, and C. Breymann, "Impact of parturition on iron status in nonanaemic iron deficiency," European Journal of Clinical Investigation, vol. 33, no. 10, pp. 919–923, 2003.

[2] M. F. Picciano, "Pregnancy and lactation: physiological adjustments, nutritional requirements and the role of dietary supplements," Journal of Nutrition, vol. 133, no. 6, pp. 1997S–2002S, 2003.

[3] A. Kumar, A. K. Rai, S. Basu, D. Dash, and J. S. Singh, "Cord blood and breast milk iron status in maternal anemia," Pediatrics, vol. 121, no. 3, pp. e673–e677, 2008.

[4] A. M. Siddappa, R. Rao, J. D. Long, J. A. Widness, and M. K. Georgieff, "The assessment of newborn iron stores at birth: a review of the literature and standards for ferritin concentrations," Neonatology, vol. 92, no. 2, pp. 73–82, 2007.

[5] R. A. El-Farrash, E. Abdel Rahman Ismail, and A. Shafik Nada, "Cord blood iron profile and breast milk micronutrients in maternal iron deficiency anemia," Pediatric Blood & Cancer, vol. 58, no. 2, pp. 233–238, 2012.

[6] T. O. Scholl, "Iron status during pregnancy: setting the stage for mother and infant," The American Journal of Clinical Nutrition, vol. 81, no. 5, pp. 1218S–1222S, 2005.

[7] C. M. Chaparro, "Setting the stage for child health and development: prevention of iron deficiency in early infancy," Journal of Nutrition, vol. 138, no. 12, pp. 2529–2533, 2008.

[8] P. N. Singla, M. Tyagi, R. Shankar, D. Dash, and A. Kumar, "Fetal iron status in maternal anemia," Acta Paediatrica, vol. 85, no. 11, pp. 1327–1330, 1996.

[9] D. G. Sweet, G. Savage, T. R. J. Tubman, T. R. J. Lappin, and H. L. Halliday, "Study of maternal influences on fetal iron status at term using cord blood transferrin receptors," Archives of Disease in Childhood: Fetal and Neonatal Edition, vol. 84, no. 1, pp. F40–F43, 2001.

[10] S. Ziaei, E. Hatefnia, and G. Togeh, "Iron status in newborns born to iron-deficient mothers," Iranian Journal of Medical Sciences, vol. 28, no. 2, pp. 62–64, 2003.

[11] F. Emamghorashi and T. Heidari, "Iron status of babies born to iron-deficient anaemic mothers in an Iranian hospital," Eastern Mediterranean Health Journal, vol. 10, no. 6, pp. 808–814, 2004.

[12] C.-T. Wong and N. Saha, "Inter-relationships of storage iron in the mother, the placenta and the newborn," Acta Obstetricia et Gynecologica Scandinavica, vol. 69, no. 7-8, pp. 613–616, 1990.

[13] R. Hadipour, A. K. Norimah, B. K. Poh, F. Firoozehchian, R. Hadipour, and A. Akaberi, "Haemoglobin and serum ferritin levels in newborn babies born to anaemic Iranian women: a cross-sectional study in an Iranian Hospital," *Pakistan Journal of Nutrition*, vol. 9, no. 6, pp. 562–566, 2010.

[14] A. de Azevedo Paiva, P. H. C. Rondó, R. A. Pagliusi, M. D. R. D. O. Latorre, M. A. A. Cardoso, and S. S. R. Gondim, "Relationship between the iron status of pregnant women and their newborns," *Revista de Saúde Pública*, vol. 41, no. 3, pp. 321–327, 2007.

[15] WHO, *Serum Ferritin Concentrations for the Assessment of Iron Status and Iron Deficiency in Populations. Vitamin and Mineral Nutrition Information System*, WHO/NMH/NHD/MNM/11.2, World Health Organization, Geneva, Switzerland, 2011, http://www.who.int/vmnis/indicators/serum_ferritin.pdf.

[16] WHO, "Haemoglobin concentrations for the diagnosis of anaemia and assessment of severity," Vitamin and Mineral Nutrition Information System, World Health Organization, Geneva, Switzerland, 2011, (WHO/NMH/NHD/MNM/11.1), http://www.who.int/vmnis/indicators/haemoglobin.pdf.

[17] D. G. Sweet, G. Savage, T. R. J. Tubman, T. R. J. Lappin, and H. L. Halliday, "Study of maternal influences on fetal iron status at term using cord blood transferrin receptors," *Archives of Disease in Childhood: Fetal and Neonatal Edition*, vol. 84, no. 1, pp. F40–F43, 2001.

[18] R. A. El-Farrash, E. A. R. Ismail, and A. S. Nada, "Cord blood iron profile and breast milk micronutrients in maternal iron deficiency anemia," *Pediatric Blood & Cancer*, vol. 58, no. 2, pp. 233–238, 2012.

[19] G. O. Walters, F. M. Miller, and M. Worwood, "Serum ferritin concentration and iron stores in normal subjects," *Journal of Clinical Pathology*, vol. 26, no. 10, pp. 770–772, 1973.

[20] R. Zetterström, "Iron deficiency and iron deficiency anaemia during infancy and childhood," *Acta Paediatrica*, vol. 93, no. 4, pp. 436–439, 2004.

[21] E. E. Ziegler, S. E. Nelson, and J. M. Jeter, "Iron supplementation of breastfed infants from an early age," *The American Journal of Clinical Nutrition*, vol. 89, no. 2, pp. 525–532, 2009.

[22] M. B. Zimmermann and R. F. Hurrell, "Nutritional iron deficiency: seminar," *The Lancet*, vol. 370, no. 9586, pp. 511–520, 2007.

[23] R. Gupta and S. Ramji, "Effect of delayed cord clamping on iron stores in infants born to anemic mothers: a randomized controlled trial," *Indian Pediatrics*, vol. 39, no. 2, pp. 130–135, 2002.

[24] E. J. Harthoorn-Lasthuizen, J. Lindemans, and M. M. A. C. Langenhuijsen, "Does iron-deficient erythropoiesis in pregnancy influence fetal iron supply?" *Acta Obstetricia et Gynecologica Scandinavica*, vol. 80, no. 5, pp. 392–396, 2001.

[25] P. F. van Rheenen and B. J. Brabin, "A practical approach to timing cord clamping in resource poor settings," *British Medical Journal*, vol. 333, no. 7575, pp. 954–958, 2006.

16

A Program of Nutritional Education in Schools Reduced the Prevalence of Iron Deficiency in Students

María Nieves García-Casal,[1] **Maritza Landaeta-Jiménez,**[2] **Rafael Puche,**[1]
Irene Leets,[1] **Zoila Carvajal,**[1] **Elijú Patiño,**[2] **and Carlos Ibarra**[1]

[1] *Laboratorio de Fisiopatología, Centro de Medicina Experimental, Instituto Venezolano de Investigaciones Científicas (IVIC), Caracas 1020-A, Venezuela*
[2] *Fundación Bengoa para la Salud y Nutrición, 8va Transversal con 7ma Avenida, Quinta Pacairigua, Altamira, Caracas 1050, Venezuela*

Correspondence should be addressed to María Nieves García-Casal, mngarcia@ivic.gob.ve

Academic Editor: Bruno Annibale

The objective was to determine the prevalence of iron, folates and retinol deficiencies in school children and to evaluate the changes after an intervention of nutritional education. The project was developed in 17 schools. The sample included 1,301 children (678 males and 623 females). A subsample of 480 individuals, was randomly selected for drawing blood for biochemical determinations before and after the intervention of nutritional education, which included in each school: written pre and post-intervention tests, 6 workshops, 2 participative talks, 5 game activities, 1 cooking course and 1 recipe contest. Anthropometrical and biochemical determinations included weight, height, body-mass index, nutritional status, hematocrit, serum ferritin, retinol and folate concentrations. There was high prevalence of iron (25%), folates (75%) and vitamin A (43%) deficiencies in school children, with a low consumption of fruit and vegetables, high consumption of soft drinks and snacks and almost no physical activity. The nutritional education intervention produced a significant reduction in iron deficiency prevalence (25 to 14%), and showed no effect on vitamin A and folates deficiencies. There was a slight improvement in nutritional status. This study shows, through biochemical determinations, that nutritional education initiatives and programs have an impact improving nutritional health in school children.

1. Introduction

Programs on nutritional education have been widely used for teaching or reinforcing knowledge on food habits or healthy life styles in children and are considered a useful strategy to prevent the appearance of nontransmissible chronic diseases at early ages. The implementation of nutritional education programs in schools may help to inculcate in children the ability of identifying a healthy food choice for themselves [1].

It has been established that the triangulation of information amongst the teacher, the children, and the family is a useful strategy for modifying negative feeding behaviors that are contributing to the recent increase in the prevalence of overweight, obesity, hypertension, diabetes, and metabolic syndrome in children, while in the opposite extreme of the spectrum, nutritional deficits persist as important nutritional problems, especially regarding micronutrient, and vitamin deficiencies such as iron, calcium, folic acid, and vitamin A, among others [2, 3].

The inclusion of nutritional education into formal education programs is one of the most used and recommended strategies, mainly because the children obtain and fix the information in a easy, fun, and permanent way, but also because they act as multipliers of the information, bringing the new information to their homes to achieve, in the best case scenario, the transmission of the information to the whole family group. Some studies indicate that to obtain a better impact on changing habits on the long term, nutritional education programs must include the whole community, to assure the permanence of changes [3].

In general, the application of nutritional education strategies obtains a limited success when implemented as an isolated strategy. In a first stage, the simultaneous application of supplementation or fortification programs with nutritional education is the ideal approach. This is in the understanding that the 2 initially mentioned interventions should be temporary measures, while the more permanent changes in nutritional habits, are achieved with the aid of nutritional education [4].

Anemia constitutes the most prevalent nutritional deficiency worldwide, especially in children and women in childbearing age. The main cause of anemia in these age groups is iron deficiency, although other nutritional deficiencies, such as folic acid, are also becoming important etiological agents [5]. Another important nutrient during growing and development periods is vitamin A, essential for vision, immunological function, development and maintenance of mucosal barriers, and so forth.

The worldwide prevalence of anemia in preschoolers is 47.4%, and 23.1 millions of those children live in the Americas [6]. In Venezuela, the prevalence of anemia for this age group is around 30% [5, 7, 8], although a study performed in groups from the marginal socioeconomic strata reported a 75% prevalence of anemia [9]. Folic acid deficiency is also high for preschool children reaching 31% in a National survey [10, 11]. Vitamin A deficiency has a prevalence of 33.3%, affecting 190 millions of children, half of which live in the Americas [6]. In Venezuela, there are few documented reports on vitamin A deficiency, which indicate a prevalence of 25–30% in children from low socioeconomic strata of the population [12, 13].

Due to the importance of these 3 nutrients for growing and development and to the higher susceptibility to suffer from these deficiencies during infancy and childhood, the objective of this study was to determine the prevalence of iron, folates, and vitamin A deficiencies in school children from 6 to 14 years and to evaluate the changes in these parameters after an intervention of nutritional education.

2. Materials and Methods

The project "Iron deficiency and anemia" was approved by Fundacion Bengoa Review Board and developed in 17 schools from 3 Venezuelan States (Aragua, Lara, and Táchira) located in the northwest region of the country. The sample was constituted by scholars from 6 to 14 years of age, selected from the inscription lists of children and adolescents to the schools of the 3 zones, during September 2007 to November 2008.

The sampling was probabilistic, in which all children from all the schools selected had a known and not null probability of being part of the sample. The sample size was 1,301 children (678 males and 623 females), and a subsample of 480 individual, were randomly selected for blood sampling and for biochemical and anthropometric determinations before and after the intervention of nutritional education. The first blood drawing had 2 objectives: 1 to determine the prevalence of iron, folic acid, and vitamin A deficiencies in

the zone and 2 to establish a baseline or time 0, before the intervention. The second blood draw, 6 months later, allowed to verify any changes in the biochemical parameters after the intervention.

Parents, children, and teachers received detailed information about the procedure and the protocol, and an informed consent was signed by all participants. After inclusion in the protocol, a detailed record with personal data, medical, and nutritional records was filled for each participant.

2.1. Nutritional Education Intervention. The nutritional education program was initiated with a written test to explore the previous nutritional knowledge of teachers, and from those results the intervention was designed. The objective was to educate teachers about the importance of a proper nutrition with emphasis on anemia and iron deficiency prevention, so they can act as multipliers transferring the information to their students.

The program contents included basic concepts in food and nutrition, how to obtain a balanced meal, anemia and iron deficiency as public health problems, growth and development according to what we eat, balanced and varied meals, food iron sources, food iron absorption enhancers and inhibitors, and menu preparation. The program in each school consisted in 6 workshops, 2 participative talks, 5 game activities, 1 cooking course, and 1 recipe contest designed and directed to teachers and/or pupils. In the workshops, different techniques were applied to obtain a harmonious and participative ambient in which interventions were encouraged and the knowledge was obtained through "learning by doing." The teachers developed original educative strategies (role-playing, songs, poetries, puppets, etc.), expositions, and participative talks. Each teacher received a set of technical notes, with the contents to teach and the transfer of knowledge was evaluated by direct supervision of the teacher, by the activities performed, the techniques used during the activities, and also by another written test at the end of the intervention

2.2. Anthropometric and Biochemical Analysis. The subsample of children and adolescents was measured in light clothes at the beginning and end of the nutritional education intervention, and weight and height were recorded by trained personnel. The measuring error was less than 1%, within expected limits. The classification according to nutritional status was performed by the combination of indicators: weight-age, height-age, and body mass index (BMI-) age. The data was grouped according to presumptive diagnosis as deficit (lower than percentile 3), at risk of deficit ($\geq$ percentile 3 and $<$ percentile 10), normal ($\geq$ percentile 10 and $\leq$ percentile 90), at risk of excess ($>$ percentile 90 and $\leq$ percentile 97), and excess ($>$ percentile 97). A 24 h food recall interview was also performed in children and adolescents from 10 to 14 years of age.

To the same group, 2 blood samples were taken at the times mentioned, to perform hemoglobin and hematocrit in blood and to determine serum concentrations of ferritin, folates, and retinol. Each sample consisted in 5 mL of blood taken from the antecubital vein of the arm after cleaning of the zone with isopropyl alcohol. From this, 4 mL were used to obtain serum and 1 mL was treated with EDTA for hemoglobin and hematocrit determinations.

Due to logistic problems and improper blood conservation and transport, it was not possible to determine hemoglobin and perform anemia prevalence analysis. Therefore, the results reported in this study include hematocrit (determined in a microcentrifuge at the place of sampling), serum ferritin, folates, and retinol concentrations and the prevalence of iron, folates, and retinol deficiencies.

Serum samples were obtained by centrifugation of blood samples, within 4 hours of extraction. Serum was kept at $-30°C$ and protected from light until analysis.

Ferritin determinations were performed by an immunoenzymatic assay [14] developed and validated in our laboratory. Polystyrene microtiter plates were coated with monoclonal antibodies to human ferritin. In each assay, ferritin standards and unknown sera were added and incubated with the same monoclonal antibody conjugated with horseradish peroxidase. The amount of enzyme retained in each well was measured by adding o-phenylenediamine dihydrochloride (OPD) and H_2O_2, and the reaction stopped by adding sulfuric acid. The absorbance in each well was measured spectrophotometrically, and ferritin concentration was calculated from a standard curve.

Serum retinol was assayed by high-performance liquid chromatography (HPLC) according to the method of Chow and Omaye [15]. Briefly, 100 μL of serum were extracted with heptane containing BHT, dried under a nitrogen stream, and suspended in methanol for separation in an HPLC system (Waters corporation, Mildford MA) with a Bondapack C18 column (3.9×300 mm), using 100% methanol as mobile phase at 0.8 mL/min. Detection was carried at 296 nm and retinol concentrations were calculated from a standard curve using Empower software from Waters.

The microbiological method for the determination of serum folates was an adaptation by the Centers for Diseases Control and Prevention (Atlanta, USA) of the method described by O'Broin and Kelleher [16] and Molloy and Scott [17]. It was based in the folate-dependent growth of a strain of *Lactobacillus*. Serum samples and bacteria were diluted in a complete nutritive medium devoid of folates. The growing of the bacteria was dependent of the presence of folates in the sample and measured by the turbidity developed in the wells at 590 nm, comparing against a standard curve.

The cutoff points used were for iron deficiency, a serum ferritin level <10 μg/L [6], for vitamin A, deficiency was classified as severe when serum concentration was <10 μg/dL, and moderate if <20 μg/dL [18]. For folic acid deficiency, it was severe for serum concentrations below 6.7 nmol/L, and moderate between 6.7 and 13.2 nmol/L [10, 11].

2.3. Statistical Analysis. Samples were analyzed for hematocrit and serum concentrations of ferritin, folates, and retinol and expressed as mean ± SD and % of prevalence of the respective deficiency. The analysis of data by sex and geographic location was performed by ANOVA with Bonfer-

TABLE 1: Changes in anthropometric and hematological parameters in children before and after the intervention of nutritional education in schools from Aragua, Táchira, and Lara States, Venezuela. ($n = 427$).

	Before intervention	After intervention
Age (years)	8.68 ± 2.31	9.44 ± 2.44*
Weight (Kg)	28.47 ± 9.69	31.12 ± 12.11*
Height (cm)	127.49 ± 13.80	131.40 ± 15.88*
Hematocrit (%)	37.42 ± 3.32	38.57 ± 2.90*
Ferritin (μg/L)	18.04 ± 12.00	22.56 ± 15.82*
Serum retinol (μg/dL)	22.09 ± 6.61	20.73 ± 5.80
Serum folate (nmol/L)	11.74 ± 7.19	10.58 ± 8.80

* Statistically significant difference between before and after intervention ($P < .05$).

TABLE 2: Classification of children according to nutritional status, by combination of indexes before and after nutritional education intervention.

Categories*	Total	Before intervention		After intervention	
		n	%	n	%
Deficit	80	41	17.1	39	16.3
At risk of deficit	65	34	14,2	31	12.9
Normal	248	120	50.0	128	53.3
At risk of excess	18	12	5.0	6	2.5
Excess	69	33	13.7	36	15.0
Total	480	240	100	240	100

* The data was grouped according to presumptive diagnosis as deficit (lower than percentile 3), at risk of deficit (≥ percentile 3 and < percentile 10), normal (≥ percentile 10 and ≤ percentile 90), at risk of excess (> percentile 90 and ≤ percentile 97), and excess (> percentile 97).

roni as a posttest. For comparisons of groups before and after nutritional education intervention, paired *t*-test was used. Differences were considered as significantly different, when $P < .05$.

3. Results

Table 1 shows the anthropometric and hematological characteristics of the children studied. At the moment of inclusion in the protocol, the group presented normal ranges, although close to lower limits, of hematocrit, ferritin, and retinol concentrations. The mean concentration of folates was below the cutoff point of 13.2 nmol/L, indicating a moderate folate deficiency in the population studied. The table also shows that after the nutritional education intervention, all parameters analyzed, except for retinol and folates, increased significantly ($P < .05$).

When classifying children according to their nutritional status before and after intervention, the percentages diminished for deficit (from 17.1 to 16.3%), at risk of deficit (from 14.2 to 12.9%), and at risk of excess categories (from 5.0 to 2.5%), while the excess category increased from 13.7% to 15.0% (Table 2). Some of the children classified as at risk of excess and excess after the intervention were in reality

TABLE 3: Changes in ferritin, retinol, and folate concentrations in children before and after the intervention of nutritional education in schools from Aragua, Táchira, and Lara States, Venezuela. Classification by State of precedence.

	n	Ferritin (μg/L)		Serum retinol μg/dL		Serum folate nmol/L	
		Before intervention	After intervention	Before intervention	After intervention	Before intervention	After intervention
Aragua	69	12.00 ± 10.17[a]	24.33 ± 18.34*	20.66 ± 6.72[a,b]	17.17 ± 3.69[a]	7.43 ± 4.99	10.34 ± 8.90[a,b]
Táchira	179	21.06 ± 12.81[b]	23.60 ± 16.48	23.72 ± 5.95[b]	22.45 ± 5.88[b]	12.99 ± 7.24	12.16 ± 9.29[b]
Lara	179	16.52 ± 10.62[a,b]	20.88 ± 13.90	20.50 ± 6.91[a]	20.48 ± 5.74[b]	11.21 ± 9.35	9.19 ± 8.07[a]
Total	427	**16.53 ± 13.17**	**22.94 ± 16.24***	**21.66 ± 6.64**	**20.09 ± 5.10**	**10.54 ± 7.19**	**10.56 ± 8.75**

* Statistically significant difference between before and after intervention ($P < .05$).
[a]Different superscript letters, statistically different between states ($P < .05$).

children with chronic undernutrition in process of weight recovery, but with a chronically diminished height.

There were no differences in the percentages of excess and deficit between the 3 states studied, and according to the 24 h food recall questionnaires, the diets were hypocaloric, with low consumption of fruit and vegetables, high consumption of soft drinks and snacks and low or no physical activity. Red meat was the main source of heme iron consumed by 57% of the children (54 g/day). Consumption of soft drinks and natural fruit juices was similar (47%), and coffee and tea was consumed by 22% of the sample. After intervention, there was a slight improvement in fruit consumption, based on the 24 h food recall questionnaires.

The intervention of nutritional education produced a significant increase in hematocrit and ferritin concentration, while retinol and folate concentrations showed no significant changes. There were also no significant differences by gender, and as shown in Table 3, when distributed by state, children from Táchira presented a better nutritional condition in terms of hematocrit (data not shown), ferritin, retinol, and folates status than children from Lara. Children from Aragua State showed no difference compared to Táchira or Lara, probably as a consequence of the smaller sample size.

The prevalence of iron deficiency was 25% at the beginning of the study and was significantly reduced to 14.3% after the intervention (Figure 1). The prevalence of severe and moderate folate deficiencies affected 39% and 36% of the sample, respectively, to reach approximately 75% of the sample being affected by some degree of folate deficiency. This degree of prevalence was not affected by the nutritional education intervention. The prevalence of serum retinol deficiency was severe in less than 3% of the cases, but moderate deficiency affected more than 40% of children. As with folates, retinol levels were not significantly affected by the intervention.

4. Discussion

The results presented in this work show a high incidence of micronutrient deficiencies in scholars from 17 schools located in 3 noncontiguous states of Venezuela, which could be indicating a problem of hidden hunger, since anthropometrical parameters were within normal ranges.

There was high prevalence of iron, folates, and vitamin A deficiencies in children and adolescents. The prevalence

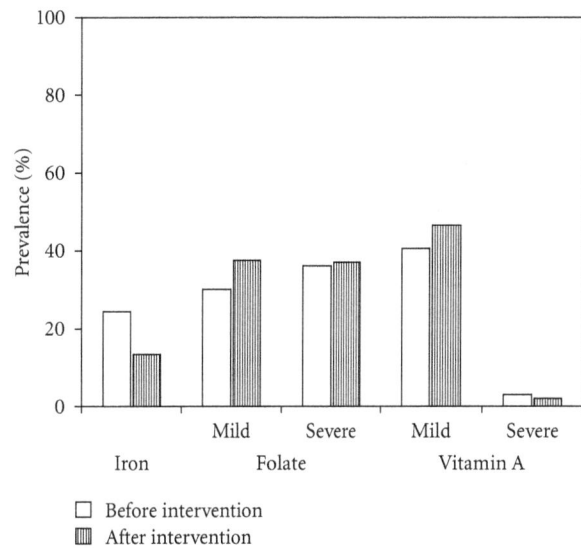

FIGURE 1: Prevalence of iron, folate, and vitamin A deficiencies in children, before and after the intervention of nutritional education in schools from Aragua, Táchira, and Lara States, Venezuela. (n = 427).

of severe folic acid deficiency affected 39% of the sample and requires immediate action, which can be achieved by a supplementation program in schools. The situation of this vitamin in Venezuela has been previously reported [10, 11], and at this point it probably could be better combated by a combined strategy, consisting in supplementation, food fortification, and nutritional education in a first stage.

The prevalence of moderate vitamin A deficiency affected 40% of the sample. If this data were extrapolated to general population, this would constitute an important Public Health problem. Regarding iron deficiency, the prevalence was 25% at the beginning of the study, a percentage similar to previously reported data for these age groups [5]. Unfortunately, due to the problems with blood and the impossibility to obtain reliable results on hemoglobin concentrations, we were unable to determine if the intervention had effects on anemia prevalence. However, a very reliable indicator of red cell volume, hematocrit, was significantly increased after the nutritional education program.

The most efficacious strategies to combat nutritional deficiencies are food fortification and supplementation programs, although it is generally recognized that nutritional education should always accompany those initiatives and also that education is the most fundamental and permanent strategy to achieve changes in food habits and to obtain a balanced nutrition that includes all the required nutrients during the different life stages [19]. However, it has been pointed out that the success of educative programs is dependent on the enthusiasm and commitment of teachers to include the suggested strategies and also of their interest in master the knowledge required and the time to implement those new contents [20].

Limitations of educational campaigns include a non-immediate, long-term effect or impact as well as a limited penetration that does not guarantee complete access or coverage [21]. Also, the impact of educational interventions is usually measured by tests that evaluate if the children received and understood the message [19, 22]. The reports in the literature about measuring biochemical parameters to evaluate the impact of a nutritional education intervention are scarce, but these evaluations are a direct measure that "the message was received, understood and put into practice," a conduct that probably would benefit not only the child or the person receiving the information, but also the whole family group.

The analysis of the impact of the nutritional intervention performed was measured not only by direct observation and supervision of activities and games, where teachers and pupils could demonstrate the acquisition of the knowledge, but also by the significant reduction in iron deficiency prevalence, measured as serum ferritin, after the intervention. There were, however, no changes in serum retinol and folate concentrations, both nutrients with high prevalence of deficiency. The lack of effect on those 2 nutrients could be due, in part, to the fact that the intervention was focused on iron and iron rich foods sources. Also, the limited access to food of animal origin and the low vegetable and fruits consumption could account for the lack of effect observed. In this group, precooked corn flour (fortified with iron) was the most consumed food (2 corn breads called "arepas" per day, 100 g/day) and constituted 96% of the iron in the diet, followed by grains. Furthermore, consumption of performed vitamin A, which should come from animal sources, was limited in this group, as well as a provitamin A carotenoids, also a good source of folates.

This study shows, through biochemical determinations, that nutritional education initiatives have an impact improving nutritional health in children. However, the permanence in time of such habit modifications that assure the maintenance of the biochemical changes achieved requires more ample interventions that involve the whole community, as well as the treatment of other external factors that affect the appearance of nutritional deficiencies [3, 20].

The combination of strategies (education, supplementation, and/or food fortification) is probably the most effective approach to combat micronutrient deficiencies, especially severe deficiencies as in the case of folic acid in this study. It would be desirable to perform strategies in nutritional education at school level, with measuring the impact through biochemical variables at the family group level. Also, existing educational campaigns should be reinforced to encourage consumption of vegetables, fruits, and other sources of folates and vitamin A.

Conflict of Interests

They also declare that they have no conflicto of interests.

Acknowledgments

Authors are thankful to children, teachers, and parents that agreed to participate in this study. The study was partially funded by NUTRIR Project (Nestlé of Venezuela SA).

References

[1] S. Olivares, C. Morón, I. Zacarías, M. Andrade, and F. Vio, "Educación en nutrición en las escuelas básicas de Chile," Food, Nutrition and Agriculture, vol. 33, pp. 64–69, 2003.

[2] E. Patino, "Educación nutricional y participación; claves del éxito en la nutrición comunitaria," Anales Venezolanos de Nutrición, vol. 18, no. 1, pp. 134–137, 2005.

[3] Y. Manios, A. Kafatos, I. Apostolaki et al., "Health and nutrition education in primary schools in Crete: 10 years' follow-up of serum lipids, physical activity and macronutrient intake," British Journal of Nutrition, vol. 95, no. 3, pp. 568–575, 2006.

[4] E. De Caballero, O. Sinisterra, F. Lagrutta, and E. Atalah, "Evaluación del impacto nutricional del programa de alimen-tación complementaria de Panamá en niños menores de 5 años," Archivos Latinoamericanos de Nutrición, vol. 54, no. 1, pp. 66–71, 2004.

[5] M. N. García-Casal, "La deficiencia de hierro como problema de salud pública. (Iron deficiency as a Public Health problem)," Anales Venezolanos de Nutrición, vol. 18, no. 1, pp. 45–48, 2005.

[6] World Health Organization, WHO, "Worldwide prevalence of anaemia 1993–2005," WHO Global Database on anemia, 2008, http://whqlibdoc.who.int/publications/2008/9789241596657_eng.pdf.

[7] J. De Abreu, S. Borno, M. Montilla, and E. Dini, "Anemia y deficiencia de vitamina A en niños evaluados en un centro de atención nutricional de Caracas.," Archivos Latinoamericanos de Nutrición, vol. 55, no. 3, pp. 226–234, 2005.

[8] S. I. Del Real, A. S. Jaeger, M. A. Barón et al., "Estado nutricional en niños preescolares que asisten a un jardín de infancia público en Valencia, Venezuela," Archivos Latinoamericanos de Nutrición, vol. 57, no. 3, pp. 248–254, 2007.

[9] J. Y. Leal, H. V. Castejón, T. Romero et al., "Interferón-gamma e interleucina-10 sérica en niños anémicos con deficiencia de vitamina A," Archivos Latinoamericanos de Nutrición, vol. 56, no. 4, pp. 329–334, 2006.

[10] M. N. García-Casal, M. Jiménez, C. Osorio et al., "Acido fólico y vitamina B12 en niños, adolescentes y mujeres embarazadas en Venezuela," Anales Venezolanos de Nutrición, vol. 18, no. 3, pp. 145–154, 2005.

[11] T. Suárez, M. Torrealba, N. Villegas, C. Osorio, and M. N. García-Casal, "Deficiencias de hierro, ácido fólico y vitamina B12 en relación a anemia, en adolescentes de una zona con alta incidencia de malformaciones congénitas en Venezuela.," Archivos Latinoamericanos de Nutrición, vol. 55, no. 2, pp. 118–123, 2005.

[12] C. Jiménez, I. Leets, R. Puche et al., "A single dose of vitamin A improves haemoglobin concentration, retinol status and phagocytic function of neutrophils in preschool children," *British Journal of Nutrition*, vol. 103, no. 6, pp. 798–802, 2010.

[13] D. Amaya-Castellanos, H. Viloria-Castejón, P. Ortega et al., "Deficiencia de vitamina A y estado nutricional antropométrico en niños marginales urbanos y rurales en el Estado Zulia, Venezuela," *Investigacion Clinica*, vol. 43, no. 2, pp. 89–105, 2002.

[14] C. A. Flowers, M. Kuizon, and J. L. Beard, "A serum ferritin assay for prevalence studies of iron deficiency," *American Journal of Hematology*, vol. 23, no. 2, pp. 141–151, 1986.

[15] F. I. Chow and S. T. Omaye, "Use of antioxidants in the analysis of vitamins A and E in mammalian plasma by high performance liquid chromatography," *Lipids*, vol. 18, no. 11, pp. 837–841, 1983.

[16] S. O'Broin and B. Kelleher, "Microbiological assay on microtitre plates of folate in serum and red cells," *Journal of Clinical Pathology*, vol. 45, no. 4, pp. 344–347, 1992.

[17] A. M. Molloy and J. M. Scott, "Microbiological assay for serum, plasma, and red cell folate using cryopreserved, microtiter plate method," *Methods in Enzymology*, vol. 281, pp. 43–53, 1997.

[18] A. Sommer and F. R. Davidson, "Assessment and control of vitamin A deficiency: the annecy accords," *Journal of Nutrition*, vol. 132, no. 9, pp. S2845–S2850, 2002.

[19] J. Kain, S. Olivares, A. M. Castillo, and D. F. Vio, "Validación y aplicación de instrumentos para evaluar intervenciones educativas en obesidad de escolares," *Revista Chilena de Pediatría*, vol. 72, no. 4, pp. 308–318, 2001.

[20] I. Kafatos, A. Peponaras, M. Linardakis, and A. Kafatos, "Nutrition education and Mediterranean diet: exploring the teaching process of a school-based nutrition and media education project in Cretan primary schools," *Public Health Nutrition*, vol. 7, no. 7, pp. 969–975, 2004.

[21] M. E. Pérez-Morales, M. Bacardí-Gascón, A. Jiménez-Cruz, and A. Armendáriz-Anguiano, "Intervenciones aleatorias controladas basadas en las escuelas para prevenir la obesidad infantil: revisión sistemática de 2006 a 2009," *Archivos Latinoamericanos de Nutrición*, vol. 59, no. 3, pp. 253–259, 2009.

[22] J. A. Kropski, P. H. Keckley, and G. L. Jensen, "School-based obesity prevention programs: an evidence-based review," *Obesity*, vol. 16, no. 5, pp. 1009–1018, 2008.

17

Nutrition and Iron Status of 1-Year Olds following a Revision in Infant Dietary Recommendations

Asa V. Thorisdottir,[1,2] Inga Thorsdottir,[1,2] and Gestur I. Palsson[3]

[1] Unit for Nutrition Research, Landspitali-The National University Hospital of Iceland, Eiríksgata 29, 101 Reykjavik, Iceland
[2] Faculty of Food Science and Nutrition, University of Iceland, 101 Reykjavik, Iceland
[3] Children's Hospital, Landspitali-The National University Hospital of Iceland, 101 Reykjavik, Iceland

Correspondence should be addressed to Inga Thorsdottir, ingathor@landspitali.is

Academic Editor: Bruno Annibale

A previous study showed low iron status in 12-month-old Icelandic infants associated most strongly with cow's milk intake and growth. Infant dietary recommendations were revised in 2003. This study investigated nutrition and iron status in a new infant cohort. *Subjects/Methods.* Randomly selected infants were prospectively investigated for diet, anthropometry, and iron status ($n = 110$–141). *Results.* Breastfeeding initiation rate was 98%; 38% of 5-month olds were exclusively and 20% of 12-month olds partially breastfed. Formula was given to 21% of 6-month olds and 64% of 12-month olds, but cow's milk to 2.5% and 54.4% of 6- and 12-month olds, respectively. Iron depletion (serum ferritin < 12 µg/L) affected 5.8%, 1.4% were also iron deficient (MCV < 74 fl), and none were anemic (Hb < 105 g/l). Iron status associated negatively with growth and breastfeeding duration and positively with meat and formula intake at 9–12 months, but not with cow's milk. *Conclusion.* Improved iron status might be explained by a shift from cow's milk to formula in the diet of Icelandic 6–12-month olds. Dietary changes altered associations between foods and iron status.

1. Introduction

Adequate iron status in infancy is important because of its effects on health and development [1]. Infants are especially susceptible to iron deficiency (ID) and iron deficiency anemia (IDA) because exogenous iron requirements increase rapidly during the second half of the first year due to high growth rate in infancy.

Iron status in infancy has been negatively associated with consumption of cow's milk [2, 3] and positively with meat intake [2, 4–6]. A prospective study on Icelandic infants in 1995–1997 also found these associations where 20% of 12-month-old Icelanders had ID (mean corpuscular volume (MCV) < 74 fl, serum ferritin (SF) < 12 µg/L), 2.7% had IDA (hemoglobin (Hb) < 105 g/L, MCV < 74 fl, SF < 12 µg/L), and 41% were iron-depleted (SF < 12 µg/L) [7]. The iron status of Icelandic infants was considerably worse compared to similar infant populations in the nineties in Denmark [2], Sweden [4], and Norway [8]. Iron-deficient 12-month olds

had been breastfed 2.5 months shorter than nondeficient infants, and a multiple regression analyses revealed that the effect on iron status was almost universally accounted for by intake of regular cow's milk at 9 and 12 months of age [7]. Higher growth velocity during the first year had an independent negative association with iron status at 1 year (y). Furthermore, low iron status was observed to negatively affect later growth and iron status [9] as well as motor developmental scores in 6-year olds in a developed affluent society such as Iceland [10].

In 2003 revised infant dietary recommendations were published in Iceland, where iron-fortified formula was recommended in the weaning period from six months of age [11]. The formula, Icelandic follow-on milk, was made available in every grocery shop ready-made in cartons at a fair price. Breastfeeding was emphasized more than before by adopting the World Health Organization (WHO) recommendation for exclusive breastfeeding until six months of age [12] instead of 4–6 months as recommended previously and also by encouraging partial breastfeeding, preferably until 1-year old or longer if it suits mother and child. Compared to regular cow's milk, the iron-fortified formula has higher iron (0.75 mg versus 0.023 mg/100 g) and lower protein (1.8 g versus 3.4 g/100 g) concentration and is complemented with other nutrients such as vitamin C (9 mg/100 g) [13] to fulfill the Codex Alimentarius, Regulation no. 735/1997 [14]. The iron content is modest and in accordance with other milk-based formulas supporting normal growth and iron status of healthy infants [15]. The revised recommendations are provided to all parents of newborns by healthcare professionals at healthcare centers. Fortification is thought to be the most effective strategy to combat nutritional deficiencies, but nutrition education interventions are also effective in improving iron status in children [16] as well as screening for iron deficiencies in more vulnerable populations [17].

The objective of this study was to investigate a prospective cohort of 12-month olds, where data collection occurred after implementation of the revised infant dietary recommendations, to evaluate iron status and its association with diet and growth. Moreover, we aim to assess the impact of the revised recommendations on infants' food and nutrient intake and iron status.

2. Subjects and Methods

2.1. Sample Recruitment. A random sample of 250 Icelandic infants born in 2005, from January to December, was collected by Statistics Iceland. The criteria for participation were the same as in the former prospective study on infant nutrition 1995–1997 [7]. The criteria were Icelandic parents, singleton birth, gestational length of 37–41 weeks, birth weight within the 10th–90th percentiles, no birth defects or congenital long-term diseases, and the mother had early and regular antenatal care. Eligible participants were 196. Informed written consent from the parents was obtained, and all individual information was processed with strict confidentiality. The study was approved by the National Bioethical Committee in Iceland (VSNb2005040019/037) and registered at the Icelandic Data Protection Authority (S2449/2005).

2.2. Dietary Assessment. Dietary data from 0–4 months of age was collected by dietary-history, including questions on breastfeeding, infant formula-feeding, other food items, and supplements. Food records were filled out monthly by the parents. Weighed food records were kept for three consecutive days (72 hours) at 9 and 12 months. All food was weighed on accurate electronic scales (PHILIPS HR 2385, Hungary; ±1 g accuracy). The breastfed infants were weighed with the same clothes before and after each breastfeeding session (Tanita model 1583, Japan or Sega model 336 7021099, Germany; both with ±10 g accuracy) to estimate the amount of breast-milk consumed as formerly described [18]. A nutrient calculation program, ICEFOOD, was used to calculate the weighed food records [19]. At 5–8 and 10-11 months of age intake was estimated by 24-hour food recall using common household measures, such as cups and spoons.

2.3. Biochemical Analysis and Anthropometric Measures. At 12 months of age blood samples were obtained for analyzing iron status. Hb, MCV, and SF were analyzed on the Coulter Counter STKS at Landspitali-The National University Hospital of Iceland. The definition for IDA includes all three indicators below cutoff points, Hb < 105 g/L, MCV < 74 fl, and SF < 12 µg/L, for ID the two latter indicators are below cutoff points and iron depletion as having SF < 12 µg/L [2, 7, 20, 21]. Anthropometry, that is, weight, length, and head circumference at birth, 1, 2, 3, 5, 6, 8, 10, and 12 months, was recorded at maternity wards and healthcare centers.

2.4. Statistical Analysis. Statistical analyses were performed with SPSS software (version 17; SPSS INC, Chicago, IL). Descriptive statistics were used for the participants' characteristics and food and nutrient intake, presented as mean and standard deviation (SD) for normally distributed variables and median with interquartile range (IQR) for skewed variables. For comparison between two groups, independent t-test, Mann-Whitney U test, or chi-square was used.

To identify predictors of the infants' iron status indices (Hb, SF, and MCV) multivariate regression models were constructed. Variables which differed between iron-depleted infants and non-iron-depleted infants were used in the model for SF. Because of skewed distribution, SF was logarithmically transformed. The model for each iron status index also included their correlating variables (Pearson's correlation coefficient), and for interrelated variables those with the weakest correlation to each iron status index were excluded from the model. Birth weight was adjusted for in the models. The sample size of 200, expecting 30% dropout, gives a power of 90% to detect the effect of 100 g weight gain on SF. To detect difference in iron status between the former (1995–1997) and current (2005–2007) cohorts the power was >90%. The level of significance in the study was $P \leq .05$.

3. Results

3.1. Study Group. A total of 141 infants (73 boys and 68 girls) participated in the study, 72% of the 196 eligible participants. The characteristics of the subjects and their parents are presented in Table 1. Dropouts did not differ significantly from participants in basic values, that is, size at birth, 3698.8 (340.6) g versus 3781.3 (368.2) g ($P = .078$), and exclusive breastfeeding duration, 3.2 (1.8) months versus 3.54 (1.8) months ($P = .073$). Characteristics, iron status and anthropometry, did not differ between children with complete ($n = 110$) and incomplete ($n = 31$) dietary data, that is, Hb values 120.4 (7.7) g/L versus 121.3 (9.8) g/L ($P = .658$), SF values 36.6 (22.1) µg/L versus 35.1 (19.7) µg/L ($P = .802$), or weight at 12 months 10038.5 (1018.4) g versus 10229.8 (1125.5) g ($P = .413$).

3.2. Diet and Nutrient Intake. In the present study 97.8% of mothers initiated breastfeeding and 38.1% of 5-month olds and 7.2% of 6-month olds were exclusively breastfed and 20.0% were still partially breastfed at 12 months of age.

TABLE 1: Infant and parental characteristics of the subjects.

Variable	Boys Mean (SD)	Girls Mean (SD)
No. of subjects [n (%)]	73 (51.8)	68 (48.2)
Infant characteristics		
Firstborn [n (%)]	20 (30.3)	24 (35.8)
Birth weight (g)	3807 (360)	3750 (369)
Birth length (cm)	52.2 (1.52)	51.7 (1.77)
Birth head circumference (cm)	36.2 (1.22)	35.4 (1.14)*
Weight at 6 mo (kg)	8.4 (0.7)	7.9 (0.75)*
Length at 6 mo (cm)	70.1 (1.7)	67.9 (1.7)*
Weight at 12 mo (kg)	10.37 (1.0)	9.76 (0.99)*
Length at 12 mo (cm)	78.0 (2.25)	76.17 (2.60)*
Hb at 12 mo (g/L)	120.96 (8.19)	120.28 (8.28)
MCV at 12 mo (fl)	76.71 (3.41)	77.69 (3.09)
log SF at 12 mo (μg/L)	3.31 (0.63)	3.57 (0.46)*
Parental and socioeconomic characteristics		
Mother's BMI (kg/m^2)	24.3 (6.09)	24.6 (5.38)
Father's BMI (kg/m^2)	26.4 (4.14)	25.1 (5.60)
Mother's age (years)	32.0 (5.25)	30.3 (4.58)
Father's age (years)	34.1 (6.13)	33.4 (5.22)
Mother's ≥12 y of schooling [n (%)]	56 (82.4)	57 (86.4)
Father's ≥12 y of schooling [n (%)]	51 (77.3)	51 (78.5)
Smoker in the household [n (%)]	14 (21.5)	13 (20)
Reside in capital and surroundings [n (%)]	60 (62.5)	60 (60)
Marital status (married/partnership) [n (%)]	63 (96.9)	62 (98.4)

* Significantly different from boys. $P \leq 0.05$ (indepedent t-test).
† Median and interquartile range (IQR).

Average food intake was similar among boys and girls, except for milk consumption (Table 2). A higher proportion of boys were exclusively breastfed at 6 months and partially at 12 months of age. A higher proportion of girls received formula at 9 and 12 months of age but consumption of regular cow's milk did not differ between the genders (Table 2). The mean (SD) intake of formula for 9–12-month olds was 156 (14.9) g/day and only 43 (9.2) g/day for regular cow's milk. Vitamin D supplementation was higher among boys than girls at 6 months of age, 60.2% among boys versus 48.1% among girls ($P = .051$). Fruit consumption was more common than vegetable consumption among 5–8-month olds, 85% or more of 6–8-month olds consumed porridge, and dairy product consumption (excluding drinking milk or formula) was modest; 1.2% of 5-month olds and 26.8% of 8-month olds consumed dairy products of some sort. The average energy intake among the subjects was close to the estimated average daily requirements (kJ/kg of body weight). The protein intake, however, exceeded the recommendations for this age group (Table 3). Nutrient intake did not differ significantly between boys and girls except for vitamin A intake at 12 months of age, which was higher for girls.

3.3. Iron Status and Associations with Diet, Growth, and Socio-demographic Factors. There were no children with IDA. ID affected 1.4% ($n = 2$) of the children, and 5.8% ($n = 8$) of the

children were iron depleted. No significant gender difference was found on MCV and Hb, but girls had significantly higher SF level, 39.2 (17.5) μg/L, compared to, 33.5 (24.6) μg/L, boys ($P = .003$).

Iron-depleted infants had lower birth weight, 3402 (255.8) g versus 3805 (361.7) g ($P = .002$), and higher growth rate than non-iron-depleted ones. Comparing iron-depleted and non-iron-depleted infants, proportional weight gain was 2.04 (0.25) versus 1.66 (0.34) ($P = .003$), absolute weight gain 4.8 (0.6) kg versus 4.3 (0.8) kg ($P = .043$) from 0 to 6 months, and 6.9 (0.8) kg versus 6.3 (1) kg ($P = .061$) from 0 to 12 months, and length growth from 0 to 12 months was 18.5 (0.82) cm versus 17.0 (1.9) cm ($P = .028$). The iron-depleted infants had longer breastfeeding duration, 9.4 (3.5) months versus 7.6 (3.3) months, although not significant, and consumed less formula, 10.5 (16.3) g/day versus 133.0 (159.9) g/day at 9 months ($P = .038$) and 33.5 (47.2) g/day versus 187.3 (199.9) g/day at 12 months ($P = .044$). Dietary vitamin and mineral intake did however, not differ significantly between iron-depleted and non-iron-depleted infants.

SF level associated negatively with growth variables in infancy, but positively with birth weight. For growth from 0 to 12 months of age proportional weight gain (which takes birth weight into account) and absolute length gain correlated most negatively with SF level. For growth from 0 to

TABLE 2: Intake of selected foods among boys and girls at 6, 9, and 12 months of age ($n = 141$ at 6 months, $n = 122$ at 9 months, and $n = 110$ at 12 months).

	Boys		Girls	
	%	Mean (SD) g/day	%	Mean (SD) g/day
6 months				
Partial breastfeeding	77.9		71.6	
Exclusive breastfeeding	11.1		3	
Iron fortified formula	21.9		19.8	
Whole milk	3.3		1.7	
9 months				
Iron-fortified formula	59.7	44.2 (243.7)*	68.3	48.8 (173.0)*
Whole milk	33.9	0 (14.7)*	36.7	0 (27.5)*
Breast milk[†]	50	21.7 (287.6)*	50	6.5 (297.5)*
Fruit & vegetables[‡]	100	99.0 (61.5)	98.3	89.5 (48.2)
Porridge	77.4	31.6 (33.1)	85	30.2 (26.0)
Dairy products[§]	50	2.9 (56.5)*	55	3.8 (58.3)*
Meat	79	8.2 (21)*	70	10.0 (26.9)*
12 months				
Iron-fortified formula	53.4	56.2 (222.6)*	75	212.9 (193.3)[‖]
Whole milk	56.9	11.8 (67.7)*	51.9	6.7 (51.3)*
Breast milk[†]	26.5	0 (25.3)*	13.4	0 (0)[1,5]
Fruits & vegetables[‡]	100	83.7 (51.3)	94.2	71.65 (46.2)
Porridge	82.8	78.6 (79.9)	92.3	93.0 (83.7)
Dairy products[§]	72.4	78.5 (81.1)	90.4	90.3 (69.7)
Meat	100	39.4 (39.5)	94.2	30.0 (26.3)

* Median and interquartile range (IQR).
[†] Mean values include nonbreastfed infants.
[‡] The food group includes infant purees and fresh fruits and vegetables. Percentage represents infants receiving either fruits or vegetables.
[§] Dairy products are milk products and cheese, excluding drinking milk.
[‖] Significantly different from boys (Mann Whitney U test; $P \leq 0.05$).

6 months weight gain correlated most negatively with SF, but growth from 6 to 12 months did not correlate significantly with the variable. After adjusting for birth weight multiple regression analysis showed that log SF level in boys decreased $0.0201\,\mu g/L$ for each 100 g of weight gain from 0 to 6 months, $0.0174\,\mu g/L$ for each 100 g of weight gain from 0 to 12 months and $0.0823\,\mu g/L$ for each cm of length gain from 0 to 12 months (Table 4). In girls, iron-fortified formula, porridge (positive), and bread (negative) consumption associated independently with log SF level after adjusting for birth weight (Table 4).

Hb level had weaker associations with growth variables (positive) than SF level. In boys Hb associated most positively with dietary iron and meat consumption and most negatively with breastfeeding duration; formula had a weaker but significant association with Hb (positive). In girls fruits and dairy products were most strongly independently associated with Hb level (Table 4). Hb level was lower in infants exclusively breastfed for 5 months or longer than in those exclusively breastfed for less than 5 months (118.6 g/L versus 121.6 g/L, $P = .034$). Exclusive breastfeeding was excluded from the regression model because partial breastfeeding duration was a stronger predictor of Hb level, and the two variables were strongly intercorrelated.

MCV did not associate with any growth variable. In boys the only variable associated independently with MCV, of borderline significance, was breastfeeding duration (negative). In girls MCV level associated most positively with dietary iron intake and a weaker association was found with dietary vitamin C intake.

No associations were found between iron status indices and sociodemographic variables, that is, habitation, parents' education, age, BMI, or smoking habits.

4. Discussion

The present study describes nutrition and iron status in well-nourished infants with low prevalence of ID and IDA, high birth weight, and breastfeeding rate. Dietary intake in infancy has changed towards the infant dietary recommendations, revised in 2003, and iron status has improved when compared to results from an earlier prospective study of a comparable nationwide cohort. Breastfeeding has increased but the main alteration in the diet is an iron-fortified formula which has replaced regular cow's milk in the latter half of the first year. The altered diet seems to have deleted cow's milk as the main variable influencing serum ferritin and iron status. The formula was developed from domestic cow's

TABLE 3: Intake of selected nutrients among boys and girls at 9 and 12 months of age as an average intake over a 3-day period ($n = 122$ at 9 months and $n = 110$ at 12 months).

	Boys	Girls	
	Mean (SD)	Mean (SD)	
9 months			RDI (6–11 mo)
Energy (kJ/kg)	344.7 (82.4)	349.4 (83.6)	355
Protein (g/kg)	2.63 (0.89)	2.46 (0.87)	1.1
Vitamin C (mg/d)	67.2 (32.3)	71.6 (28.3)	20
Vitamin D (μg/d)	9.7 (6.2)	9.4 (9.9)*	10
Vitamin A (RJ/d)	854.9 (678.1)*	947.6 (584.6)	300
Zinc (mg/d)	3.32 (1.78)	3.23 (1.42)	5
Iron (mg/d)	6.28 (3.19)	6.27 (2.73)	8
Calcium (mg/d)	510.8 (242.2)	488.2 (212.7)	540
12 months			RDI (12–23 mo)
Energy (kJ/kg)	351.1 (74.7)	353.8 (80.4)	355
Protein (g/kg)	3.04 (0.99)*	3.03 (0.95)	1.0
Vitamin C (mg/d)	58.1 (25.0)	60.2 (32.1)	25
Vitamin D (μg/d)	9.1 (6.8)	8.3 (5.2)	10
Vitamin A (RJ/d)	785.3 (999.0)*	768.8 (492.1)[†]	300
Zinc (mg/d)	3.91 (2.01)	2.86 (2.28)*	5
Iron (mg/d)	6.82 (3.97)	5.77 (1.97)*	8
Calcium (mg/d)	565.2 (238.6)	576.0 (186.3)	600

* Median and interquartile range (IQR).
[†] Significantly different from boys (Mann Whitney U test; $P \le 0.05$).

milk to diminish the change for the infants' population as Icelandic cow's milk has some characteristics different from major brands [22]. Calculated nutrient intake showed that mean intake of iron, zinc, and calcium was below RDI. However, iron status was acceptable irrespective of the low iron intake. This may partially be explained by incomplete nutrient information in the database, such as for organic infant porridges which were commonly consumed by the study population. The RDI is estimated to meet the needs of 97.5% of the total population and RDI for zinc and calcium is extrapolated from the adult RDI, which can result in unnecessarily high recommendations for infants. Therefore the risk of deficiency might be small. However, further studies are needed on young children's vitamin and mineral status.

In comparison with the former study on infant nutrition (1995–1997), iron status of 12-month-old Icelandic infants has improved significantly (Figure 1). The prevalence of ID decreased from 20% to 1.4%, iron depletion from 41% to 5.8%, and IDA from 2.7% to 0. The participants in the two studies were nationwide random samples of healthy term infants and analogous with respect to sociodemographic factors, that is, habitation, number of siblings, parents' age, and education [7], and therefore comparable. Iron status in the 1995–1997 infant study was worse than in the neighboring countries [7] but according to the latest data from the Scandinavian countries there seems to be a lower prevalence of ID infants in Iceland than in the other Nordic countries. In a Swedish and a Norwegian study 18% and 10% of 12-month-old infants, respectively, were iron depleted

(SF $< 12\,\mu$g/L) [4, 8], compared with 5.8% in the 2005–2007 infant cohort now presented. In the present study the threshold for Hb level was 105 g/L and for MCV it was 74 fl, as it was also used in the previous Icelandic infant study and other Nordic studies for this age group [2, 7, 20, 21]. The thresholds for infants are, however, controversial, and the World Health Organization recommends the use of 110 g/L for Hb in children between the ages of 6 to 59 months and 79 fl for MCV in children between the ages of 1 to 1.9 years. Changing the thresholds for Hb and MCV in our cohorts towards WHO standards did not change the result or the conclusion of the study, the difference between the two cohorts was even larger.

In the present study the negative association between iron status and regular cow's milk seen in the 1995–1997 infant study had disappeared as the consumption had decreased and been replaced by the iron-fortified formula (Figure 2). Iron-fortified formula had a weak positive association with iron status. Breastfeeding rates have increased since the previous study, both partial and exclusive breastfeeding, but exclusive breastfeeding rates among 6-month olds are still low. That may partly be explained by the fact that the data for exclusive breastfeeding was collected from the recorded food intake at monthly birthdays. The value for exclusive breastfeeding among 5-month olds might therefore be more representative for exclusive breastfeeding rate for the first 6 months as the infants received complementary diet between the ages of 5 and 6 months. This has also been seen in other European countries with high initiation rates [23]. There are numerous benefits of long breastfeeding

TABLE 4: Multiple regression analysis of weight growth and food factors influencing change in iron status indices.

| Dependent variable At 12 months | Independent variable | Boys | | | Girls | | |
| | | | 95% Conf interval of B | | | 95% Conf interval of B | |
		B	Lower Bound	Upper Bound	B	Lower Bound	Upper Bound
Log SF	Length gain, cm (0–12 months)	−0.0823	−0.150	−0.014	—	—	—
	Weight gain, 100 g (0–6 months)	−0.0201	−0.040	−0.001	−0.0122	−0.027	0.003
	Weight gain, 100 g (0–12 months)	−0.0174	−0.032	−0.003	0.00454	−0.016	0.007
	Formula g/per day at 12 months	0.00077	−0.000062	0.0016	0.00077	0.00019	0.0014
	Porridge g/per day at 9 months	—	—	—	0.0124	0.002	0.023
	Bread g/per day at 9 months	—	—	—	−0.0113	−0.017	−0.005
Hb	Meat intake g/per day at 9 months	0.127	0.043	0.211	—	—	—
	Breastfeeding duration (mo)	−0.919	−1.473	−0.365	—	—	—
	Formula g/per day at 12 months	0.0145	0.004	0.025	—	—	—
	Fruit intake g/per day at 12 months	—	—	—	0.0384	0.009	0.068
	Dairy intake g/per day at 12 months	—	—	—	0.0319	0.003	0.061
	Iron intake mg/per day at 9 months	0.879	0.224	1.534	—	—	—
MCV	Breastfeeding duration (mo)	−0.261	−0.515	0.003	—	—	—
	Iron intake mg/per day at 12 months	—	—	—	0.297	0.061	0.534
	Vitamin C intake mg/per day at 9 months	—	—	—	0.0359	0.008	0.064

Adjusted for birth weight.
—No association found.

duration and it has even been associated with lower adiposity at 15 years of age [24]. Therefore, more attention has to be given to increase breastfeeding rates in accordance to WHO recommendations [12]. In the present study partial breastfeeding duration was negatively associated with both Hb and MCV in boys, and exclusive breastfeeding for 5 months or longer was also associated with lower Hb level, although within the normal range, this might support the suggestion about reconsideration of the optimal length of exclusive breastfeeding [25]. In the previous Icelandic study, longer duration of breastfeeding was positively associated with iron status. This can be explained by the change in the total diet. The main substitute for breast-milk in the previous study was regular cow's milk, but in the present study it was iron-fortified formula. Furthermore, low iron content of breast-milk and an insufficient additional source of iron in the diet have been shown to affect iron status negatively [26, 27]. Iron concentration of breast-milk has though been suggested to increase during the weaning period

[28]. The breast-milk as such does not seem to be the important component in this context but the total diet; sufficient iron intake from the complementary diet and the substitute for breastfeeding, that is, milk or formula, are the most important factors for good iron status in infancy.

Meat consumption was most strongly independently associated with Hb in the present study's multiple regression analysis. This association is consistent with the 1995–1997 study, and meat consumption did not differ between the two studies. Meat is an important source of iron and a known enhancer of good iron status [4–6], and it apparently affects iron status even though meat consumption is very low in this age group.

Another factor negatively associated with iron status, which was consistent in both studies, was growth rate. In the present study, iron-depleted children had markedly faster weight and length gain than non-iron-depleted ones. This difference was also seen in the 1995–1997 study between iron-deficient children and non-iron-deficient ones [7].

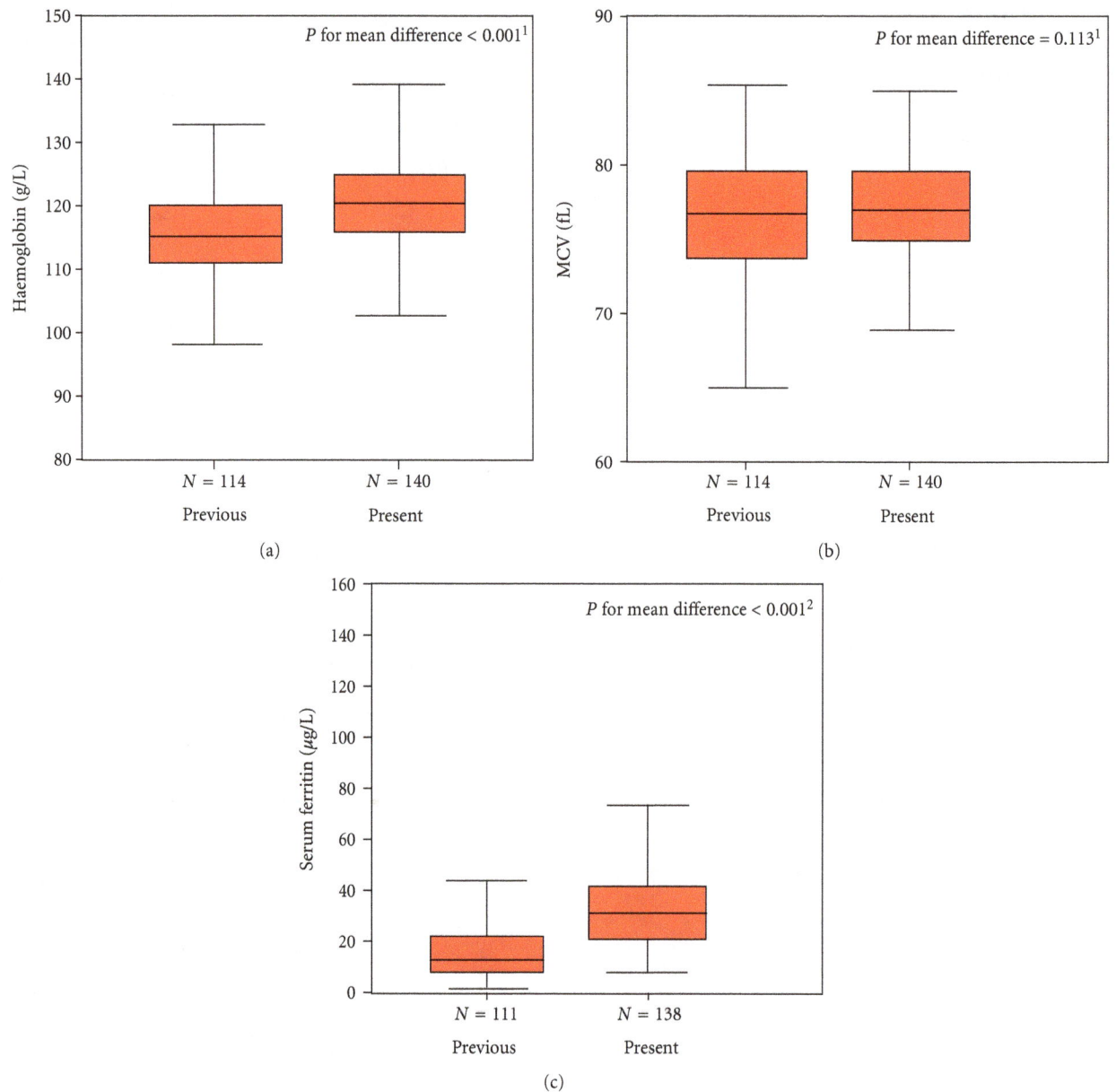

FIGURE 1: Box plots of iron status indices in 12-month olds, from previous (1995–1997) and present (2005–2007) studies. The box plots show the median, quartiles, maximum, and minimum values. Independent t-test was used for hemoglobin ($P = .001$), and MCV ($P = .113$), data were normally distributed and Mann-Whitney test for serum ferritin ($P = .001$) data were not normally distributed.

Furthermore, a study from the USA showed that 20% of overweight toddlers had ID versus 7% of normal-weight toddlers [29]. Faster growth during the first year has been proposed to affect iron status negatively [9] and BMI positively [30] at 6 years of age. This is probably attributed to the higher iron demands from a higher growth velocity [31]. Iron requirements are relatively the greatest during the rapid growth of infancy, especially from 6 months to 2 years of age, since full-term infants of non-iron-deficient mothers are born with sufficient iron storage to last for the first 4–6 months of life [18]. However, chronic iron deficiency over a long period has been shown to negatively affect growth in developing countries and some vulnerable

groups in developed countries [10, 32, 33]. Limitations to the present study might be the incomplete data set for 31 of the 141 participants and lack of information on iron status at birth. However, iron status or other measures such as anthropometry and social status did not differ between those with complete and incomplete dietary data sets. In healthy full-term infants of normal birth weight it is unlikely that iron status at birth is influencing the status at the age of 12 months. Thus these possible limits are unlikely to influence the results and conclusion of the present study.

Iron stores were worse among boys; their SF levels were significantly lower than in girls and 9.9% of boys were below the cut-off values versus 1.5% of girls, which can not

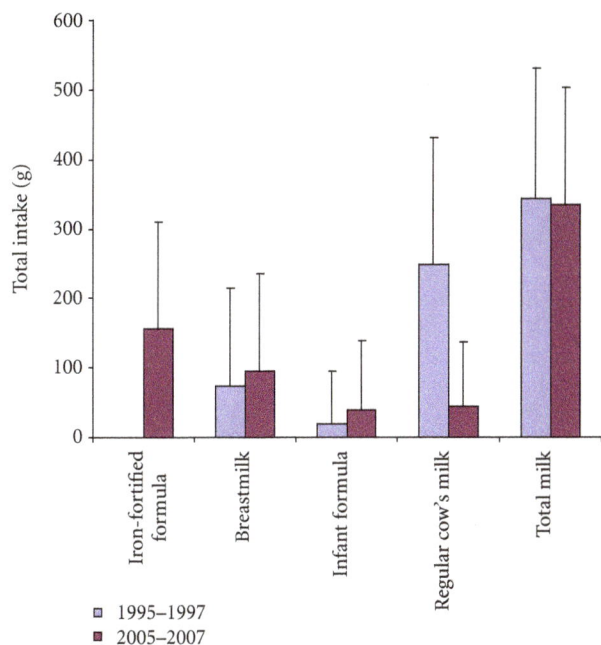

FIGURE 2: Difference in milk consumption between previous, (1995–1997) and present (2005–2007) studies, showed as mean and SD.

be attributed simply to differences in growth rate. Dietary factors and growth had more impact on iron status in boys than in girls (Table 4). A gender difference in SF level has also been seen in other studies, and Domellöf et al. concluded that it was possibly attributed to difference in iron metabolism because of hormonal differences between the sexes [34]. Furthermore, a higher proportion of boys were breastfed, and they had lower intake of iron-fortified formula at 12 months of age compared with girls in the present study, which might also partly explain the gender difference in iron status.

5. Conclusion

Iron status among 12-month-old Icelanders has improved enormously since the previous infant study. The largest alteration in the infants' diet between the two studies is the replacement of regular cow's milk by iron-fortified formula. The study demonstrates altered associations between iron status indices and food when the diet is changed. The lower intake of cow's milk deleted former association with ferritin. The association with duration of breastfeeding, although weak changed from being positive in the former cohort study to being negative in the present study. The effect of breastfeeding may mainly be derived from the other food used, that is, milk or formula, but not the breastfeeding as such. The findings also show the effect and importance of seeking solutions for public health problems with better dietary advice.

Conflict of Interests

The authors declare no conflict of interests.

Acknowledgments

This study was supported by the Icelandic Research Fund (050424031) and the Icelandic Research Fund for graduate students (080740008). The authors are most grateful to the participating children and their parents and to the two Master's students, Gudrun L. Gudmundsdottir and Ragnheidur Gudjonsdottir, for their assistance in collecting and analyzing data. They would also like to thank the staff at the Landspitali-The National University Hospital laboratories in Reykjavik, Iceland, for blood analysis.

References

[1] B. Lozoff, E. Jimenez, J. Hagen, E. Mollen, and A. W. Wolf, "Poorer behavioral and developmental outcome more than 10 years after treatment for iron deficiency in infancy," *Pediatrics*, vol. 105, no. 4, p. E51, 2000.

[2] K. F. Michaelsen, N. Milman, and G. Samuelson, "A longitudinal study of iron status in healthy Danish infants: effects of early iron status, growth velocity and dietary factors," *Acta Paediatrica*, vol. 84, no. 9, pp. 1035–1044, 1995.

[3] K. Dube, J. Schwartz, M. J. Mueller, H. Kalhoff, and M. Kersting, "Iron intake and iron status in breastfed infants during the first year of life," *Clinical Nutrition*, vol. 29, no. 6, pp. 773–778, 2010.

[4] I. Öhlund, T. Lind, A. Hörnell, and O. Hernell, "Predictors of iron status in well-nourished 4-y-old children," *American Journal of Clinical Nutrition*, vol. 87, no. 4, pp. 839–845, 2008.

[5] C. W. Fitch, M. S. Cannon, G. E. Seidel, and D. A. Krummel, "Dietary factors affecting iron status of children residing in rural West Virginia," *The West Virginia Medical Journal*, vol. 104, no. 3, pp. 19–22, 2008.

[6] C. W. Thane, C. M. Walmsley, C. J. Bates, A. Prentice, and T. J. Cole, "Risk factors for poor iron status in British toddlers: further analysis of data from the National Diet and Nutrition Survey of children aged 1.5–4.5 years," *Public Health Nutrition*, vol. 3, no. 4, pp. 433–440, 2000.

[7] I. Thorsdottir, B. S. Gunnarsson, H. Atladottir, K. F. Michaelsen, and G. Palsson, "Iron status at 12 months of age-effects of body size, growth and diet in a population with high birth weight," *European Journal of Clinical Nutrition*, vol. 57, no. 4, pp. 505–513, 2003.

[8] G. Hay, B. Sandstad, A. Whitelaw, and B. Borch-Iohnsen, "Iron status in a group of Norwegian children aged 6–24 months," *Acta Paediatrica*, vol. 93, no. 5, pp. 592–598, 2004.

[9] B. S. Gunnarsson, I. Thorsdottir, and G. Palsson, "Iron status in 6-y-old children: association with growth and earlier iron status," *European Journal of Clinical Nutrition*, vol. 59, no. 6, pp. 761–767, 2005.

[10] B. S. Gunnarsson, I. Thorsdottir, G. Palsson, and S. J. Gretarsson, "Iron status at 1 and 6 years versus developmental scores at 6 years in a well-nourished affluent population," *Acta Paediatrica*, vol. 96, no. 3, pp. 391–395, 2007.

[11] "The Icelandic nutrition council and centre for child health services," in *Icelandic Infant Nutrition Recommendation (IINR)*, The Icelandic Nutrition Council, Reykjavík, Iceland, 2003.

[12] World Health Organization, "Infant and young child nutrition. Global strategy on infant and young child feeding. Report by the Secretariat," in *Proceedings of the 55th World Health Assembly A55/15 Provisional Agenda Item 13.10 16*, World Health Organization, 2002.

[13] ISGEM, (The Icelandic Food Composition Database), 2008, http://www.matis.is/ISGEM/is/leit/.

[14] "Regulation on infant formulas and follow-on milk 735/1997," Ministry of the Interior, Reykjavík, Iceland, 1997, http://www.reglugerd.is.

[15] C. K. Bradley, L. Hillman, A. R. Sherman et al., "Evaluation of two iron-fortified, milk-based formulas during infancy," *Pediatrics*, vol. 91, no. 5, pp. 908–914, 1993.

[16] M. N. García-Casal, M. Landaeta-Jiménez, R. Puche et al., "A program of nutritional education in schools reduced the prevalence of iron deficiency in students," *Anemia*, vol. 2011, Article ID 284050, 6 pages, 2011.

[17] T. Hokama, C. Yogi, C. W. Binns, and A. H. Lee, "Community-based screening for infantile anemia in an Okinawan village, Japan," *Anemia*, vol. 2011, Article ID 278371, 3 pages, 2011.

[18] H. Atladottir and I. Thorsdottir, "Energy intake and growth of infants in Iceland," *European Journal of Clinical Nutrition*, vol. 54, no. 9, pp. 695–701, 2000.

[19] L. Steingrimsdottir, H. Thorgeirsdottir, and A. S. Olafsdottir, *The Diet of Icelanders. Dietary Survey, Main Findings* , The Icelandic Nutrition Council, Reykjavík, Iceland, 2003.

[20] M. A. Siimes, L. Salmenpera, and J. Perheentupa, "Exclusive breast-feeding for 9 months: risk of iron deficiency," *Journal of Pediatrics*, vol. 104, no. 2, pp. 196–199, 1984.

[21] D. G. Gill, S. Vincent, and D. S. Segal, "Follow-on formula in the prevention of iron deficiency: a multicentre study," *Acta Paediatrica*, vol. 86, no. 7, pp. 683–689, 1997.

[22] I. Thorsdottir, B. E. Birgisdottir, I. M. Johannsdottir et al., "Different β-casein fractions in icelandic versus Scandinavian cow's milk may influence diabetogenicity of cow's milk in infancy and explain low incidence of insulin-dependent diabetes mellitus in Iceland," *Pediatrics*, vol. 106, no. 4 I, pp. 719–724, 2000.

[23] A. Cattaneo, T. Burmaz, M. Arendt et al., "Protection, promotion and support of breast-feeding in Europe: progress from 2002 to 2007," *Public Health Nutrition*, vol. 13, no. 6, pp. 751–759, 2010.

[24] A. M. Grjibovski, B. Ehrenblad, and A. Yngve, "Infant feeding in Sweden: socio-demographic determinants and association with adiposity in childhood and adolescence," *International Breastfeeding Journal*, vol. 3, article 23, 2008.

[25] M. S. Fewtrell, J. B. Morgan, C. Duggan et al., "Optimal duration of exclusive breastfeeding: what is the evidence to support current recommendations?" *American Journal of Clinical Nutrition*, vol. 85, no. 2, pp. 635S–638S, 2007.

[26] R. J. Moy, "Prevalence, consequences and prevention of childhood nutritional iron deficiency: a child public health perspective," *Clinical and Laboratory Haematology*, vol. 28, no. 5, pp. 291–298, 2006.

[27] P. Oti-Boateng, R. Seshadri, S. Petrick, R. A. Gibson, and K. Simmer, "Iron status and dietary iron intake of 6–24-month-old children in Adelaide," *Journal of Paediatrics and Child Health*, vol. 34, no. 3, pp. 250–253, 1998.

[28] M. Domellöf, B. Lönnerdal, K. G. Dewey, R. J. Cohen, and O. Hernell, "Iron, zinc, and copper concentrations in breast milk are independent of maternal mineral status," *American Journal of Clinical Nutrition*, vol. 79, no. 1, pp. 111–115, 2004.

[29] J. M. Brotanek, J. Gosz, M. Weitzman, and G. Flores, "Iron deficiency in early childhood in the United States: risk factors and racial/ethnic disparities," *Pediatrics*, vol. 120, no. 3, pp. 568–575, 2007.

[30] I. Gunnarsdottir and I. Thorsdottir, "Relationship between growth and feeding in infancy and body mass index at the age of 6 years," *International Journal of Obesity and Related Metabolic Disorders*, vol. 27, no. 12, pp. 1523–1527, 2003.

[31] K. F. Michaelsen, "Nutrition and growth during infancy. The Copenhagen cohort study," *Acta Paediatrica*, vol. 420, no. 420, supplement, pp. 1–36, 1997.

[32] J. M. Schneider, M. L. Fujii, C. L. Lamp, B. Lönnerdal, K. G. Dewey, and S. Zidenberg-Cherr, "The use of multiple logistic regression to identify risk factors associated with anemia and iron deficiency in a convenience sample of 12–36-mo-old children from low income families," *American Journal of Clinical Nutrition*, vol. 87, no. 3, pp. 614–620, 2008.

[33] S. P. Walker, T. D. Wachs, J. M. Gardner et al., "Child development: risk factors for adverse outcomes in developing countries," *Lancet*, vol. 369, no. 9556, pp. 145–157, 2007.

[34] M. Domellöf, B. Lönnerdal, K. G. Dewey, R. J. Cohen, L. Landa Rivera, and O. Hernell, "Sex differences in iron status during infancy," *Pediatrics*, vol. 110, no. 3, pp. 545–552, 2002.

18

Frequency of Anemia and Iron Deficiency among Children Starting First Year of School Life and their Association with Weight and Height

Mirza Sultan Ahmad ⓘ, Hadia Farooq, Sumaira Noor Maham, Zonaira Qayyum, Abdul Waheed, and Waqar Nasir

Fazle Omar Hospital Rabwah, Chenab Nagar, Pakistan

Correspondence should be addressed to Mirza Sultan Ahmad; ahmadmirzasultan@gmail.com

Academic Editor: Aurelio Maggio

The objectives of the study were to ascertain frequency of anemia and iron deficiency among children starting first year of school life and test association with height and weight. One in four children starting first year of school life in five schools of Rabwah, Pakistan, was included. Full blood counts and ferritin levels of the children included in the study were checked. Status of their height and weight was determined according to Z-score charts. Chi-square test was used to test association. Two hundred and ninety-five children with median age of 67 months were included in the study. Out of 295, 240 (81.4%) had normal Hb and 55 (18.6%) had anemia. Ferritin levels were found to be below normal level in 242 (82%) children. There was no significant difference between hemoglobin and ferritin levels of children belonging to different categories of height and weight. Spearman test showed that there was very weak correlation between ferritin and hemoglobin levels (r_s = .163). Our conclusions were that iron deficiency without anemia is very frequent among children starting first year of school. Regression models show that ferritin levels cannot be predicted by independent variables like status of height and weight on Z-score charts, age, gender, and anemia.

1. Introduction

Iron deficiency is the commonest nutrient deficiency in the world and a major public health risk in both the developing and industrialized countries. It affects more than a billion people of different age groups around the world [1–4]. It is the commonest cause of anemia and is also a common deficiency among nonanemic children, especially among children of resource limited countries. A study by Ekwochi et al. showed that iron deficiency was present in 27.5% of nonanemic children under 5 [5]. Iron is necessary for healthy function and development of brain. There is evidence that its deficiency without anemia causes fatigue. It can affect visual and auditory functioning and is weakly associated with poor cognitive development in children [6–9].

This makes it important to study frequency of iron deficiency among children starting the first year of school.

Serum ferritin is the preferred initial diagnostic test for iron deficiency. It depicts the status of iron stores in body [10, 11]. The first year of school life is important because it is the start of academic career. Usually children start their school life at 5 years age. Like any other age group different nutritional problems are common at this age.

The objectives of this study were

(1) To ascertain the frequency of iron deficiency and anemia among the children starting first year of school

(2) To ascertain whether value of dependent variable, that is, ferritin, can be predicted based on independent variables like age, gender, anemia, status of height according to WHO (World Health Organization) Z-score charts, and status of weight according to WHO Z-score charts.

2. Methods

Five schools, belonging to the largest school system of the town, that is, Nazarat Taleem school system, out of a total of 11 schools providing primary level education in Rabwah were selected for this study. One in four children was selected by computer randomization. The children having fever and any sign or symptom of infectious disease or inflammation and the children receiving iron therapy were excluded from the study. Names of all children admitted in prep class (first year of school) were entered in software, and one in four children was selected by computer randomization. Five milliliter of the blood of the selected children was drawn for full blood count and ferritin levels. Full blood count (FBC) was checked by Medonic M 20 analyzer, and ferritin levels were checked by Elisa method (Statfox 200). Name, age in months, sex, hemoglobin levels (Hb), and ferritin levels were entered in a data form and pro forma. SPSS 20 was used for data analysis. For children below 5 years of age hemoglobin (Hb) level of <11.0 was categorized as anemia, and for children > 5 years of age Hb level <11.5 gm/dl was labeled as anemia. For children below 5 years of age ferritin levels below 12 ng/ml were labeled as low ferritin levels and for children above 5 years of age ferritin level <10 ng/ml was defined as low ferritin level. Those with both hemoglobin and ferritin levels below normal were categorized as having iron deficiency anemia.

Weight and height of these children were checked with a single combined height and weight scale of RE 160 type. These parameters were plotted on World Health Organization (WHO) Z-score charts for height and weight. WHO charts were used for male and female children of different ages included in this study: (i) Z-score weight for age chart for boys from birth to 5 years of age; (ii) Z-score weight for age chart for boys from 5 to 10 years; (iii) Z-score weight for age chart for girls from birth to 5 years; (iv) Z-score weight for age charts for girls from 5 to 10 years; (v) Z-score height for age chart for boys from birth to 5 years; (vi) Z-score height for age charts for boys from 5 to 19 years; (vii) Z-score height for age chart for girls from birth to 5 years; (viii) Z-score height for age chart for girls from 5 to 19 years. These charts were used to categorize weight for age and height for age and sex of the children. According to weight for age children were divided into 5 categories, that is, (1) obese $\geq$ +3 SD (standard deviation), (2) overweight $\geq$ +2 SD, (3) normal < +2 SD $\rightarrow$ −2 SD, (4) underweight $\leq$ −2 SD, and (5) severe underweight $\leq$ −3 SD. According to their height for age, children were divided into 5 categories, that is, (1) very tall $\geq$ +3 SD, (2) tall $\geq$ +2 SD, (3) normal < +2 SD $\rightarrow$ −2SD, (4) stunted $\leq$ −2 SD, and (5) severely stunted $\leq$ −3 SD. Study was conducted in August and September 2015. Informed consent was taken from the parents, and one of the parents was present during measurement of height and weight.

Name, age on the day of test, sex, hemoglobin levels, ferritin levels, weight in Kilogram, status of weight according to WHO Z-score chart for weight for age, height in centimeters (cm.), and status of height according to WHO Z-score chart for height for age were entered on a data form.

Shapiro–Wilk test was used to test the normality of continuous variables. Mean values ± standard deviation were used to show central tendency and spread of normally distributed data, and Median value (interquartile range [IQR]) was used to show central tendency and spread of nonnormal data. Chi-square test was used to test association. Spearman test was used to test correlation between two continuous variables. Value of Spearman coefficient (r_s) from 0 to 0.19 was taken as very weak, from 0.20 to 0.39 as weak, from 0.40 to 0.59 as moderate, from 0.60 to 0.79 as strong, and from 0.80 to 1.0 as very strong correlation. Multiple linear regression analysis was applied to find out correlates of ferritin. For this purpose 3 models were made. In Model 1, ferritin level was taken as dependent variable, and status of height according to Z-score charts, age, and gender were taken as independent variables. In Model 2, ferritin was taken as dependent variable and status of weight according to Z-score charts, age, and gender were taken as independent variables. In Model 3, ferritin was taken as dependent variable and age, gender, status of weight according to Z- score, status of height according to Z-score charts, and anemia were taken as independent variables. Results were reported for these models as standardized beta coefficient (β) and level of significance (p value).

3. Results

One thousand and eighty students got admitted to prep class (first year of school) of five schools of Nazarat Taleem school system, in Rabwah. One in every four students was selected to be included in the study by computer randomization. One child had sore throat, so he was excluded from the study. Full blood count and ferritin levels of the remaining 295 children were checked. Out of these 295 children 164 (55.6%) were female and 131 (44.6%) were male. Among the continuous variables height had normal distribution. And age, weight, ferritin levels, and hemoglobin levels had nonnormal distribution. Median age was 67 (IQR: 9.0) months. Baseline characteristics and hemoglobin and ferritin levels of males, females, and all subjects included in the study are shown in Table 1. Out of 295, 240 (81.4%) had normal Hb and 55 (18.6%) had anemia. The difference between frequency of anemia among male and female subjects was nonsignificant (p = 0.26). See Table 2. Ferritin level was found to be normal in 49 (16.6%) children and it was found to be below normal level in 246 (83.4%) children. The difference between frequencies of low ferritin levels among male and female subjects was found to be nonsignificant (p = 0.47). See Table 2. Among those with anemia 81.8% had low ferritin levels, and among those with normal hemoglobin levels 83.4% had low ferritin levels. See Table 3. According to WHO Z-score weight for age chart 3 (1%), 238 (80.7%), 36 (12.2%), and 18 (6.1%) children were categorized as obese, having normal weight, underweight, and severely underweight, respectively. According to WHO Z-score height for age chart 2 (0.7%), 260 (88.1%), 26 (8.8%), and 7 (2.4%) children were categorized as tall, having normal height, stunted, and severely stunted, respectively.

Spearman test showed that there was very weak correlation between ferritin and hemoglobin levels (r_s = .163). Table 3 shows that median ferritin levels among the patients with normal hemoglobin and anemia were 5.1 ng/ml and

TABLE 1: Baseline characteristics of males, females, and all subjects.

Variable	Males	Females	All subjects
Number (%)	139 (44.6%)	164 (55.6%)	295 (100%)
Median age in months (IQR)	67 (62–70)	67 (61–70)	67 (61–70)
Median weight in kilogram (IQR)	17.50 (16–19.50)	17.0 (15–19)	17.0 (15.5–19.0)
Mean height in centimeter (±SD)	109.02 (±6.01)	108.01 (±5.29)	108.4 (±5.63)
Median Hb gm/dl (IQR)	11.90 (11.50–12.50)	12.10 (11.50–12.78)	12.0 (11.5–12.7)
Median ferritin ng/ml (IQR)	4.40 (2.8–7.3)	5.10 (3.03–7.30)	4.90 (4.9–12.4)

TABLE 2: Frequency of anemia and low ferritin in males, females, and all subjects.

	Males	Females	Total	p value
Normal hemoglobin level	104 (79.4%)	136 (82.9%)	240 (81.3%)	0.26
Anemia	27 (20.6%)	28 (17.1%)	55 (18.7%)	
Normal ferritin levels	21 (16%)	28 (17%)	49 (16.6%)	0.47
Low ferritin levels	110 (84%)	136 (83%)	246 (83.4%)	

TABLE 3: Status of ferritin among subjects with anemia and normal hemoglobin.

Status of hemoglobin	Normal ferritin	Low ferritin
Normal hemoglobin	39 (16.2%)	201 (83.8%)
Anemic	10 (18.2%)	45 (81.8%)

$p = 0.72$.

3.9 ng/ml, respectively. Mann–Whitney U test showed that the difference was nonsignificant. ($p = 0.112$)

Table 4 shows results of regression Model 1. None of the independent variables, that is, status of height, age, and gender had significant p value. Table 5 shows results of regression Model 2. None of the independent variables, that is, status of height, age, and gender had significant p value. Table 6 shows results of regression Model 3. None of the independent variables had significant p value. This shows that level of ferritin cannot be predicted by status of height and weight, presence of anemia, age, and gender.

4. Discussion

Iron deficiency anemia and iron deficiency without anemia are common nutritional problems in pediatric age group worldwide. A study by Killip et al. showed that, in Pakistan among children from 6 months to five years of age, 62.3% were anemic (hemoglobin levels <110 g/L), while 33.2% had iron deficiency anemia (defined as having both hemoglobin levels <110 g/L and ferritin levels <12 μg/L). Ferritin deficiency (ferritin levels <12 μg/L) was present in 47.1% cases, and 13.9% had ferritin deficiency without anemia [10, 11].

Our study focused on children who were starting first year of school. It showed that frequency of anemia was present in 18.6% cases, out of these 81.8% had low ferritin levels. Low ferritin levels were present in 88% of children, and 66.7% of the children included in this study had nonanemic iron deficiency (defined as ferritin < 10 ug/L). As compared with the study by Killip et al., our study showed low frequency

of anemia and high frequency of iron deficiency. There can be different possible explanations for the difference in frequencies found in the two studies. Our study included only children starting the first year of school while the study by Killip et al. included the children from six months to five years of age. Our study included children from a single small urban community, and later study included children from a nationwide survey. It highlights the possibility that there can be communities and age groups with prevalence of anemia which is less than half the national average, but high frequency of low ferritin levels is present like silent hunger. Another study in Pakistan by Zeeshan et al., which included children presenting in a tertiary care hospital with anemia from 2 months to 2 years of age, showed that only 4% of the children had low ferritin levels, 60% had low folic acid, and 45% had low Vit B 12 levels [12]. It is worth noting that our study included patients with median age of 67 (IQR: 9.0) months; on the other hand the study by Zeeshan et al. included children from 2 months to 2 years of age. This difference can be a possible reason that in our study 81.8% anemic children had low ferritin levels, while in the study by Zeeshan et al. only 4% of the anemic children had low ferritin levels.

Our study showed that ferritin levels have got weak correlation with hemoglobin levels. Some other studies have analyzed correlation between hemoglobin and ferritin. Study by Khan et al. showed that among overweight and obese people, ferritin had negative correlation with Hb, iron, TIBC, and transferrin saturation ($p < 0.001$) [13]. Another study including pregnant women in third trimester showed that ferritin had weak correlation with hemoglobin (with Spearman coefficient of 0.21) [14]. Study by Kusumastuti et al. showed that, among children 6–59 months of age, ferritin had weak negative correlation with hemoglobin (Spearman constant = −0.220) [15].

The abovementioned studies show that correlation between ferritin and hemoglobin varies from being weak negative to weak positive. Despite the fact that iron deficiency is the commonest cause of anemia, according to our research no study has shown moderate or strong correlation between

TABLE 4: Linear regression Model 1. Ferritin as dependent variable and status of height, age, and gender as independent variables.

Factor	Standardized coefficient beta	p value
Status of height according to Z-score chart	−.028	.634
Age	.044	.454
Gender	.067	.251

TABLE 5: Linear regression Model 2. Ferritin as dependent variable and status of weight, age, and gender as independent variables.

Factor	Standardized coefficient beta	p value
Status of weight according to Z-score charts	.051	.382
Age	.043	.466
Gender	.07	.223

TABLE 6: Linear regression Model 3. Ferritin as dependent variable and anemia, status of height, status of weight, age, and gender as independent variable.

Factor	Standardized coefficient beta	p value
Anemia	−.084	.156
Status of height according to Z-score charts	−.059	.352
Status of weight according to Z-score charts	.083	.193
Age	.052	.377
Gender	.070	.234

ferritin and hemoglobin levels. Keeping in view the fact that iron deficiency is the commonest cause of anemia and ferritin level is the measure of iron stores, more strong correlation is expected between ferritin and hemoglobin levels. Different possible causes can be considered responsible for this scenario. Study by Kate et al. showed that iron content of ferritin molecules varies under different conditions. This leads to the conclusion that merely ferritin level may not depict true status of iron stores [16]. Moreover release of iron from core of iron molecules is another step before iron is made available for use by different cells. Different factors can affect release of iron by ferritin molecules in vivo [17].

Some other studies have analyzed association of anemia and low ferritin levels with nutritional status. Study by Nodoshan et al. showed that children, from 6 to 60 months of age, who were having malnutrition according to Gomez classification, had significantly low hemoglobin, MCV, and MCH as compared with nutritionally normal children. Frequency of anemia was high among children with malnutrition. But there was no significant difference between ferritin levels and frequency of low ferritin levels among the two groups [18]. A meta-analysis, conducted among children from 6 months to 59 months of age, showed that anemia was associated with both underweight and stunting in majority of the studies [19]. Secondary analysis was performed on the National Nutrition Survey in Pakistan 2011-2012 conducted by Killip et al. which showed that stunting was associated with iron deficiency anemia among the children from 6 months to 5 years of age [10, 11]. Regression model of our study showed that ferritin level was not predictable by status of height and weight, gender, age, and presence of anemia.

It is important to study prevalence of iron and anemia at the start of school life because a number of studies have

shown that children who had anemia or iron deficiency without anemia demonstrated psychomotor retardation, cognitive delays, lower cognitive scores later on, and lower academic performance, especially in mathematics [20–22].

Some studies have shown that early recognition and treatment of iron deficiency with or without anemia can reverse psychomotor delay and improves psychomotor development [23, 24]. On the other hand, other studies have shown that children who suffered chronic iron deficiency in infancy did not catch up to the group with good iron status in cognitive scores over time [20]. This highlights the importance of timely recognition and treatment of iron deficiency in early childhood. Otherwise this can lead to permanent consequences. Our study has shown very high frequency of low ferritin levels among children starting first year of their school life.

5. Conclusions

Low ferritin levels are frequent among children starting first year of school life. Low ferritin levels are equally frequent among children with or without anemia. There is weak correlation between ferritin and hemoglobin levels.

Additional Points

Key Points. (i) Iron deficiency is very common among children starting school. Iron deficiency without anemia is more common as compared with iron deficiency with anemia. (ii)

Ferritin level cannot be predicted by independent variables like status of height, weight, age, and anemia.

Conflicts of Interest

The authors declare that they have no conflicts of interest.

References

[1] B. Grosbois, O. Decaux, B. Cador, C. Cazalets, and P. Jego, "Human iron deficiency," *Bull Acad Natl Med*, vol. 189, pp. 1649–1663, 2005.

[2] R. Akramipour, M. Rezaei, and Z. Rahimi, "Prevalence of Iron deficiency Anemia among adolescent schoolgirls from Kermanshah, Western Iran," *International Journal of Hematology*, vol. 13, no. 6, pp. 352–355, 2008.

[3] K. B. Shill, P. Karmakar, M. G. Kibria et al., "Prevalence of iron-deficiency anaemia among university students in Noakhali Region, Bangladesh," *Journal of Health, Population and Nutrition*, vol. 32, no. 1, pp. 103–110, 2014.

[4] M. R. Kadivar, H. Yarmohammadi, A. R. Mirahmadizadeh, M. Vakili, and M. Karimi, "Prevalence of iron deficiency anemia in 6 months to 5 years old children in Fars, Southern Iran," *Medical Science Monitor*, vol. 9, no. 2, pp. CR100–CR104, 2003.

[5] U. Ekwochi, O. Odetunde, I. Maduka, J. Azubuike, and I. Obi, "Iron deficiency among non-anemic under-five children in Enugu, South-East, Nigeria," *Annals of Medical and Health Sciences Research*, vol. 3, no. 3, pp. 402–406, 2013.

[6] C. Algarín, P. Peirano, F. Garrido, F. Pizarro, and B. Lozoff, "Iron deficiency anemia in infancy: Long-lasting effects on auditory and visual system functioning," *Pediatric Research*, vol. 53, no. 2, pp. 217–223, 2003.

[7] F. Verdon, B. Burnand, C.-L. Stubi et al., "Iron supplementation for unexplained fatigue in non-anaemic women: Double blind randomised placebo controlled trial," *British Medical Journal*, vol. 326, no. 7399, pp. 1124–1126, 2003.

[8] J. L. Beard and J. R. Connor, "Iron status and neural functioning," *Annual Review of Nutrition*, vol. 23, pp. 41–58, 2003.

[9] B. Lozoff, "Iron deficiency and child development," *Food and Nutrition Bulletin*, vol. 28, 4, pp. S560–S571, 2007.

[10] S. Killip, J. M. Bennett, and M. D. Chambers, "Iron deficiency anemia," *American Family Physician*, vol. 75, no. 5, pp. 671–678, 2007.

[11] M. A. Habib, K. Black, S. B. Soofi et al., "Prevalence and predictors of iron deficiency anemia in children under five years of age in Pakistan, a secondary analysis of national nutrition survey data 2011–2012," *PLoS ONE*, vol. 11, no. 5, Article ID 0155051, 2016.

[12] F. Zeeshan, A. Bari, S. Farhan, U. Jabeen, and A. W. Rathore, "Correlation between maternal and childhood VitB12, folic acid and ferritin levels," *Pakistan Journal Of Medical Sciences*, vol. 33, no. 1, pp. 162–166, 2017.

[13] A. Khan, W. M. Khan, M. Ayub, M. Humayun, and M. Haroon, "Ferritin Is a Marker of Inflammation rather than Iron Deficiency in Overweight and Obese People," *Journal of Obesity*, vol. 2016, Article ID 1937320, 7 pages, 2016.

[14] K. Tam and T. T. Lao, "Hemoglobin and Red Cell Indices Correlated With Serum Ferritin Concentration in Late Pregnancy," *Obstetrics & Gynecology*, vol. 93, no. 3, pp. 427–431, 1999.

[15] F. D. T. Kusumastuti, S. Sutaryo, and S. Mulatsih, "Correlations between hemoglobin, serum ferritin, and soluble transferrin receptor levels in children aged 6-59 months," *Paediatrica Indonesiana*, vol. 54, no. 2, pp. 122–126, 2013.

[16] J. T. Kate, A. Wolthuis, B. Westerhuis, and C. van Deursen, "The Iron Content of Serum Ferritin: Physiological Importance and Diagnostic Value," *Clinical Chemistry and Laboratory Medicine*, vol. 35, no. 1, pp. 53–56, 1997.

[17] T. Z. Kidane, E. Sauble, and M. C. Linder, "Release of iron from ferritin requires lysosomal activity," *American Journal of Physiology-Cell Physiology*, vol. 291, no. 3, pp. C445–C455, 2006.

[18] A. H. J. Nodoshan, A. Hashemi, A. Golzar, F. Karami, and R. Akhondzaraini, "Hematological Indices in Children with Non-organic Failure to Thrive: a Case-Control Study," *Iranian Journal of Pediatric Hematology and Oncology*, vol. 6, no. 1, pp. 38–42, 2016.

[19] R. Engle-Stone, G. J. Aaron, J. Huang et al., "Predictors of anemia in preschool children: Biomarkers Reflecting Inflammation and Nutritional Determinants of Anemia (BRINDA) project," *The American Journal of Clinical Nutrition*, vol. 106, 1, pp. 402S–415S, 2017.

[20] B. Lozoff, E. Jimenez, and J. B. Smith, "Double burden of iron deficiency in infancy and low socioeconomic status: A longitudinal analysis of cognitive test scores to age 19 years," *JAMA Pediatrics*, vol. 160, no. 11, pp. 1108–1113, 2006.

[21] M. M. Black, "Micronutrient Deficiencies and Cognitive Functioning," *Journal of Nutrition*, vol. 133, 2, no. 11, pp. 3927S–3931S, 2003.

[22] J. S. Halterman, J. M. Kaczorowski, C. A. Aligne, P. Auinger, and P. G. Szilagyi, "Iron deficiency and cognitive achievement among school-aged children and adolescents in the United States," *Pediatrics*, vol. 107, no. 6, pp. 1381–1386, 2001.

[23] P. Idjradinata and E. Pollitt, "Reversal of developmental delays in iron-deficient anaemic infants treated with iron," *The Lancet*, vol. 341, no. 8836, pp. 1–4, 1993.

[24] M. A. Aukett, Y. A. Parks, P. H. Scott, and B. A. Wharton, "Treatment with iron increases weight gain and psychomotor development," *Archives of Disease in Childhood*, vol. 61, no. 9, pp. 849–857, 1986.

19

Efficacy and Tolerability of Intravenous Ferric Carboxymaltose in Patients with Iron Deficiency at a Hospital Outpatient Clinic: A Retrospective Cohort Study of Real-World Clinical Practice

António Robalo Nunes,[1] Ana Palricas Costa,[2] Sara Lemos Rocha,[2] and Ana Garcia de Oliveira[2]

[1]Hospital de Dia de Imuno-Hemoterapia, Hospital Pulido Valente, Centro Hospitalar Lisboa Norte (CHLN), Alameda das Linhas de Torres 117, 1769-001 Lisboa, Portugal

[2]Hospital de Dia de Imuno-Hemoterapia, Hospital de Santa Maria, CHLN, Avenida Prof. Egas Moniz, 1649-035 Lisboa, Portugal

Correspondence should be addressed to Antonio Robalo Nunes; robalonunes@gmail.com

Academic Editor: Ajit C. Gorakshakar

Ferric carboxymaltose (FCM) is an intravenous iron formulation to correct iron deficiency. Although its use has been extensively studied in clinical trials, real-world evidence regarding FCM treatment is scarce. Our aim was to evaluate the efficacy and tolerability of FCM treatment in patients with iron deficiency, with or without anemia, at a hospital outpatient clinic. Data was collected retrospectively from medical records. During this 2-year study, 459 patients were included. Mean age was 58.6 ± 17.5 years and most patients received cumulative FCM doses of 501–1000 mg (63.2%). Six weeks after administration of FCM, efficacy endpoints hemoglobin increase ≥2 g/dL, hemoglobin increase ≥3 g/dL, and transferrin saturation > 20% were attained by 41%, 20%, and 63% of patients, respectively. Patients who received higher FCM doses showed significant reduced odds of not achieving hemoglobin increase ≥2 g/dL (501–1000 mg, adjusted odds ratio [OR]: 0.34, 95% confidence interval [CI] 0.18–0.62; 1001–3000 mg, OR: 0.19, 95% CI 0.07–0.49), compared to 500 mg doses. Treatment-emergent adverse events were documented in <4% of patients. In conclusion, FCM treatment was effective and well-tolerated by outpatients with iron deficiency at a hospital clinic, and its dosage should be adjusted to improve iron deficiency management in clinical practice.

1. Introduction

Iron deficiency is the most common nutritional deficiency worldwide. It has been estimated to affect at least 30–40% of preschool children and pregnant women and about one-sixth of the total population in developed countries [1–3]. Iron deficiency is frequently associated with fatigue, susceptibility to infections, and poorer work capacity and quality of life and is a major cause for anemia in both developing and developed countries [1, 2]. Moreover, comorbidity of iron deficiency and anemia with other diseases have been described to increase the risk of morbidity and mortality [2, 4].

Iron deficiency can occur in two main types: absolute, associated with low total body iron stores due to decreased dietary intake or blood loss, or functional, which occurs when the iron absorption or release from storage areas is inadequate, despite normal or increased total body iron stores [4–6]. Functional iron deficiency may be caused by chronic inflammation, associated with several conditions such as renal failure, congestive heart failure, inflammatory bowel disease, cancer, or autoimmune conditions, which contributes to the onset of the anemia of chronic diseases [7, 8].

Treatment for iron deficiency involves the restoration of iron stores to normal levels and the increase of hemoglobin values, as well as addressing its underlying causes [9]. Oral iron supplementation is the first-line therapy for iron deficiency [6]. However, oral iron therapy presents disadvantages, such as low absorption of iron, drug interactions, increased oxidative stress in the gastrointestinal tract, or high incidence of gastrointestinal adverse events, which can reduce patient compliance [4]. Thus, oral iron has limited efficacy in treating chronic iron deficiency anemia (IDA), hence being more adequate for short periods of iron requirements [6, 10]. Intravenous iron formulations such as ferric carboxymaltose, iron dextran, ferric gluconate, and iron sucrose may potentially solve these issues and may be more convenient both to healthcare providers and patients, if oral iron therapy does not provide the required correction of iron deficiency or is not well-tolerated by patients [4, 6, 9].

Ferric carboxymaltose (FCM) is a relatively recent intravenous iron formulation, which can be administered in short periods of time and at large single doses (up to 1000 mg) [4, 11]. Its efficacy in correcting iron deficiency has been evaluated in several adult populations, namely, patients with gastrointestinal disorders, chronic kidney disease, chronic heart failure, gynecological and obstetrics disorders, and neoplasms [4, 5, 7–10, 12]. Indeed, these studies highlighted the advantages of using intravenous FCM in detriment of oral iron, in terms of both efficacy and tolerability [4, 8–10, 12].

In clinical trials, FCM was associated with rapid hematopoietic improvement by increasing hemoglobin levels, refurnishing iron stores (i.e., changes in ferritin levels), and increasing available iron for erythropoiesis (i.e., raise in transferrin saturation) [9, 12]. Administration of FCM was also well-tolerated by patients, with most drug-related adverse events considered to be mild to moderate in severity [4, 10, 12]. However, real-world data on the efficacy of intravenous FCM therapeutics in current clinical practice are still scarce [5, 8, 13, 14]. Therefore, the purpose of this study was to evaluate the efficacy and tolerability of intravenous FCM treatment of iron deficiency, in patients with or without anemia, attending an outpatient hospital clinic setting.

2. Materials and Methods

2.1. Study Design. This was a retrospective cohort study, conducted at the Immunohemotherapy (transfusion medicine) outpatient clinic of Hospital Pulido Valente and Hospital de Santa Maria, both hospitals of Centro Hospitalar Lisboa Norte. Data was collected retrospectively from medical records on all consecutive patients with iron deficiency attending the hospital outpatient clinic, who were treated with intravenous FCM from January 2014 to December 2015. For each patient included in this study, data was only collected regarding treatment of first episode with a follow-up period of six weeks (±1 week), and no subsequent episodes were included.

2.2. Patients. Eligible patients were adult individuals (≥18 years old) who had iron deficiency with or without anemia and were submitted to intravenous FCM therapeutics at the hospital outpatient clinic. Iron deficiency was defined as transferrin saturation <20% [15]. Anemia was defined as hemoglobin ≤12 g/dL in women, and ≤13 g/dL in men, according to the World Health Organization threshold hemoglobin concentrations [1]. Patients were excluded if they had missing data regarding any of the hematological or

iron laboratory tests or did not complete the first episode treatment with FCM.

Patients were assigned to FCM dose levels according to their individual potential iron requirement, as recommended by the Summary of Product Characteristics (SmPC) or calculated using the Ganzoni formula [16]. According to this formula, individual potential iron requirement is a function of the patient's hemoglobin level and body weight: total iron deficit (mg) = body weight (kg) × (target hemoglobin – actual hemoglobin) (g/dL) × 2.4 + depot iron of 500 mg.

Patients received single doses of FCM from 500 mg or 15 mg/kg up to a maximum dose of 1000 mg per week, given as intravenous infusions over 15 to 30 min.

2.3. Data Collection. Demographic, clinical, laboratory, and safety data were retrospectively collected from patients' medical records, at admission (before treatment) and follow-up visits (after treatment). Demographic data included age and gender, while clinical data included primary diagnosis, cumulative iron dose levels, and adverse events. Primary diagnoses were coded using the high-level classification of the 10th revision of the International Statistical Classification of Diseases and Related Health Problems (ICD-10) [17]. Patients were stratified by cumulative iron dose levels in three categories: 500 mg, 501–1000 mg, and 1001–3000 mg. Laboratory test results data included pretreatment and posttreatment serum hemoglobin, hematocrit, mean corpuscular volume (MCV), mean corpuscular hemoglobin (MCH), ferritin, and transferrin saturation. Reference ranges of the local laboratory were 12.0–15.3 g/dL (female) or 13.0–17.5 g/dL (male) for hemoglobin; 36–46% (female) or 40–50% (male) for hematocrit; 80–97 fL (female or male) for MCV; 27–33 pg (female or male) for MCH; and 13–150 ng/mL (female) or 30–400 ng/mL (male) for ferritin.

2.4. Endpoints. The primary efficacy endpoint of the data analysis was the proportion of patients with a hemoglobin increase of ≥2.0 g/dL after treatment (i.e., achieving a hematopoietic response). Secondary efficacy endpoints were the proportion of patients attaining a hemoglobin increase of ≥3.0 g/dL after treatment, and the proportion of patients attaining a transferrin saturation >20% after treatment (i.e., achieving an iron bioavailability response).

Safety endpoint was the incidence of treatment-emergent adverse events (TEAEs) occurring during or after administration of intravenous FCM. All safety data were collected during clinical care, without a systematic method, which means some data might not have been registered in the patient files.

2.5. Statistical Analysis. Continuous variables were summarized by mean and standard deviation or median and 1st quartile-3rd quartile as applicable. Categorical variables were summarized by relative and absolute frequencies. The variation in the hematological and iron parameters was assessed using the paired t-test or Wilcoxon signed-rank test as applicable.

Primary diagnoses were coded using the high-level classification of ICD-10. For the analyses of the efficacy endpoints, classes with less than 10 patients were merged into a single class named "other diseases," to ensure an adequate statistical power for the comparisons. The remaining classes (i.e., neoplasms, diseases of the genitourinary system, diseases of the circulatory system, and diseases of the digestive system) were analyzed individually.

Due to the study design, no reference group was established. Therefore, pairwise exploratory comparisons regarding diagnoses groups were performed against all the remaining subjects (e.g., the group of patients with neoplasms was compared against the group of subjects who did not have neoplasms). As for the dosage groups, pairwise exploratory comparisons were performed against the lower dose (i.e., 500 mg), used as reference dose.

To assess the treatment efficacy, a logistic regression model was used to determine the probability of clinical failure in each endpoint (i.e., not achieving the efficacy endpoint after treatment with intravenous FCM). The odds ratio (OR) and 95% confidence intervals (CIs) were estimated. The computed OR were adjusted for age and pretreatment hemoglobin for the endpoints related to hemoglobin increase and for age and pretreatment transferrin saturation for the endpoint related to the increase of transferrin saturation.

Due to the low incidence of adverse events, no statistical inference was performed.

3. Results

3.1. Patients Characteristics. A total of 459 patients who received intravenous FCM treatment were included in the study. Demographic and clinical characteristics of the patients are shown in Table 1. Mean age was 58.6 ± 17.5 years and most patients were female (78%). In all, anemia was recorded in 82.4% of patients, iron deficiency was recorded in 98% of patients, and IDA was recorded in 81.3% of patients. The majority of patients received a single FCM dose between 501 mg and 1000 mg (63.2%). Only 10.2% of patients received cumulative iron doses from 1001 mg to 3000 mg in divided doses (one per week). Most common primary diagnoses were diseases of the digestive system (43.4%), diseases of the genitourinary system (26.4%), neoplasms (10.2%), and diseases of the circulatory system (8.3%). Other diseases comprised the following categories: diseases of the blood and blood-forming organs and certain disorders involving the immune mechanism (3.3%); endocrine, nutritional, and metabolic diseases (2.0%); diseases of the musculoskeletal system and connective tissue (1.7%); diseases of the nervous system (1.5%); diseases of the eye and adnexa (1.3%); pregnancy, childbirth, and the puerperium (1.1%); diseases of the respiratory system (0.7%); and certain infectious and parasitic diseases (0.2%). After 6 weeks (±1 week) following FCM treatment, all hematological and iron measurements significantly increased from baseline (Table 2).

3.2. Efficacy Endpoints. The primary (i.e., hemoglobin increase ≥ 2 g/dL) and secondary (i.e., hemoglobin increase ≥ 3 g/dL and transferrin saturation > 20%) efficacy endpoints, following intravenous FCM treatment, are shown in Table 3.

TABLE 1: Demographic and clinical characteristics of the study population.

Characteristic	Patients ($N = 459$)
Age (years), mean (SD)	58.6 (17.5)
Elderly > 65 years, n (%)	187 (40.7)
Male, n (%)	101 (22.0)
Anemia, n (%)	378 (82.4)
Iron deficiency, n (%)	450 (98.0)
Iron deficiency anemia, n (%)	373 (81.3)
Iron deficiency without anemia, n (%)	77 (16.8)
Cumulative FCM treatment dose, n (%)	
500 mg	122 (26.6)
501–1000 mg	290 (63.2)
1001–3000 mg	47 (10.2)
Diagnosis per ICD-10 high level category, n (%)	
Diseases of the digestive system	199 (43.4)
Diseases of the genitourinary system	121 (26.4)
Neoplasms	47 (10.2)
Diseases of the circulatory system	38 (8.3)
Other diseases	54 (11.8)

FCM: ferric carboxymaltose; ICD-10: International Classification of Diseases 10th Revision.

After 6 weeks, hemoglobin increase of ≥ 2 g/dL was attained by 41% of all patients, 40% in the IDA group, 40% in the diseases of the digestive system group, 55% in the diseases of the genitourinary system group, 26% in the neoplasms group, and 29% in the diseases of the circulatory system group. Moreover, our analysis indicated that patients with diseases of the genitourinary system presented significant decreased odds of clinical failure (OR: 0.46, 95% CI 0.25, 0.87), whereas patients with diseases of the circulatory system showed about three times higher odds of clinical failure (OR: 3.34, 95% CI 1.31–8.98). Regarding cumulative FCM treatment dose, we found significant decreased odds of clinical failure in patients who received doses ranging from 501 to 1000 mg (OR: 0.34, 95% CI 0.18–0.62) or 1001–3000 mg doses (OR: 0.19, 95% CI 0.07–0.49), compared to patients who received doses of 500 mg (Table 3).

Hemoglobin increase of ≥ 3 g/dL after 6 weeks after FCM dose was attained by 20% of all patients, 24% of the patients in the IDA group, 22% in the diseases of the digestive system group, 26% in the diseases of the genitourinary system group, 11% in the neoplasms group, and 16% in the diseases of the circulatory system group. Furthermore, our analysis indicated that patients with IDA presented significant lower odds of clinical failure (OR: 0.07, 95% CI 0.01–0.24). Concerning total FCM treatment dose, our analysis showed significant lower odds of clinical failure in patients who received doses ranging from 501 to 1000 mg (OR: 0.36, 95% CI 0.12–0.92) or 1001–3000 mg doses (OR: 0.23, 95% CI 0.06–0.73), compared to patients who received doses of 500 mg (Table 3).

Finally, transferrin saturation > 20% after 6 weeks after FCM dose was attained by 63% of all patients, 69% of patients

TABLE 2: Hematological laboratory tests before and after treatment with intravenous ferric carboxymaltose (FCM).

Variables	Before treatment	After treatment	p value
Hemoglobin (g/dL)	10.67 (1.67)	12.65 (1.26)	<0.001
Hematocrit (%)	33.32 (4.48)	38.57 (3.81)	<0.001
MCV (fL)	80.67 (8.94)	86.75 (6.56)	<0.001
MCH (pg)	25.62 (3.63)	28.30 (2.37)	<0.001
Ferritin (μg/dL)	9.60 (5.70–24.00)	137.00 (59.95–243.10)	<0.001
Transferrin saturation (%)	8.70 (4.76)	25.02 (10.16)	<0.001

Values are expressed as mean (standard deviation) or median (1st quartile-3rd quartile). Laboratory reference ranges in normal adults: hemoglobin, 12.0–15.3 g/dL (female) and 13.0–17.5 g/dL (male); hematocrit, 36–46% (female) and 40–50% (male); MCV, 80–97 fL; MCH, 27–33 pg; ferritin, 13–150 μg/dL (female) and 30–400 μg/dL (male); MCH: mean corpuscular hemoglobin; MCV: mean corpuscular volume.

in both IDA and iron deficiency without anemia groups, 63% in the diseases of the digestive system group, 68% in the diseases of the genitourinary system group, 67% in the neoplasms group, and 47% in the diseases of the circulatory system group. Our analysis indicated significant lower odds of clinical failure in patients who received doses ranging from 501 to 1000 mg (OR: 0.57, 95% CI 0.36–0.88) or 1001–3000 mg doses (OR: 0.25, 95% CI 0.10–0.55), compared to patients who received doses of 500 mg (Table 3).

3.3. Safety Endpoint. A total of 17 TEAEs were recorded in 15 (3.3%) patients. The most common documented TEAEs were nausea ($n = 4$), rash ($n = 4$), and urticaria ($n = 2$). Additionally, patients also experienced diarrhea ($n = 1$), chill ($n = 1$), myalgia ($n = 1$), abdominal pain ($n = 1$), wheeze ($n = 1$), arthralgia ($n = 1$), and hyperthermia ($n = 1$).

4. Discussion

This study evaluated the efficacy and tolerability of intravenous FCM treatment for the correction of iron deficiency, with or without anemia, in patients with diverse diagnoses, who were attending a hospital outpatient Immunohemotherapy clinic. The rationale for studying the complete population of patients under FCM treatment and not only some subgroups as most studies report [8, 14, 18–21] was to improve the prescription standards of the intravenous FCM in clinical practice.

Treatment efficacy with FCM considering the primary endpoint of hemoglobin increase ≥2 g/dL at week 6 was 41% in all patients, in agreement with previous studies performed in various populations of patients with IDA [4, 5, 8, 9]. For patients with IDA, no differences in treatment efficacy were found for hemoglobin increase of ≥2 g/dL and transferrin saturation > 20%, compared with patients without IDA. However, we found a significant difference in hemoglobin increase of ≥3 g/dL. This finding was expected, as achieving such a high increase is more challenging for patients with normal hemoglobin levels.

Efficacy of FCM was lower in patients with neoplasms and diseases of the circulatory system. This might be due to the increased inflammatory states commonly caused by these diseases (e.g., cancer, acute or chronic congestive heart failure), which are known to impair patients' ability to absorb

iron and hence to achieve a rapid hemoglobin increase [8]. To illustrate, neoplasms patients achieved lower efficacy in hemoglobin increase, but higher efficacy in transferrin saturation >20%. This finding is consistent with the presence of anemia of chronic disease rather than absolute iron deficiency (i.e., low body iron stores), which makes these patients less respondent to iron supplementation [7, 8, 11, 22]. In contrast, FCM efficacy was significantly higher in patients with diseases of the genitourinary system for hemoglobin increase, as most of the diagnoses included in this group were heavy uterine bleeding, a condition that presents a good response to iron treatment due to its pathophysiology [5, 8, 10, 21, 22]. Accordingly, male patients presented an apparent lower efficacy rate, although not significant. Finally, efficacy of FCM treatment in patients with diseases of the digestive system was comparable to the ones of other subgroups. This finding is consistent with the pathophysiology of most diseases in this subgroup, which include either food disorders or acute bleedings. Other diseases had a low presence to allow any conclusion.

The incidence of TEAEs was low in this study (<4%). Rash and nausea were the most common TEAEs, and no serious adverse events were found in the medical records. Although these events might be underreported, it was not expected that FCM would present a high toxicity, as other studies also reported FCM as a well-tolerated therapy [6, 9–12, 23, 24] with an acceptable safety profile in patients with diverse diagnoses [5, 8, 10, 11, 23]. Nevertheless, the conservativeness in the cumulative FCM treatment doses might also be a factor that explains the low incidence of TEAEs.

Not so surprisingly, higher cumulative doses of FCM (i.e., 501–1000 mg and 1001–3000 mg) showed a significant higher efficacy compared to the lower dose (i.e., 500 mg), used as reference. In this study, doses of 500 mg were on average 75% less effective than doses above 1000 mg, even when adjusted for age and predose hemoglobin or transferrin saturation serum levels. Although no data on body weight was collected, we may assume that patients were frequently treated with lower doses than the ones recommended in the SmPC due to the high frequency of cumulative FCM doses of 500 mg (26.6%). This lower dosage profile might affect overall treatment efficacy in our clinical setting, as demonstrated by the lower efficacy rates associated with lower cumulative FCM doses shown in this study.

TABLE 3: Odds ratio of clinical failure in primary and secondary efficacy endpoints for intravenous FCM treatment.

Characteristic	Hemoglobin increase ≥2 g/dL		Hemoglobin increase ≥3 g/dL		Transferrin saturation > 20%[a]	
	n (%)	OR (95% CI)	n (%)	OR (95% CI)	n (%)	OR (95% CI)
All	190 (41)	—	94 (20)	—	285 (63)	—
Male	35 (35)	1.7 (0.94–3.13)	20 (20)	1.01 (0.50–2.10)	54 (55)	1.45 (0.91–2.31)
Iron deficiency anemia	184 (40)	1.27 (0.42–3.45)	92 (24)	**0.07 (0.01–0.24)**	53 (69)	1.29 (0.77–2.23)
Iron deficiency without anemia	—	—	—	—	53 (69)	0.77 (0.45–1.30)
Diseases of the digestive system	79 (40)	0.88 (0.54–1.42)	43 (22)	0.57 (0.31–1.04)	123 (63)	0.95 (0.63–1.4)
Diseases of the genitourinary system	67 (55)	**0.46 (0.25–0.87)**	31 (26)	1.22 (0.59–2.54)	82 (68)	0.88 (0.52–1.48)
Neoplasms	12 (26)	2.19 (0.98–5.19)	5 (11)	1.63 (0.57–5.72)	30 (67)	0.70 (0.35–1.38)
Diseases of the circulatory system	11 (29)	**3.34 (1.31–8.98)**	6 (16)	2.1 (0.72–6.86)	18 (47)	1.82 (0.91–3.65)
Other diseases	21 (40)	0.94 (0.45–1.97)	9 (17)	1.12 (0.47–2.90)	32 (62)	1.13 (0.61–2.06)
Cumulative FCM treatment dose[b]						
500 mg	18 (15)	—	5 (4)	—	58 (51)	—
501–1000 mg	141 (49)	**0.34 (0.18–0.62)**	70 (24)	**0.36 (0.12–0.92)**	189 (65)	**0.57 (0.36–0.88)**
1001–3000 mg	31 (66)	**0.19 (0.07–0.49)**	19 (40)	**0.23 (0.06–0.73)**	38 (81)	**0.25 (0.10–0.55)**

Significant odds ratio in boldface; CI: confidence interval; FCM: ferric carboxymaltose; OR: odds ratio; [a]N = 450, only patients who had transferrin saturation <20% before treatment were considered for this endpoint. [b]Reference group: cumulative iron dose of 500 mg.

Although most clinical trials and studies reported low toxicity for FCM, clinicians might be still using the traditionally lower doses of oral iron therapy, which is less tolerated by the patients [6, 9–12, 23, 24]. Therefore, our results suggest that patients might be undertreated due to treatment conservativeness of the clinicians prescribing intravenous iron therapeutics. Indeed, we found better hematological responses with the use of higher cumulative FCM doses. Hence, our study provides additional data supporting the indication of higher cumulative FCM doses for the treatment of iron deficiency, across patients with diverse diagnoses. As previously reported by other authors [10, 18, 22, 23, 25], higher FCM doses may benefit the patients in terms of treatment efficacy and quality of life, without significantly impacting treatment tolerability and safety. In addition, administration of single large doses up to 1000 mg, instead of multiple lower iron dosages, is more convenient for the patients and may result in cost savings for healthcare systems and society [5, 8].

To our knowledge, this is one of the first observational studies reporting the efficacy of intravenous FCM treatment in a real-world setting, across a population of patients with a considerable dimension ($n = 459$) [5, 8, 13, 14]. Moreover, this study presents data on a single drug formulation, prescribed to patients with diverse ages and primary diagnoses. Therefore, we may assume that the results of this study are representative of FCM treatment efficacy in patients with iron deficiency in current clinical practice. Nevertheless, due to its retrospective and observational nature, this study presents some limitations. First, our analyses were based on the clinical and hematological data collected during routine clinical practice, which might have led to an apparent underreporting of adverse events and exclusion of some valid cases. Moreover, as several clinicians were involved in the prescription of FCM dosage, some patients were treated as recommended by the SmPC, while other patients were treated according to the Ganzoni formula. In addition, the lack of a clearly defined reference group limited our conclusions regarding the overall FCM treatment efficacy. Therefore, findings of this study, although valid, may only be considered as exploratory. Additional prospective studies should be performed, using appropriate populations and systematic documentation of hematological and TEAEs data. Future research should also address the efficacy and safety of intravenous FCM in different real-world clinical settings.

5. Conclusions

Our study showed that the use of FCM increases hemoglobin levels ≥2 g/dL after 6 weeks in 41% of all iron deficiency patients, with or without anemia, in a hospital day setting and was associated with a low incidence of TEAEs. Moreover, treatment efficacy was significantly higher in patients who received higher cumulative FCM doses, that is, 501–1000 and 1001–3000 mg, compared to patients who received doses of 500 mg. Our findings indicate that intravenous FCM dosage should be adjusted to improve treatment efficacy of iron deficiency in different clinical practice settings.

Conflicts of Interest

António Robalo Nunes has received fees from OM Pharma for advice on intravenous ferric carboxymaltose treatment. Ana Palricas Costa, Sara Lemos Rocha, and Ana Garcia de Oliveira declare that there are no conflicts of interest regarding the publication of this article.

Authors' Contributions

António Robalo Nunes was responsible for study design. António Robalo Nunes, Ana Palricas Costa, Sara Lemos Rocha, and Ana Garcia de Oliveira were responsible for study conduct. António Robalo Nunes, Ana Palricas Costa, Sara Lemos Rocha, and Ana Garcia de Oliveira were responsible for data collection. António Robalo Nunes and Ana Palricas Costa were responsible for data analysis. António Robalo Nunes, Ana Palricas Costa, Sara Lemos Rocha, and Ana Garcia de Oliveira were responsible for data interpretation. António Robalo Nunes was responsible for drafting manuscript. António Robalo Nunes, Ana Palricas Costa, Sara Lemos Rocha, and Ana Garcia de Oliveira were responsible for revising manuscript content. António Robalo Nunes, Ana Palricas Costa, Sara Lemos Rocha, and Ana Garcia de Oliveira approved final version of manuscript.

Acknowledgments

OM Pharma provided a grant to support statistical analysis and medical writing services. The authors acknowledge Scientific Toolbox Consulting for providing consulting services in the following areas: statistical analysis and medical writing.

References

[1] E. McLean, M. Cogswell, I. Egli, D. Wojdyla, and B. De Benoist, "Worldwide prevalence of anaemia, WHO Vitamin and Mineral Nutrition Information System, 1993–2005," *Public Health Nutrition*, vol. 12, no. 4, pp. 444–454, 2009.

[2] World Health Organization, *Iron Deficiency Anaemia: Assessment, Prevention and Control. A Guide for Programme Managers*, World Health Organization, Geneva, Switzerland, 2001.

[3] C. Fonseca, F. Marques, A. Robalo Nunes, A. Belo, D. Brilhante, and J. Cortez, "Prevalence of anaemia and iron deficiency in Portugal: the EMPIRE study," *Internal Medicine Journal*, vol. 46, no. 4, pp. 470–478, 2016.

[4] C. Rognoni, S. Venturini, M. Meregaglia, M. Marmifero, and R. Tarricone, "Efficacy and Safety of Ferric Carboxymaltose and Other Formulations in Iron-Deficient Patients: A Systematic Review and Network Meta-analysis of Randomised Controlled Trials," *Clinical Drug Investigation*, vol. 36, no. 3, pp. 177–194, 2016.

[5] J. E. Toblli and M. Angerosa, "Optimizing iron delivery in the management of anemia: patient considerations and the role of

ferric carboxymaltose," *Drug Design, Development and Therapy*, vol. 8, pp. 2475–2491, 2014.

[6] G. R. Bailie, N. A. Mason, and T. G. Valaoras, "Safety and tolerability of intravenous ferric carboxymaltose in patients with iron deficiency anemia," *Hemodialysis International*, vol. 14, no. 1, pp. 47–54, 2010.

[7] G. C, "Doron Schwartz, Should a search for iron deficiency be part of the regular screening in all patients, whether anemic or not?" *Journal of Hematology & Thromboembolic Diseases*, vol. 02, no. 05, 2014.

[8] G. M. Keating, "Ferric carboxymaltose: a review of its use in iron deficiency," *Drugs*, vol. 75, no. 1, pp. 101–127, 2015.

[9] K. A. Lyseng-Williamson and G. M. Keating, "Ferric carboxymaltose: a review of its use in iron-deficiency anaemia," *Drugs*, vol. 69, no. 6, pp. 739–756, 2009.

[10] G. R. Bailie, "Efficacy and safety of ferric carboxymaltose in correcting iron-deficiency anemia: a review of randomized controlled trials across different indications.," *Arzneimittel-Forschung*, vol. 60, no. 6 a, pp. 386–398, 2010.

[11] J. E. Onken, D. B. Bregman, R. A. Harrington et al., "A multicenter, randomized, active-controlled study to investigate the efficacy and safety of intravenous ferric carboxymaltose in patients with iron deficiency anemia," *Transfusion*, vol. 54, no. 2, pp. 306–315, 2014.

[12] R. A. Moore, H. Gaskell, P. Rose, and J. Allan, "Meta-analysis of efficacy and safety of intravenous ferric carboxymaltose (Ferinject) from clinical trial reports and published trial data," *BMC Blood Disorders*, vol. 11, article 4, 2011.

[13] M. Kuster and D. N. Meli, "Treatment of iron deficiency with intravenous ferric carboxymaltose in general practice: a retrospective database study," *Journal of Clinical Medicine Research*, vol. 7, no. 1, pp. 37–40, 2015.

[14] M. Varcher, S. Zisimopoulou, O. Braillard, B. Favrat, and N. J. Perron, "Iron deficiency intravenous substitution in a Swiss academic primary care division: Analysis of practices," *International Journal of General Medicine*, vol. 9, pp. 221–227, 2016.

[15] L. Peyrin-Biroulet, N. Williet, and P. Cacoub, "Guidelines on the diagnosis and treatment of iron deficiency across indications: A systematic review," *American Journal of Clinical Nutrition*, vol. 102, no. 6, pp. 1585–1594, 2015.

[16] A. M. Ganzoni, "Intravenous iron-dextran: therapeutic and experimental possibilities," *Schweizerische Medizinische Wochenschrift*, vol. 100, no. 7, pp. 301–303, 1970.

[17] World Health Organization, *International statistical classification of diseases and related health problems. - 10th revision*, World Health Organization, Geneva, Switzerland, 2016.

[18] R. Mahey, A. Kriplani, K. D. Mogili, N. Bhatla, G. Kachhawa, and R. Saxena, "Randomized controlled trial comparing ferric carboxymaltose and iron sucrose for treatment of iron deficiency anemia due to abnormal uterine bleeding," *International Journal of Gynecology and Obstetrics*, vol. 133, no. 1, pp. 43–48, 2016.

[19] S. Garcia-Lopez, J. M. Bocos, J. P. Gisbert et al., "High-dose intravenous treatment in iron deficiency anaemia in inflammatory bowel disease: early efficacy and impact on quality of life," *Blood Transfusion = Trasfusione del Sangue*, vol. 14, no. 2, pp. 199–205, 2016.

[20] M. Bach, T. Geisel, J. Martin et al., "Efficacy and Safety of Intravenous Ferric Carboxymaltose in Geriatric Inpatients at a German Tertiary University Teaching Hospital: A Retrospective Observational Cohort Study of Clinical Practice," *Anemia*, vol. 2015, Article ID 647930, 2015.

[21] R. Herfs, L. Fleitmann, and I. Kocsis, "Treatment of iron deficiency with or without anaemia with intravenous ferric carboxymaltose in gynaecological practices—a non-interventional study," *Geburtshilfe und Frauenheilkunde*, vol. 74, no. 1, pp. 81–88, 2014.

[22] T. A. Koch, J. Myers, and L. T. Goodnough, "Intravenous Iron Therapy in Patients with Iron Deficiency Anemia: Dosing Considerations," *Anemia*, vol. 2015, Article ID 763576, 2015.

[23] B. Favrat, K. Balck, C. Breymann et al., "Evaluation of a single dose of ferric carboxymaltose in fatigued, iron-deficient women—PREFER a randomized, placebo-controlled study," *PLoS ONE*, vol. 9, no. 4, Article ID e94217, 2014.

[24] C. F. Barish, T. Koch, A. Butcher, D. Morris, and D. B. Bregman, "Safety and efficacy of intravenous ferric carboxymaltose (750 mg) in the treatment of iron deficiency anemia: two randomized, controlled trials," *Anemia*, vol. 2012, Article ID 172104, 9 pages, 2012.

[25] P. Geisser and J. Banké-Bochita, "Pharmacokinetics, safety and tolerability of intravenous ferric carboxymaltose: a dose-escalation study in volunteers with mild iron-deficiency anaemia," *Arzneimittel-Forschung*, vol. 60, no. 6a, pp. 362–372, 2010.

20

Using Soluble Transferrin Receptor and Taking Inflammation into Account When Defining Serum Ferritin Cutoffs Improved the Diagnosis of Iron Deficiency in a Group of Canadian Preschool Inuit Children from Nunavik

Huguette Turgeon O'Brien,[1] **Rosanne Blanchet,**[2] **Doris Gagné,**[3] **Julie Lauzière,**[4] **and Carole Vézina**[5]

[1]*School of Nutrition, Laval University, 2425 rue de l'Agriculture, Québec City, QC, Canada G1V 0A6*
[2]*Interdisciplinary School of Health Sciences, University of Ottawa, 35 University Private THN140, Ottawa, ON, Canada K1N 6N5*
[3]*Nutrition DG, 1187 rue du Saint-Brieux, Québec City, QC, Canada G1Y 2B9*
[4]*Department of Family Medicine and Emergency Medicine, University of Sherbrooke, 150 place Charles-Le Moyne, Longueuil, QC, Canada J4K 0A8*
[5]*Inuulitsivik Health and Social Services Centre, Puvirnituq, QC, Canada J0M 1P0*

Correspondence should be addressed to Huguette Turgeon O'Brien; huguette.turgeon-obrien@fsaa.ulaval.ca

Academic Editor: Bruno Annibale

The prevalence of iron depletion, iron deficient erythropoiesis (IDE), and iron deficiency anemia (IDA) was assessed in preschool Inuit children using soluble transferrin receptor (sTfR) and traditional indicators of iron status while disregarding or taking inflammation into account when defining SF cutoffs. Iron depletion was defined as follows: (1) SF < 15 μg/L regardless of the C-reactive protein (CRP) level and (2) SF < 15 or <50 μg/L with CRP ≤ 5 or >5 mg/L, respectively. IDE corresponded to iron depletion combined with total iron binding capacity > 72 μmol/L and/or transferrin saturation < 16%. Iron depletion and IDE affected almost half of the children when accounting for inflammation, compared to one-third when the SF cutoff was defined regardless of CRP level ($P < 0.0001$). The prevalence of IDE adjusted for inflammation (45.1%) was very similar to the prevalence observed when sTfR was used as a sole marker of IDE (47.4%). The prevalence of anemia was 15%. The prevalence of IDA (IDE + hemoglobin < 110 g/L) was higher when accounting for than when disregarding inflammation (8.0% versus 6.2%, $P = 0.083$). Using sTfR and different SF cutoffs for children with versus without inflammation improved the diagnosis of iron depletion and IDE. Our results confirm that Inuit children are at particularly high risk for iron deficiency.

1. Introduction

Iron deficiency (ID) typically exists in three overlapping stages: depletion of storage iron, decreased iron transport within the body resulting in iron deficient erythropoiesis (IDE), and iron deficiency anemia (IDA) when IDE is combined with low hemoglobin. ID can have several adverse effects on children's health including impaired growth, poor cognitive and motor development, lethargy, and alterations of immune defense mechanisms [1].

Anemia from all causes affects almost 50% of preschool-aged children worldwide [2] and, according to the WHO, IDA is the most common type of anemia [3]. Although in industrialized countries the prevalence of ID among young children has been greatly reduced with the advent of food fortification, it continues to be an important public health problem among young Aboriginal children from Canada's remote north. There are only a few studies available on the prevalence of anemia and ID among preschool children. Recent data from a nationally representative sample of 3- to

5-year-old Canadian children revealed that 0.5% were anemic and 3.3% had depleted iron stores [4] compared with 16.8% and 18% for a group of Inuit children recruited at random from 16 Nunavut communities [5].

However, the impact of a concomitant inflammatory state which can increase serum ferritin (SF) levels in spite of depleted iron stores has received little attention in Inuit children. One approach to ensure a more accurate assessment of iron status is to measure an acute phase protein such as C-reactive protein or α1-acid glycoprotein and exclude persons with inflammation from the analysis [5, 6]. This approach can potentially underestimate the prevalence of ID [7] and can also be impracticable where the prevalence of inflammation is extensive [7], such as in Canadian Inuit children [8]. A higher cutoff value for SF, extending the normal 12–15 μg/L limit to 30–50 μg/L, has also been used in the presence of inflammation [9, 10]. More recently, the measurement of soluble transferrin receptor (sTfR), a transmembrane glycoprotein that transfers circulating iron into developing red blood cells [11] and is thought to be unaffected by inflammation [12, 13], has been proposed as a novel approach to diagnose ID in patients with concurrent inflammation [14]. Moreover, the combination of measurements of iron stores and of functional tissue iron as represented by sTfR/log ferritin (sTfR-ferritin index: sTfR-FI) is thought to have a higher diagnostic power than sTfR or SF alone in detecting ID with concomitant inflammation [14, 15].

To our knowledge, no studies have reported the impact of adjusting SF cutoffs to take into account the influence of inflammation or used sTfR and sTfR-FI in the diagnosis of ID among preschool Inuit children. The purpose of this study was to determine the prevalence of ID in a group of preschool Inuit children attending childcare centres in Nunavik using sTfR and traditional laboratory indicators of iron status while taking into account or disregarding the influence of inflammation on SF cutoffs.

2. Methods

2.1. Study Population and Data Collection. The study methods have been described in detail elsewhere [16]. Briefly, this prospective research project was part of a Nutrition Program implemented in childcare centres of Nunavik (northern Québec, Canada). The Nutrition Program, whose main purpose is to provide a balanced diet and reduce ID among Inuit preschool children, includes a four-week cycle menu (breakfast, lunch, and midafternoon snack) rich in absorbable iron. Information regarding total iron, bioavailable iron, and vitamin C content of the menu can be found elsewhere [16]. Data collection took place during the fall season between 2006 and 2010, and childcare centres located in ten of the fourteen Nunavik communities were visited. Parents or respondents of Inuit children aged 1–4 years and attending a childcare centre were invited to participate. Information on the study was provided individually, orally, or through a DVD available in Inuktitut, English, and French. Parents or respondents of participating children gave their written informed consent. This study was approved by the Research Ethics Board of the Centre Hospitalier de l'Université Laval

du Centre Hospitalier Universitaire de Québec (CHUL-CHUQ), Québec (Canada). A total of 245 children were recruited between 2006 and 2010. The respondent for the child at the time of the interview was the biological mother (78.8%, $n = 193$) or father (2.8%, $n = 7$), the adoptive mother (15.5%; $n = 38$), the foster mother (2.4%, $n = 6$), or the foster father (0.4%, $n = 1$). Of the 245 children recruited for this study, a smaller number of participants had at least one laboratory indicator of iron status ($n = 180$) due to challenges related to drawing blood from young children [17]. Also, 162 children had a complete set of traditional laboratory indicators of iron status, whereas 149 had a sTfR measurement.

2.2. Blood Sampling and Laboratory Analyses. A nonfasting venipuncture blood sample was drawn into a vacutainer tube containing EDTA (BD 367863, Becton Dickinson and Co.) and into an iron free plastic tube. Blood samples were kept at room temperature, kept in an insulated container with ice packs, or refrigerated at 4°C for a maximum of 20 min prior to processing. For the determination of the complete blood count, whole blood aliquots of 0.5 mL (Sarstedt 2 mL tubes) were prepared, refrigerated, and sent to Inuulitsivik or Tulattavik hospitals located in Nunavik. Analyses were performed within 24 hours (exceptionally within 48 hours) using a Cell-Dyn 3200 haematology analyser (Abbott, Abbott Park, IL, USA).

The iron-free plastic tubes were centrifuged and the serum was isolated and aliquoted in Sarstedt 2 mL tubes. Within 3 h of collection, serum aliquots were frozen and stored at −18/−20°C. Frozen aliquots were kept in insulated containers with ice packs during transportation to laboratories in Québec City and Montreal. Serum iron (SI) and transferrin were measured on a Roche Modular system (Roche Diagnostics, Basel, Switzerland) using, respectively, the Ferrozine method without deproteinization and a standard particle-enhanced immunoturbidimetric assay. The coefficients of variation (intermediate precision) for transferrin and SI were, respectively, 1.4% and 1.8%. Percent transferrin saturation (TS) was calculated as follows: SI (μmol/L)/TIBC (μmol/L) × 100, where TIBC is total iron binding capacity, calculated as 25.1 × serum transferrin (g/L). SF was measured by electrochemiluminescence immunoassay using the Roche Modular E170 automated analyser (Roche Diagnostics, Basel, Switzerland). The precision was determined using Elecsys reagents in a protocol (EP5-A2) of the CLSI (Clinical and Laboratory Standards Institute) and corresponded to a coefficient of variation of 8.1%. High-sensitivity C-reactive protein (CRP) was determined by particle-enhanced immunonephelometry on a BN ProSpec nephelometer (Dade Behring, Siemens Healthcare Diagnostics, Liederbach, Germany). The total coefficient of variation for CRP was 5.8%. SI, transferrin, SF, and CRP were all measured at the Biochemistry Department, CHUL-CHUQ, Québec City. sTfR was performed with a nephelometric technique on a BN ProSpec System (Dade Behring, Siemens, Marburg, Germany) at the Immunology-Inflammation Laboratory, Notre-Dame Hospital, CHUM, Montreal. The total coefficient of variation of the sTfR method varied between 1.5 and 2.1% at concentrations between 0.14

TABLE 1: Diagnostic criteria defining iron depletion, IDE, and IDA based on traditional indicators of iron status and CRP.

	Traditional indicators of iron status and CRP[*]					
	Hb (g/L)	CRP (mg/L)	SF (μg/L)	TIBC (μmol/L)	and/or[†]	TS
SF cutoff < 15 μg/L regardless of CRP level						
Iron depletion[†]	—	—	<15	—		—
IDE	—	—	<15	>72	or	<16
IDA	<110	—	<15	>72	or	<16
SF cutoffs < 15 or <50 μg/L w/o or w/ inflammation, respectively[‡]						
Iron depletion w/o inflammation[§]	—	≤5	<15	—		—
Iron depletion w/ inflammation[§]	—	>5	<50	—		—
IDE w/o inflammation	—	≤5	<15	>72	or	<16
IDE w/ inflammation	—	>5	<50	>72	or	<16
IDA w/o inflammation	<110	≤5	<15	>72	or	<16
IDA w/ inflammation	<110	>5	<50	>72	or	<16

IDE: iron deficient erythropoiesis; IDA: iron deficiency anemia; CRP: C-reactive protein; Hb: hemoglobin; SF: serum ferritin; TIBC: total iron binding capacity; TS: transferrin saturation; w/o: without; w/: with.
[*] Reference sources for the cutoffs were as follows: Hb [19]; CRP [7, 31–33]; SF [6, 30]; TIBC [22, 23]; TS [14, 19, 23].
[†] The choice "and/or" applies to the last two biochemical parameters.
[‡] SF cutoffs were adjusted for inflammation using the C-reactive protein (CRP): w/o inflammation: CRP < 5 mg/L; w/ inflammation: CRP ≥ 5 mg/L.
[§] Without or with concomitant IDE and IDA.

and 4.4 mg/L. The sTfR-FI corresponded to the sTfR level divided by the log 10 of SF [18].

2.3. References Values and Iron Deficiency States.

Anemia was defined as a Hb concentration < 110 g/L [19]. The cutoff values for red blood cell indices indicating, respectively, microcytosis and hypochromia were as follows: MCV < 72 fL [20] and MCHC (<320 g/L) [21]. SI < 9 μmol/L [22, 23], TIBC > 72 μmol/L [22, 23], and TS < 16% [14, 19, 23] are indicative of IDE. Elevated sTfR and sTfR-FI also reflect IDE [11, 24]. According to Vendt et al. every method used for measuring sTfR needs its own cutoff value [25]. The reference value recommended by the laboratory where our analyses were done was based on Raya et al. who showed that the 95th percentile of sTfR in children aged 3 to 10 years when measured on a Dade Behring nephelometer was 1.95 [26]. A sTfR-FI of 1.5 has been used as cutoff for ID in numerous studies [18, 27–29] and was taken in the current study. As summarized in Table 1, two methods based on traditional indicators of iron status (SF, TIBC, and TS) were used to define iron depletion, IDE, and IDA. In the first method, a SF cutoff < 15 μg/L was used irrespective of the CRP level. In the second method, two different cutoffs were used for SF to take into account the absence (SF < 15 μg/L) [30] or presence of inflammation (SF < 50 μg/L) [6], which were defined as a CRP ≤ 5 mg/L or >5 mg/L, respectively [7, 31–33].

2.4. Data Analysis.

Statistical analyses were conducted with SAS (version 9.2; SAS Institute Inc., Cary, NC, USA). Values are given as percentages (n), arithmetic means (SD), or medians with interquartile range (IQR: 25th–75th percentiles). The normality of distribution was revised both graphically and with the Shapiro-Wilk test. The spread of results was not normally distributed; thus, nonparametric statistical tests were used in this study. Because the Hb concentration was one of the most measured laboratory indicators among our participants, we used this parameter to compare the demographic and clinical characteristics of participants with ($n = 180$) or without ($n = 65$) an iron status indicator. The median test was used to compare the medians of breastfeeding duration, whereas the Wilcoxon rank-sum test and the chi-square test were used for continuous and categorical variables, respectively. We considered the following participant characteristics: age (months); sex (% male); coast of residence (% Hudson); breastfeeding status (% ever breastfed), breastfeeding duration (months); maternal age during pregnancy (years); supplement use during pregnancy (% yes); respondent's education (% secondary completed or more); and working status (% working). Breastfeeding duration was calculated only for breastfed children and was expressed as the median (IQR). For children who were still breastfed when the interview was conducted, it was equal to the child's age at the time of the interview. The McNemar test was used to compare differences in the prevalence of iron depletion, IDE, and IDA between the two methods (one SF cutoff versus two cutoffs). Spearman's correlation coefficients between different indicators of iron status were calculated. P value < 0.05 was considered a significant level.

3. Results

3.1. Population Characteristics.

Demographic and clinical characteristics of participants with or without a Hb test are shown in Table 2. The mean age (SD) of children was 24.6 (9.8) months; about half of them were boys and lived on the Hudson coast. About seventy percent of these children had ever been breastfed (i.e., breastfed for some period). The median breastfeeding duration (IQR) in children who

TABLE 2: Demographic and clinical characteristics of preschool Inuit children with or without a Hb test.

Characteristics	With a Hb test[*] (n)	Without a Hb test[*] (n)	p[†]
Age (months)	24.6 (9.8) (180)	25.0 (9.5) (65)	0.64
Sex (% male)	52.2 (180)	52.3 (65)	0.99
Coast of residence (% Hudson)[‡]	52.8 (180)	55.4 (65)	0.72
Any breastfeeding			
Ever breastfed (% yes)	70.8 (178)	70.8 (65)	0.99
Breastfeeding duration (months)[§]	7.0 (2.5–15.0) (126)	6.2 (2.0–15.0) (46)	0.58
Maternal age during pregnancy (years)	23.7 (5.2) (163)	23.7 (5.7) (58)	0.74
Supplement use during pregnancy (% yes)	81.3 (155)	82.5 (57)	0.85
Respondent education level (secondary completed or more (%))[‖]	37.8 (180)	44.6 (65)	0.43
Respondent working status (% working)[‖]	83.9 (180)	81.5 (65)	0.66

Values are given as arithmetic means (±SD) or percentages unless otherwise specified.

[*]180 participants had a Hb test, while 65 had none. Some characteristics, namely, breast feeding status, maternal age, and supplement use during pregnancy, were not available for all the children.

[†]Differences were assessed using a Wilcoxon rank-sum test for continuous variables, chi-square statistics for categorical variables, and the median two-sample test for breastfeeding duration.

[‡]Nunavik occupies a third of the province of Quebec (Canada) north of the 55th parallel and is bordered by the Ungava Bay (east), Hudson Strait (north), and Hudson Bay (west).

[§]Breastfeeding duration in breastfed children. Duration was equal to the child's age for children who were still breastfed at the time of the interview. Median (IQR: interquartile range).

[‖]The respondent for the child at the time of the interview was the biological mother (78.8%, n = 193) or father (2.8%, n = 7), the adoptive mother (15.5%; n = 38), the foster mother (2.4%, n = 6), or the foster father (0.4%, n = 1).

TABLE 3: Prevalence of abnormal values for iron status indicators regardless of inflammation and C-reactive protein (CRP) in preschool Inuit children.

	Mean (SD)	Median (IQR)	Cutoff point[*]	Prevalence of abnormal values % (n)
Hb (g/L)	120.2 (11.0)	120 (114–128)	<110	15.0 (27/180)
MCV (fL)	74.5 (5.7)	75.4 (72.3–77.9)	<72	22.8 (41/180)
MCHC (g/L)	330.0 (17.0)	329 (319–344)	<320	27.7 (49/177)
SI (μmol/L)	8.7 (4.7)	8.0 (5.0–11.0)	<9	54.7 (93/170)
TIBC (μmol/L)	81.3 (13.8)	80.6 (71.3–89.4)	>72	74.1 (126/170)
TS (%)	11.1 (6.5)	10.0 (6.3–14.0)	<16	81.8 (139/170)
SF (μg/L)	24.5 (18.6)	21.0 (11.8–30.0)	<15	32.9 (56/170)
sTfR (mg/L)	2.1 (0.7)	1.9 (1.7–2.3)	>1.95	47.4 (73/154)
sTfR-FI	1.9 (1.8)	1.5 (1.2–1.9)	>1.5	49.7 (74/149)
CRP (mg/L)	5.9 (12.6)	0.9 (0.5–4.8)	>5	24.7 (42/170)

SD: standard deviation; IQR: interquartile range.

Hb: hemoglobin; MCV: mean corpuscular volume; MCHC: mean corpuscular hemoglobin concentration; SI: serum iron; TIBC: total iron binding capacity; TS: transferrin saturation; SF: serum ferritin; sTfR: soluble transferrin receptor; sTfR-FI: soluble transferrin receptor-ferritin index.

[*]Reference sources for the cutoffs were as follows: Hb [19]; MCV [20]; MCHC [21]; SI and TIBC [22, 23]; TS [14, 19, 23]; SF [6, 30]; sTfR [26]; sTfR-FI [18, 27–29]; CRP [7, 31–33].

had been breastfed was 7.0 (2.5–15.0) months. The mean age (SD) of biological mothers during pregnancy was 23.7 (5.2) years. Eighty-one percent of mothers took a prenatal supplement during pregnancy. Almost two-thirds of mothers took a prenatal vitamin and mineral supplement (PVMS), while nearly a quarter of them took an iron supplement in addition to the PMMS (results not shown). About 38% of respondents had completed secondary schooling or more and 84% were working at the time of the interview. There were no significant differences in demographic and clinical characteristics of children who had at least one iron status indicator and those who had none (Table 2).

3.2. Iron Status. The mean (SD) Hb and SF concentrations were 120.2 (11.0) g/L and 24.5 (18.6) μg/L, respectively (Table 3). The median (IQR) SF concentration was 21.0 (11.8–30.0) μg/L. Among the other iron indicators, the mean sTfR-FI was 1.9 (1.8) and the median (IQR) was 1.5 (1.2–1.9). The prevalence of anemia from all causes (Hb < 110 g/L) was 15%. Microcytosis and hypochromia were found, respectively,

TABLE 4: Prevalence of iron depletion, IDE, and IDA in preschool Inuit children while disregarding or accounting for the influence of inflammation on SF cutoffs.

Iron status	n	Prevalence (%)	95% CI	P^*
Iron depletion[†]				
SF < 15 μg/L regardless of CRP level	53	32.7	25.4, 40.0	<0.0001
SF < 15 or <50 μg/L w/o or w/ inflammation, respectively[‡]	75	46.3	38.5, 54.0	
IDE[§]				
SF < 15 μg/L regardless of CRP level	51	31.5	24.2, 38.7	<0.0001
SF < 15 or <50 μg/L w/o or w/ inflammation, respectively[‡]	73	45.1	37.3, 52.8	
IDA[§]				
SF < 15 μg/L regardless of CRP level	10	6.2	2.4, 9.9	0.083
SF < 15 or <50 μg/L w/o or w/ inflammation, respectively[‡]	13	8.0	3.8, 12.2	

IDE: iron deficient erythropoiesis; IDA: iron deficiency anemia; SF: serum ferritin; w/o: without, w/: with.
[*]The McNemar test was used to compare differences in the prevalence of iron depletion, IDE, and IDA between the two methods in children with a complete set of traditional indicators of iron status ($n = 162$).
[†]Without ($n = 2$) or with concomitant IDE and, in some cases, IDA.
[‡]SF cutoffs were adjusted for inflammation using the C-reactive protein (CRP): w/o inflammation: CRP < 5 mg/L; w/ inflammation: CRP ≥ 5 mg/L.
[§]IDE and IDA as defined in Table 1.

TABLE 5: Spearman's correlation coefficients (R) between the different iron status indicators[*].

	Hb	MCV	MCHC	SI	TIBC	TS	sTfR	sTfR-FI	SF	CRP
Hb	1.0									
MCV	0.451[*]	1.0								
MCHC	0.592[*]	0.414[*]	1.0							
SI	0.295[*]	0.501[*]	0.196[§]	1.0						
TIBC	−0.227[‡]	−0.450[*]	−0.297[*]	−0.123	1.0					
TS	0.352[*]	0.598[*]	0.280[†]	0.952[*]	−0.390[*]	1.0				
sTfR	−0.348[*]	−0.650[*]	−0.371[*]	−0.547[*]	0.499[*]	−0.670[*]	1.0			
sTfR-FI	−0.252[‡]	−0.552[*]	−0.365[*]	−0.294[†]	0.630[*]	−0.473[*]	0.782[*]	1.0		
SF	0.098	0.310[*]	0.205[‡]	−0.007	−0.537[*]	0.158[§]	−0.340[*]	−0.828[*]	1.0	
CRP	−0.167[§]	−0.252[‡]	−0.173[§]	−0.625[*]	−0.080	−0.545[*]	0.268[†]	0.019	0.328[*]	1.0

Abbreviations are as defined in Table 3.
[*]With the exception of correlation coefficients involving sTfR and sTfR-FI for which the n varied between 141 and 149 participants and MCHC between 159 and 177, the n for all the other correlation coefficients varied between 162 and 180 participants.
P (P value): [*]$P \le 0.0001$; [†]$P \le 0.001$; [‡]$P < 0.01$; [§]$P < 0.05$.

in 22.8% and 27.7% of the study population. Low TS and increased TIBC, sTfR, and sTfR-FI, all indicative of IDE, were found in 81.8%, 74.1%, 47.4%, and 49.7% of children, respectively. Almost 25% of participants had a CRP concentration higher than the clinical cut-point for inflammation. Also, 32.9% of participants had depleted iron stores (SF < 15 μg/L) irrespective of the CRP level.

As indicated in Table 4, almost half of the children had depleted iron stores when the absence or presence of inflammation was taken into account, whereas this proportion only reached one-third when SF was used irrespective of the CRP level ($P < 0.0001$). Similar results were observed for IDE and the difference between both methods was also statistically significant ($P < 0.0001$). With the exception of two participants, all the children with iron depletion also suffered from IDE. The prevalence of anemia from all causes was 15%. The prevalence of IDA was higher when two cutoffs were used for SF compared to using only one cutoff regardless of the CRP level (8.0% versus 6.2%, $P = 0.083$). It is

noteworthy to mention that 3 of the remaining 13 children not classified as having IDA were very close to suffering from IDA in the absence of inflammation, except for their SF level that was slightly above the cutoff limit of <15 μg/L (SF: 15 μg/L, 15.3 μg/L, and 17 μg/L (results not shown)). Two other participants could not be classified as having IDA with coexistent inflammation due to the fact that their SF level was not <50 μg/L, but rather 51 and 53 μg/L (results not shown). In clinical practice, this would represent an additional 3% of participants classified as having IDA.

As shown in Table 5, there were significant correlations between Hb, MCV, and MCHC and all the other iron status indicators with the exception of Hb that was not significantly related to SF. Hb, MCV, and MCHC were negatively associated with TIBC, sTfR, and sTfR-FI. TIBC was negatively correlated with TS and SF but positively related to sTfR and sTfR-FI. TS was negatively related to sTfR and sTfR-FI but positively associated with SF. CRP was negatively correlated to Hb, MCV, MCHC, SI, and TS, whereas it was positively associated with sTfR and SF. Also of interest, sTfR and sTfR-FI were negatively correlated to SF.

4. Discussion

To our knowledge, this study is the first to determine the prevalence of iron deficiency in a group of young Inuit children using sTfR and sTfR-FI as well as a variety of conventional laboratory indicators of iron status while taking into account the absence or presence of inflammation.

4.1. Iron Depletion. Iron depletion, the initial stage of ID, is characterized by a low SF level. The mean SF concentration (SD) observed in our study was higher than the level reported in preschool Nunavut children (24.5 versus 19.1 μg/L in Nunavut) [5]. This can be partially explained by a higher prevalence of inflammation in our study (CRP $\geq$ 8 mg/L: 18.8% (result not shown) versus 5.1% in Nunavut) which is associated with increased SF levels [34, 35]. The impact of CRP levels on SF values has also been observed in a group of Australian Aboriginal children from 6 to 60 months of age whose mean SF concentration was 56.3 μg/L while 69.9% had a CRP level above 8 mg/L [36].

The prevalence of iron depletion irrespective of the CRP level affected one-third of our participants (Table 3). This is identical to the prevalence observed in older Inuit children (mean age: 11.3 years) from Nunavik [37]. However, we found a higher prevalence of iron depletion without inflammation than that found in a group of preschool Inuit children from Nunavut (SF < 12 μg/L and CRP level < 8 mg/L: 29% (result not shown) versus 18% in Nunavut) [5]. This can partially be explained by the fact that preschoolers from Nunavik were twice as young as the ones from Nunavut (2.1 versus 4.4 years) and, thus, more susceptible to developing ID. Indeed, it has been reported in low income families that 1- to 2-year-old children were at higher risk of ID than 3- to 4-year-olds [38]. Moreover, a large database of 32,000 patients aged 12 to 59 months from Alberta (Canada) revealed that the peak age for IDA was 19 months [39].

In agreement with other studies [34, 35], we found that the use of two cutoffs for SF enabled us to identify significantly more children with depleted iron stores than when SF was used irrespective of the CRP level (Table 4). According to Wieringa et al., "using indicators of micronutrient status without considering the effects of the acute phase response results in a distorted estimate of micronutrient deficiencies, whose extent depends on the prevalence of infection in the population" [34]. We found that a quarter of our participants had an elevated CRP level confirming the high infection rate observed in many Canadian Inuit children [8]. However, the prevalence of inflammation observed in the present study was probably greater than revealed due to the fact that CRP detects acute inflammation while α1-acid glycoprotein, not measured in our participants, better detects chronic inflammation [7, 9, 35]. Considering that infections are more likely to occur in ID children [40], the exclusion of subjects with inflammation can reduce the prevalence of iron depletion aside from preventing the use of valuable data [34] making comparison with other studies more difficult.

4.2. Iron Deficient Erythropoiesis. When storage iron becomes depleted, the second stage of ID known as IDE develops. It is characterized by a decrease in iron being transported within the body resulting in low SI, increased TIBC, and reduced TS [23]. In agreement with other studies [41], we found that the proportions of children who were iron deficient based on these indicators used separately varied considerably (Table 3).

In the present study, elevated sTfR levels were found in almost half of the participants indicating that iron stores were low which was followed by an increase in sTfR. Indeed, during the process of iron depletion, sTfR concentration remains stable [15]. However, when iron stores are depleted, as indicated by a subnormal SF level, the concentration of sTfR increases [15]. Calculation of the sTfR-FI has been proposed to take advantage of the reciprocal relationship between SF and sTfR [42]. Yet, the proportion of abnormal values using the sTfR-FI and sTfR alone was similar in our study (49.7% versus 47.4%, Table 3) indicating that both indices were good indicators of IDE among our participants. Kamer et al. also reported in 6- to 36-month-old children that both sTfR and the sTfR-FI were good indicators of ID and could be useful in the differential diagnostics of anemia, especially in young children [43]. On the contrary, the log of sTfR-SF ratio has been described as a better criterion than either sTfR or sTfR-FI for defining the iron status of children, although the sTfR-SF ratio was not able to exclude IDA in the presence of inflammation [14]. Interestingly, Cook et al. used the sTfR-SF ratio to define an algorithm for estimating body iron in adult subjects [44]. However, the use of the sTfR-SF ratio to estimate body iron has certain limitations. Indeed, the extent to which this algorithm can be applied in school-aged and preschool-aged children is uncertain, whereas one of its main limitations is the influence of inflammation on SF levels independent of body iron stores [44]. Considering the high prevalence of inflammation found among our participants, the use of sTfR-SF ratio to assess the iron status based on the quantitative measurement of body iron would have been premature.

We also observed that the prevalence of IDE based on three traditional indicators of iron status in addition to CRP was similar to the proportion found when sTfR was used as a sole marker of IDE (45.1% (Table 4) versus 47.4% (Table 3)). When using traditional indicators of iron status, we raised the cutoff value for SF from 15 to 50 μg/L with an elevated CRP level, whereas sTfR has been shown to be unaffected by concomitant infectious or inflammatory conditions [18, 45]. Even though sTfR assay is not available everywhere [46] (as is the case in Nunavik), it is set to become a useful diagnostic tool in clinical settings [11]. Until sTfR is more easily available, using different cutoffs for SF in the absence or presence of inflammation can significantly improve the diagnosis of IDE.

4.3. Iron Deficiency Anemia. In the present study, the prevalence of anemia from all causes (15%) (Table 3) was similar to that reported in Inuit preschool-aged children from Nunavut [5] but slightly more elevated than the one found among Québec Cree infants screened between 2002 and 2007 (12.5%) [47]. Nevertheless, before screening for anemia was initiated in 1995 in the Cree region of Québec, the prevalence of anemia was much higher reaching 31.7% [47].

In agreement with other studies [3], we found that IDA was the most common type of anemia among our participants. Indeed, there were 8% of children with IDA when using different cutoffs for children with versus without inflammation (Table 4), whereas an additional 3% of participants would have been classified as having IDA except for a borderline SF. Determining a cutoff limit for SF in the presence of inflammation is problematic and values between 10 and 100 μg/L have been suggested to represent a diagnostic grey zone [48].

The prevalence of IDA observed in these preschool Inuit children from Nunavik (8%) was almost identical to the level reported in older children and adolescents also from Nunavik (8- to 10-year-olds) (8.7%) [37]. Although the determinants of anemia in children seem to vary according to the age bracket [49], the prevalence of IDA in Nunavik appears to remain stable throughout childhood and adolescence.

To our knowledge, there are currently no national statistics for the prevalence of IDA in Canadian children. However, a study carried out by Obaid in Edmonton (Alberta) (cited by Hartfield) and using a large database of more than 32,000 patients 12 to 59 months of age, between 2002 and 2008, indicated that the prevalence of IDA was 7.7% [39], which is almost identical to the rate observed in the current study. In USA, the prevalence of IDA in toddlers is estimated to be 1.2% [50], although higher prevalence has been observed in American children from high-risk population and low income families (3–6%) [38, 51]. Nevertheless, in the studies just mentioned above, children with an elevated CRP concentration ($\geq$10 mg/L) were excluded from the analyses [38], or an acute phase protein such as CRP was neither measured [50, 51] nor reported [39]; thus the real prevalence of IDA might be higher than reported.

IDA is the most common cause of microcytosis and hypochromia [52, 53]. Microcytosis develops either ahead of or at the same time as any reduction in the Hb level [54]. A low MCV could indicate early ID that has not yet resulted in anemia [54]. This seems to be the case in our study as almost a quarter of the children had a low MCV (Table 3) while the prevalence of anemia was 15%. A decrease in MCH and MCHC, reflecting red cell hypochromia, can also be used to diagnose IDA. However, since hypochromia normally accompanies microcytosis, MCH [54] and MCHC are not more reliable than the MCV for detecting iron deficiency.

4.4. Correlation Coefficients between Iron Status Indicators. In our study, correlations were observed between traditional laboratory indicators of iron status and sTfR. As expected, there was a positive association between sTfR, sTfR-FI, and TIBC confirming results from previous studies which have shown that ID unquestionably leads to a significant rise of sTfR levels and TIBC [11, 22]. However, sTfR was negatively related to TS, SI, and MCV and, to a lower extent, to SF. The weakest correlation observed between SF and sTfR is not surprising since SF is a measure of iron stores whereas sTfR is

a measure of tissue iron. The correlation found between sTfR and MCHC is not as strong as the one observed between sTfR and MCV. This is likely due to the fact that MCHC tends to be the last indicator to fall as ID worsens [55]. As reported by other authors, we observed a positive association between CRP and sTfR [9], as well as CRP and SF [9, 12, 32]. We also found a negative association between CRP and Hb [9, 12, 32], as well as CRP and SI [56].

5. Conclusion

The prevalence of anemia from all causes was 15%, thus near the upper limit defined by the WHO for mild anemia (5% to 19.9%) [3]. As expected, ID was the main cause of anemia among our participants. Moreover, accounting for the elevating effect of inflammation on SF significantly improved the diagnosis of iron depletion and IDE which affected almost half of the children compared to one-third when disregarding inflammation. Interestingly, taking inflammation into account when using traditional indicators of iron status resulted in a prevalence of IDE that was almost identical to the prevalence observed when sTfR, thought to be unaffected by inflammation [12, 13], was used as a sole marker of IDE. Although ID remains a public health concern in Canadian children, our results confirm that Aboriginal children are at particularly high risk [57]. However, the iron status of participating children could be better than that of Nunavimmiut children not enrolled in childcare since nonattendance to childcare has been identified as a risk factor for ID and IDA [57]. Strategies for preventing or reducing ID in preschool Inuit children from Nunavik are therefore needed.

Additional Points

Certain limitations of our study need to be considered. First, data comparison between studies using sTfR is hampered by the lack of comparability of results across manufacturer assays [45, 58]. According to the WHO, there is an urgent need for a reference material with a certified concentration of transferrin receptor to standardize sTfR assays [30]. Another limitation is the fact that we only measured CRP which better detects acute inflammation as opposed to α1-acid glycoprotein which is a more sensitive indicator of chronic inflammation. Also, our participants have not been randomly selected in childcare facilities of Nunavik. Nevertheless, this study provides valuable insight concerning the iron status of these children considering that 245 participants have been recruited between 2006 and 2010 in 10 of the 14 Nunavik communities. Even though laboratory indicators of iron status were not available for the 245 participants, no significant differences were observed between demographic and clinical characteristics of participants with at least one laboratory indicator of iron status and those who had none.

Competing Interests

The authors declare that there are no competing interests regarding the publication of this paper.

Authors' Contributions

Carole Vézina was responsible for the coordination of all the laboratory analyses; Huguette Turgeon O'Brien and Rosanne Blanchet conducted the statistical analyses. Huguette Turgeon O'Brien interpreted the results with the contribution of Rosanne Blanchet, Julie Lauzière, and Doris Gagné; Huguette Turgeon O'Brien prepared the first draft of the paper; Doris Gagné and Carole Vézina were responsible for the Nutrition Program idea and design. All the authors read and approved the final paper.

Acknowledgments

The authors are grateful to the Nunavik parents and children for their participation. They wish to thank all educators, cooks, and directors of childcare centres in Nunavik, who were very supportive of the project. They give special thanks to Margaret Gauvin and Julie-Ann Berthe from the Kativik Regional Government for their constant support. They are thankful to the Nunavik Nutrition and Health Committee for their expertise and support and to nurses and dietitians who worked on this project. They also want to thank Chantal Vinet-Lanouette, Émilie Vaissière, Marthe Paris, Annie Augiak, Lizzie Anne Esperon, Maryse Turcot, and Sylvie St-Hilaire for their great involvement in the nutrition program. They also benefited from the expertise of Hélène Crépeau (Service de Consultation Statistique, Université Laval) for statistical analysis. They are very grateful to Dr. Jean-Marc Gagné (Biochemistry Department, CHUL-CHUQ, Québec City) and Dr. Jean-Pierre Émond (Immunology-Inflammation Laboratory, Notre-Dame Hospital, CHUM, Montreal) for the laboratory analyses. They also wish to thank Edward James O'Brien for ensuring English language support. This study was made possible through funding by the Aboriginal Affairs and Northern Development Canada, Canada, Northern Contaminants Program, Kativik Regional Government, and Health Canada.

References

[1] J. L. Beard, "Iron biology in immune function, muscle metabolism and neuronal functioning," *Journal of Nutrition*, vol. 131, no. 2, pp. 568S–580S, 2001.

[2] E. McLean, M. Cogswell, I. Egli, D. Wojdyla, and B. De Benoist, "Worldwide prevalence of anaemia, WHO Vitamin and Mineral Nutrition Information System, 1993–2005," *Public Health Nutrition*, vol. 12, no. 4, pp. 444–454, 2009.

[3] World Health Organization, *Worldwide Prevalence of Anaemia 1993–2005*, World Health Organization, Geneva, Switzerland, 2008.

[4] M. Cooper, L. Greene-Finestone, H. Lowell, J. Levesque, and S. Robinson, "Iron sufficiency of Canadians," *Health Reports*, vol. 23, pp. 41–48, 2012.

[5] A. Pacey, H. Weiler, and G. M. Egeland, "Low prevalence of iron-deficiency anaemia among Inuit preschool children: Nunavut Inuit Child Health Survey, 2007–2008," *Public Health Nutrition*, vol. 14, no. 8, pp. 1415–1423, 2011.

[6] J. L. Beard, L. E. Murray-Kolb, F. J. Rosales, N. W. Solomons, and M. L. Angelilli, "Interpretation of serum ferritin concentrations as indicators of total-body iron stores in survey populations: the role of biomarkers for the acute phase response," *The American Journal of Clinical Nutrition*, vol. 84, no. 6, pp. 1498–1505, 2006.

[7] D. I. Thurnham, L. D. McCabe, S. Haldar, F. T. Wieringa, C. A. Northrop-Clewes, and G. P. McCabe, "Adjusting plasma ferritin concentrations to remove the effects of subclinical inflammation in the assessment of iron deficiency: a meta-analysis," *American Journal of Clinical Nutrition*, vol. 92, no. 3, pp. 546–555, 2010.

[8] P. H. Orr, "Respiratory tract infections in Inuit children: 'set thine house in order'," *Canadian Medical Association Journal*, vol. 177, no. 2, pp. 167–168, 2007.

[9] F. K. E. Grant, P. S. Suchdev, R. Flores-Ayala et al., "Correcting for inflammation changes estimates of iron deficiency among rural Kenyan preschool children," *Journal of Nutrition*, vol. 142, no. 1, pp. 105–111, 2012.

[10] K. Abraham, C. Müller, A. Grüters, U. Wahn, and F. J. Schweigert, "Minimal inflammation, acute phase response and avoidance of misclassification of vitamin A and iron status in infants—importance of a high-sensitivity C-Reactive Protein (CRP) assay," *International Journal for Vitamin and Nutrition Research*, vol. 73, no. 6, pp. 423–430, 2003.

[11] S. H. Yoon, D. S. Kim, S. T. Yu, S. R. Shin, and D. Y. Choi, "The usefulness of soluble transferrin receptor in the diagnosis and treatment of iron deficiency anemia in children," *Korean Journal of Pediatrics*, vol. 58, no. 1, pp. 15–19, 2015.

[12] F. S. Asobayire, P. Adou, L. Davidsson, J. D. Cook, and R. F. Hurrell, "Prevalence of iron deficiency with and without concurrent anemia in population groups with high prevalences of malaria and other infections: a study in Côte d'Ivoirel-3," *American Journal of Clinical Nutrition*, vol. 74, no. 6, pp. 776–782, 2001.

[13] A. E. Mast, M. A. Blinder, A. M. Gronowski, C. Chumley, and M. G. Scott, "Clinical utility of the soluble transferrin receptor and comparison with serum ferritin in several populations," *Clinical Chemistry*, vol. 44, no. 1, pp. 45–51, 1998.

[14] B. I. Malope, A. P. MacPhail, M. Alberts, and D. C. Hiss, "The ratio of serum transferrin receptor and serum ferritin in the diagnosis of iron status," *British Journal of Haematology*, vol. 115, no. 1, pp. 84–89, 2001.

[15] G. L. Chouliaras, E. Premetis, G. Tsiftis et al., "Serum transferrin receptors: distribution and diagnostic performance in preschool children," *Blood Cells, Molecules, and Diseases*, vol. 43, no. 2, pp. 163–168, 2009.

[16] D. Gagné, R. Blanchet, J. Lauzière et al., "Traditional food consumption is associated with higher nutrient intakes in Inuit children attending childcare centres in Nunavik," *International Journal of Circumpolar Health*, vol. 71, Article ID 18401, 2012.

[17] S. Lunder, L. Hovander, I. Athanassiadis, and Å. Bergman, "Significantly higher polybrominated diphenyl ether levels in young U.S. children than in their mothers," *Environmental Science and Technology*, vol. 44, no. 13, pp. 5256–5262, 2010.

[18] K. Punnonen, K. Irjala, and A. Rajamäki, "Serum transferrin receptor and its ratio to serum ferritin in the diagnosis of iron

deficiency," *Blood*, vol. 89, no. 3, pp. 1052–1057, 1997.

[19] World Health Organization, UNICEF, and UNU, *Iron Deficiency Anemia: Assessment, Prevention, and Control. A Guide for Programme Managers*, World Health Organization, Geneva, Switzerland, 2001.

[20] I. Öhlund, T. Lind, A. Hörnell, and O. Hernell, "Predictors of iron status in well-nourished 4-y-old children," *The American Journal of Clinical Nutrition*, vol. 87, no. 4, pp. 839–845, 2008.

[21] F. A. Oski, "Iron deficiency in infancy and childhood," *The New England Journal of Medicine*, vol. 329, no. 3, pp. 190–193, 1993.

[22] A. N. R. Lakshmi and P. Paramjyothi, "Association of serum iron and total iron binding capacity in rural children," *International Journal of Biological and Medical Research*, vol. 4, no. 1, pp. 2717–2719, 2013.

[23] A. C. F. Vieira, A. S. Diniz, P. C. Cabral et al., "Nutritional assessment of iron status and anemia in children under 5 years old at public daycare centers," *Jornal de Pediatria*, vol. 83, no. 4, pp. 370–376, 2007.

[24] J. Chang, R. Bird, A. Clague, and A. Carter, "Clinical utility of serum soluble transferrin receptor levels and comparison with bone marrow iron stores as an index for iron-deficient erythropoiesis in a heterogeneous group of patients," *Pathology*, vol. 39, no. 3, pp. 349–353, 2007.

[25] N. Vendt, T. Talvik, S. Leedo et al., "The reference limits and cut-off value for serum soluble transferrin receptors for diagnosing iron deficiency in infants," *International Journal of Laboratory Hematology*, vol. 31, no. 4, pp. 440–446, 2009.

[26] G. Raya, J. Henny, J. Steinmetz, B. Herbeth, and G. Siest, "Soluble transferrin receptor (sTfR): biological variations and reference limits," *Clinical Chemistry and Laboratory Medicine*, vol. 39, no. 11, pp. 1162–1168, 2001.

[27] R. Goyal, R. Das, P. Bambery, and G. Garewal, "Serum transferrin receptor-ferritin index shows concomitant iron deficiency anemia and anemia of chronic disease is common in patients with rheumatoid arthritis in north India," *Indian Journal of Pathology and Microbiology*, vol. 51, no. 1, pp. 102–104, 2008.

[28] S. Jain, S. Narayan, J. Chandra, S. Sharma, S. Jain, and P. Malhan, "Evaluation of serum transferrin receptor and sTfR ferritin indices in diagnosing and differentiating iron deficiency anemia from anemia of chronic disease," *Indian Journal of Pediatrics*, vol. 77, no. 2, pp. 179–183, 2010.

[29] C. W. Choi, W. R. Cho, K. H. Park et al., "The cutoff value of serum ferritin for the diagnosis of iron deficiency in community-residing older persons," *Annals of Hematology*, vol. 84, no. 6, pp. 358–361, 2005.

[30] World Health Organization, *Assessing the Iron Status of Population: Including Literature Reviews: Report of a Joint World Health Organization/Centers for Disease Control and Prevention Technical Consultation on the Assessment of Iron Status at the Population Level*, World Health Organization, Geneva, Switzerland, 2nd edition, 2007.

[31] A. Demir, N. Yarali, T. Fisgin, F. Duru, and A. Kara, "Most reliable indices in differentiation between thalassemia trait and iron deficiency anemia," *Pediatrics International*, vol. 44, no. 6, pp. 612–616, 2002.

[32] K. A. Bresnahan, J. Chileshe, S. Arscott et al., "The acute phase response affected traditional measures of micronutrient status in rural zambian children during a randomized, controlled feeding trial," *Journal of Nutrition*, vol. 144, no. 6, pp. 972–978, 2014.

[33] L. Uijterschout, M. Domellöf, J. Vloemans et al., "The value of Ret-Hb and sTfR in the diagnosis of iron depletion in healthy, young children," *European Journal of Clinical Nutrition*, vol. 68, no. 8, pp. 882–886, 2014.

[34] F. T. Wieringa, M. A. Dijkhuizen, C. E. West, C. A. Northrop-Clewes, and Muhilal, "Estimation of the effect of the acute phase response on indicators of micronutrient status in Indonesian infants," *Journal of Nutrition*, vol. 132, no. 10, pp. 3061–3066, 2002.

[35] E. Nel, H. S. Kruger, J. Baumgartner, M. Faber, and C. M. Smuts, "Differential ferritin interpretation methods that adjust for inflammation yield discrepant iron deficiency prevalence," *Maternal and Child Nutrition*, vol. 11, supplement 4, pp. 221–228, 2015.

[36] B. Ritchie, Y. McNeil, and D. R. Brewster, "Soluble transferrin receptor in Aboriginal children with a high prevalence of iron deficiency and infection," *Tropical Medicine and International Health*, vol. 9, no. 1, pp. 96–105, 2004.

[37] C. M. Pirkle, M. Lucas, R. Dallaire et al., "Food insecurity and nutritional biomarkers in relation to stature in inuit children from Nunavik," *Canadian Journal of Public Health*, vol. 105, no. 4, pp. e233–e238, 2014.

[38] J. M. Schneider, M. L. Fujii, C. L. Lamp, B. Lönnerdal, K. G. Dewey, and S. Zidenberg-Cherr, "Anemia, iron deficiency, and iron deficiency anemia in 12-36-mo-old children from low-income families," *The American Journal of Clinical Nutrition*, vol. 82, no. 6, pp. 1269–1275, 2005.

[39] D. Hartfield, "Iron deficiency is a public health problem in Canadian infants and children," *Paediatrics and Child Health*, vol. 15, no. 6, pp. 347–350, 2010.

[40] V. Kumar and V. P. Choudhry, "Iron deficiency and infection," *Indian Journal of Pediatrics*, vol. 77, no. 7, pp. 789–793, 2010.

[41] D. A. Lacher, J. P. Hughes, and M. D. Carroll, "Biological variation of laboratory analytes based on the 1999–2002 National Health and Nutrition Examination Survey," *National Health Statistics Reports*, no. 21, pp. 1–7, 2010.

[42] B. S. Skikne, K. Punnonen, P. H. Caldron et al., "Improved differential diagnosis of anemia of chronic disease and iron deficiency anemia: a prospective multicenter evaluation of soluble transferrin receptor and the sTfR/log ferritin index," *American Journal of Hematology*, vol. 86, no. 11, pp. 923–927, 2011.

[43] B. Kamer, E. Dółka, R. Pasowska, and E. Światkowska, "The usefulness of soluble transferrin receptor (sTfR) in differentiating anemia occurring in young children," *Folia Histochemica et Cytobiologica*, vol. 50, no. 3, pp. 473–479, 2012.

[44] J. D. Cook, C. H. Flowers, and B. S. Skikne, "The quantitative assessment of body iron," *Blood*, vol. 101, no. 9, pp. 3359–3363, 2003.

[45] I. Infusino, F. Braga, A. Dolci, and M. Panteghini, "Soluble transferrin receptor (sTfR) and sTfR/log ferritin index for the diagnosis of iron-deficiency anemia: a meta-analysis," *American Journal of Clinical Pathology*, vol. 138, no. 5, pp. 642–649, 2012.

[46] D. W. Thomas, R. F. Hinchliffe, C. Briggs, I. C. Macdougall, T. Littlewood, and I. Cavill, "Guideline for the laboratory diagnosis of functional iron deficiency," *British Journal of Haematology*, vol. 161, no. 5, pp. 639–648, 2013.

[47] N. Willows, D. Dannenbaum, and S. Vadeboncoeur, "Prevalence of anemia among Quebec Cree infants from 2002 to 2007 compared with 1995 to 2000," *Canadian Family Physician*, vol. 58, no. 2, pp. e101–e106, 2012.

[48] D. H. Shin, H. S. Kim, M. J. Park, I. B. Suh, and K. S. Shin, "Utility of access soluble transferrin receptor (sTfR) and sTfR/log ferritin index in diagnosing iron deficiency anemia," *Annals of Clinical and Laboratory Science*, vol. 45, no. 4, pp. 396–402, 2015.

[49] R. M. Cotta, F. D. C. Oliveira, K. A. Magalhães et al., "Social and biological determinants of iron deficiency anemia," *Cadernos de Saúde Pública*, vol. 27, supplement 2, pp. S309–S320, 2011.

[50] S. E. Cusick, Z. Mei, D. S. Freedman et al., "Unexplained decline in the prevalence of anemia among US children and women between 1988–1994 and 1999–2002," *American Journal of Clinical Nutrition*, vol. 88, no. 6, pp. 1611–1617, 2008.

[51] K. Park, M. Kersey, J. Geppert, M. Story, D. Cutts, and J. H. Himes, "Household food insecurity is a risk factor for iron-deficiency anaemia in a multi-ethnic, low-income sample of infants and toddlers," *Public Health Nutrition*, vol. 12, no. 11, pp. 2120–2128, 2009.

[52] M. van Vranken, "Evaluation of microcytosis," *American Family Physician*, vol. 82, no. 9, pp. 1117–1122, 2010.

[53] J. J. Irwin and J. T. Kirchner, "Anemia in children," *American Family Physician*, vol. 64, no. 8, pp. 1379–1386, 2001.

[54] D. N. Subramanian, S. Kitson, and A. Bhaniani, "Microcytosis and possible early iron deficiency in paediatric inpatients: a retrospective audit," *BMC Pediatrics*, vol. 9, article 36, 2009.

[55] J. P. Greer, *Wintrobe's Clinical Hematology*, Wolters Kluwer Health/Lippincott Williams & Wilkins, Philadelphia, Pa, USA, 13th edition, 2014.

[56] V. De la Cruz-Góngora, S. Villalpando, R. Rebollar, T. Shamah-Levy, and I. M.-G. Humarán, "Nutritional causes of anemia in Mexican children under 5 years. Results from the 2006 National Health And Nutrition Survey," *Salud Publica de Mexico*, vol. 54, no. 2, pp. 108–115, 2012.

[57] K. Abdullah, S. Zlotkin, P. Parkin, and D. Grenier, *Iron-Deficiency Anemia in Children. Canadian Paediatric Surveillance Program Resource*, Public Health Agency of Canada and the Canadian Paediatric Society, Ottawa, Canada, 2011.

[58] World Health Organization, "Serum transferrin receptor levels for the assessment of iron status and iron deficiency in populations," Tech. Rep. WHO/NMH/NHD/EPG/14.6, World Health Organization, Geneva, Switzerland, 2014.

21

Absolute Reticulocyte Count and Reticulocyte Hemoglobin Content as Predictors of Early Response to Exclusive Oral Iron in Children with Iron Deficiency Anemia

Emilia Parodi,[1] Maria Teresa Giraudo,[2] Fulvio Ricceri,[3] Maria Luigia Aurucci,[4] Raffaela Mazzone,[5] and Ugo Ramenghi[4]

[1]*Pediatric and Neonatology Unit, Ordine Mauriziano Hospital, Largo Turati 62, 10128 Turin, Italy*
[2]*Department of Mathematics "G. Peano", University of Turin, Via Carlo Alberto 10, 10123 Turin, Italy*
[3]*Unit of Epidemiology, Regional Health Service ASL TO3, Via Sabaudia 164, Grugliasco, 10095 Turin, Italy*
[4]*Hematology Unit, Department of Sciences of Public Health and Pediatrics, University of Turin, Piazza Polonia 94, 10126 Turin, Italy*
[5]*Hematology and Coagulation Laboratory, Città della Scienza e della Salute Hospital, Piazza Polonia 94, 10126 Turin, Italy*

Correspondence should be addressed to Emilia Parodi; emilia.parodi@unito.it

Academic Editor: Maria Stella Figueiredo

We report data regarding kinetic of response to oral iron in 34 iron deficiency anemia children. Twenty-four/34 patients (70.5%) reached reference value of hemoglobin (Hb) concentration for age and sex at day + 30 from the beginning of treatment (complete early responders (CERs)), and 4/34 (12%) reached an Hb concentration at least 50% higher than the original (partial early responders (PERs)). CHr at T1 (within 7 days from the beginning of treatment) was significantly different in the different groups (22.95 in CERs versus 18.41 in other patients; $p = 0.001$; 22.42 in early responders versus 18.07 in NERs; $p = 0.001$). Relative increase of CHr from T0 to T1 resulted significantly higher in CERs than in other patients (0.21 versus 0.11, $p = 0.042$) and in early responders than in NERs (0.22 versus 0.004, $p = 0.006$). Multivariate logistic models revealed a higher probability of being a complete early responder due to relative increase of ARC from T0 to T1 [OR (95% CI) = 44.95 (1.54–1311.98)] and to CHr at T1 [OR (95% CI) =3.18 (1.24–8.17)]. Our preliminary data confirm CHr as early and accurate predictor of hematological response to oral iron.

1. Introduction

Reticulocytes are the youngest erythrocytes released from the bone marrow into circulating blood. Under normal conditions, after maturing for 1–3 days within the bone marrow, they are released into peripheral blood where they circulate for 1-2 days before becoming mature erythrocytes. The reticulocyte hemoglobin content (CHr) provides an indirect measure of the functional iron available for new red blood cell production over the previous 3-4 days [1]. CHr in peripheral blood samples has been proven to be a useful marker for diagnosis of iron deficiency and iron deficiency anemia (IDA) both in children [2–4] and adults [5].

Brugnara et al. [6] demonstrated that CHr also provides an early measure of the response to parenteral iron therapy increasing within 2–4 days of the initiation of intravenous iron therapy.

The goal of therapy for IDA, the most common hematological disease of infancy and childhood, is to supply sufficient iron to repair the hemoglobin (Hb) deficit and replenish storage iron [7]. Oral iron administration is a well-established effective and worldwide accepted treatment for anemia derived from inadequate dietary iron intake because of its efficacy, safety, and cost-effectiveness [8]. Thus, in our Pediatric Hematology Unit, oral iron treatment is the first-line therapy for all children with IDA with anamnestic suspicion of inadequate iron intake, independently of base Hb level. Recently, we have identified absolute reticulocyte count (ARC) and CHr as accurate and precocious markers in order to early detect early responders to exclusive oral iron therapy in a small cohort of pediatric patients with severe iron deficiency anemia (IDA) [9]. These preliminary results in children with very low base Hb levels (median Hb level before treatment 6.3 g/dL; range 4.5–7.0) prompted us to investigate the efficacy of reticulocyte parameters in monitoring the response to oral iron supplementation in a larger cohort of pediatric patients.

2. Materials and Methods

2.1. Patients and Hematological Evaluation. Clinical records of patients referred to our Pediatric Hematology Unit for IDA between July 1, 2012, and June 30, 2014, were retrospectively analyzed.

Patients who matched inclusion criteria and did not present exclusion criteria were included in the study. Data about patients with an age between 6 months and 16 years, a hemoglobin level more than 2 standard deviations below the mean reference value for age and gender, a transferrin saturation < 15%, and a high anamnestic suspicion of inadequate iron intake were analyzed. Patients with diagnosis of celiac disease, positivity of fecal occult blood test, or positivity of *Helicobacter pylori* fecal antigen test were excluded. Patients from our preliminary report were not included in the present study [9].

All children with these characteristics had started a first-line treatment with exclusive oral iron supplementation at a dosage equivalent to 2 mg/kg/die of elemental iron. In all patients but one, who underwent therapy with liposomial iron, bisglycinate chelate iron was administered.

Data about Hb levels and reticulocyte parameters (ARC and CHr) at diagnosis, before treatment (T0), within 7 days (T1), and at day +30 (T2) from the beginning of iron supplementation, were extrapolated from clinical records of each patient and analyzed with analytical methods.

Hb and reticulocyte parameters on peripheral blood samples had been measured with an automated flow cytometer (Advia 120 Bayer®) with optic measure; reticulocytes had been stained with dye oxazine 750. Approximately 50.000 cells had been counted for each red blood cell and reticulocyte determinations.

2.2. Statistical Analysis. We described data as number and frequencies or mean and standard deviation for qualitative and quantitative variables, respectively.

Differences between different groups of patients were tested using Fisher's exact test or Wilcoxon sum rank test (due to the not normal distribution of all the values as established by means of Shapiro-Wilks normality tests), as appropriate.

To account for possible confounding variables, we performed a multivariate logistic model, adjusting for age, sex, and Hb value at diagnosis.

Relative increase of ARC and CHr from T0 to T1 was computed as (T1 value – T0 value)/T0 value.

All tests were two-sided and a p value lower than 0.050 was considered significant. Analyses were performed using SAS V9.4.

2.3. Definitions. Response was defined as early and complete if patients reached mean Hb reference value for age at day +30 (T2) from the onset of iron therapy (complete early responders (CERs)).

Response at T2 was defined as early and partial if patients reached an Hb concentration at least 50% higher than the original one, computed as (Hb T2 – Hb T0)/Hb T0 (partial early responders, PERs).

Patients who at T2 did not achieve an Hb concentration at least 50% higher than the original one were classified as not early responders (NERs).

3. Results and Discussion

3.1. Patients. Thirty-four pediatric patients, 22 males and 12 females, with a mean (SD) age at diagnosis of 52 (61) months, matched inclusion criteria and were enrolled in the study. Patients' characteristics at diagnosis are set out in Table 1.

3.2. Hemoglobin and Reticulocyte Parameters at T0, T1, and T2. Data regarding values of Hb, ARC, and CHr at T0, T1, and T2 are set out in Table 2.

Mean (SD) Hb level before treatment (T0) was 6.84 (1.22) g/dL. It increased to 7.36 g/L (1.31) and 10.56 g/L (1.62) at T1 and T2, respectively.

Mean (SD) ARC before treatment (T0) was 72799/mmc (35155). It increased to 168583/mmc (101196) at T1 and then decreased again to 76317/mmc (38924) at T2, respectively.

CHr could be fully monitored only for 28 patients. Mean CHr before treatment was 18.20 pg (2.32). It increased to 21.48 pg (3.04) and 25.43 pg (4.49) at T1 and T2, respectively.

Twenty-four/34 patients (70.5%) were classified as complete early responders (CERs), 4/34 (12%) as partial early responders (PERs), and the remaining 6 (17.5%) as not early responders (NERs).

Data about mean Hb, ARC, and CHr at T0, T1, and T2 in different groups of patients are set out in Tables 3(a) and 3(b).

Trends of mean values of Hb, ARC, and CHr in the different groups of children are graphically represented in Figure 1.

3.3. Factors Predictive of Response at Day +30: Comparison between Complete Early Responders and Other Patients. No differences were detected regarding gender and hemoglobin values at diagnosis (T0).

CHr at T0 was significantly higher in CERs than in remaining patients (19.94 pg versus 16.73 pg; $p = 0.020$).

Analysis of Hb values at T1 revealed no difference between the two different groups (7.67 g/dL versus 6.63 g/dL, $p = 0.05$).

CHr at T1 was significantly different between CERs and other patients (22.95 versus 18.41; $p = 0.001$).

Relative increase of CHr from T0 to T1, computed as (T1 CHr – T0 CHr)/T0 CHr, resulted significantly higher in CERs than in other patients (0.21 versus 0.11, $p = 0.042$).

Results from multivariate logistic models revealed a higher probability of being a complete early responder due

TABLE 1: Patients' characteristics at diagnosis.

Patient (id)	Sex (M/F)	Age at diagnosis (months)	Hb T0 (g/dL)	ARC T0 (n/mmc)	CHr T0 (pg)
1	M	9	5.8	82800	15.3
2	M	9	5.5	79800	15.4
3	M	12	5.1	54100	15.4
4	M	48	5.0	82200	15.7
5	M	7	5.7	148100	15.7
6	M	24	4.5	145700	15.8
7	F	24	6.8	89200	16.1
8	F	24	6.1	66700	16.4
9	F	144	7.0	126000	16.7
10	F	96	6.3	92300	16.9
11	F	72	6.3	85400	17.2
12	M	36	7.9	78300	17.5
13	M	48	8.1	94000	18.0
14	M	7	8.7	43700	18.2
15	M	9	6.0	56800	18.2
16	F	36	7.8	69500	18.5
17	F	7	5.8	78000	18.8
18	M	11	9.3	53600	18.8
19	F	8	8.9	15500	19.0
20	F	180	7.4	63500	19.4
21	M	60	7.2	47700	19.7
22	M	192	8.5	40500	20.4
23	M	24	7.4	46600	20.4
24	F	156	6.8	78600	20.5
25	F	180	6.5	56100	20.6
26	M	48	7.9	59700	21.2
27	M	36	8.0	19800	21.8
28	M	4	8.8	57700	24.8
29	M	192	6.3	68000	na
30	M	24	6.7	18600	na
31	M	6	6.3	132000	na
32	M	24	6.0	152000	na
33	M	5	6.8	50000	na
34	F	8	5.5	42000	na

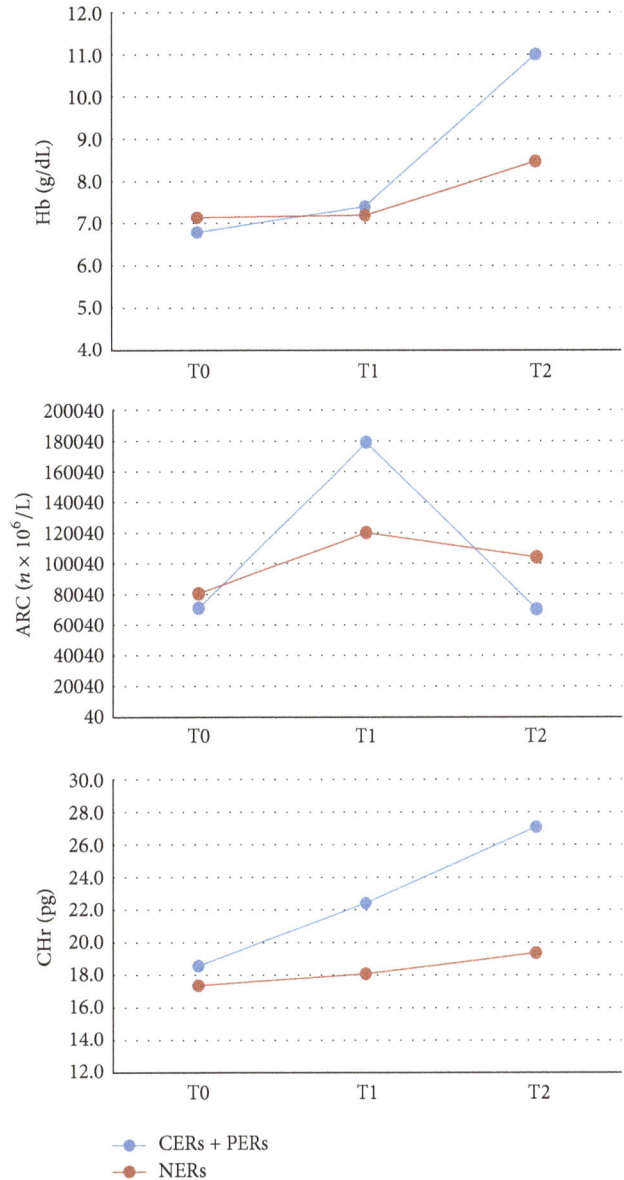

FIGURE 1: Trends of mean Hb, ARC, and CHr values (y-axis) in early responding patients (CERs + PERs) and not early responding patients (NERs) at T0: diagnosis, T1: within 7 days from the beginning of oral iron supplementation, and T2: at +30 from the onset of therapy (x-axis).

to relative increase of ARC from T0 to T1 [OR (95% CI) = 44.95 (1.54–1311.98); $p < 0.030$] and to CHr at T1 [OR (95% CI) = 3.18 (1.24–8.17); $p = 0.016$]. Both models were adjusted by age at diagnosis, sex, and level of Hb at T0.

Differences between CERs and other patients are reported in Table 3(a).

3.4. Factors Predictive of Response at Day +30: Comparison between Early Responders and Not Early Responders. When the distinction between early responders and not responders was taken into account, CHr at T1 was significantly different in the two groups (22.42 versus 18.07; $p = 0.001$).

Relative increase of CHr from T0 to T1, computed as (T1 CHr − T0 CHr)/T0 CHr, resulted significantly higher, too (0.22 versus 0.004, $p = 0.006$).

Differences between early responders and not responders are reported in Table 3(b).

3.5. Discussion. Our data confirm the efficacy of oral iron administration in promptly improving Hb values in patients with severe anemia, too.

More than 70% of patients retrospectively enrolled in the study reached mean hemoglobin (Hb) reference value for age and gender within one month from the initiation

TABLE 2: Hemoglobin and reticulocyte parameters at T0 (before treatment), T1 (within 7 days from the beginning of oral iron), and at T2 (day +30 from the beginning of treatment).

Patient (id)	T0 Hb (g/dL)	T1 Hb (g/dL)	T2 Hb (g/dL)	T0 ARC (n/mmc)	T1 ARC (n/mmc)	T2 ARC (n/mmc)	T0 CHr (pg)	T1 CHr (pg)	T2 CHr (pg)
1	5.8	6.3	9.1	82800	182200	84200	15.3	21.0	26.0
2	5.5	5.7	8.4	79800	137300	141300	15.4	15.8	19.6
3	5.1	5.9	11.1	54100	99100	44000	15.4	18.7	29.8
4	5.0	4.9	7.0	82200	126300	78900	15.7	16.8	16.4
5	5.7	5.9	8.0	148100	232000	154100	15.7	17.5	17.7
6	4.5	4.5	9.4	145700	209400	122200	15.8	20.5	24.9
7	6.8	7.6	12.9	89200	190000	47400	16.1	21.9	25.2
8	6.1	7.2	13.2	66700	155300	31500	16.4	24.2	30.1
9	7.0	7.2	12.4	126000	201400	106200	16.7	19.9	29.0
10	6.3	7.1	11.8	92300	315000	79400	16.9	22.3	27.2
11	6.3	6.1	7.4	85400	134500	107000	17.2	18.3	19.3
12	7.9	8.1	9.8	78300	110600	66000	17.5	20.8	23.7
13	8.1	8.6	10.5	94000	148200	54300	18.0	23.8	27.6
14	8.7	9.7	9.4	43700	71600	67100	18.2	18.8	18.1
15	6.0	7.0	12.2	56800	108200	60000	18.2	19.7	26.6
16	7.8	7.4	9.5	69500	71500	69500	18.5	19.3	23.6
17	5.8	6.3	12.4	78000	232000	43800	18.8	21.0	31.3
18	9.3	9.1	9.5	53600	84200	148300	18.8	17.7	21.0
19	8.9	9.3	10.5	15500	262500	61900	19.0	25.6	22.5
20	7.4	8.8	10.8	63500	148100	44800	19.4	27.3	27.6
21	7.2	7.2	12.5	47700	155900	71100	19.7	22.7	28.9
22	8.5	8.4	10.5	40500	44600	70100	20.4	25.7	26.2
23	7.4	8.8	10.5	46600	240300	42200	20.4	26.7	32.1
24	6.8	7.7	13.7	78600	105500	26100	20.5	24.3	32.0
25	6.5	8.9	10.7	56100	149900	188500	20.6	22.6	22.3
26	7.9	7.5	10.4	59700	93900	35400	21.2	22.0	26.3
27	8.0	8.9	11.8	19800	42000	63500	21.8	22.9	30.9
28	8.8	9.2	10.8	57700	59200	75500	24.8	23.9	26.2
29	6.3	6.9	10.0	68000	101340	82800	na	na	na
30	6.7	8.0	10.0	18600	345700	26400	na	na	na
31	6.3	6.7	12.4	132000	294100	37000	na	na	na
32	6.0	6.7	9.3	152000	233000	103000	na	na	na
33	6.8	6.7	9.8	50000	110000	94500	na	na	na
34	5.5	6.0	11.2	42000	537000	66800	na	na	na

of treatment, independently from base Hb level. Only a negligible percentage of children did not reach an Hb concentration at least 50% higher than the original after one month of therapy and was therefore classified as unresponsive to therapy. As our patients have not been tested for alpha and beta thalassemia at diagnosis or during the first month of therapy, we cannot rule out the possibility that these children have not responded to iron because of a concomitant hemoglobinopathy.

Measurement of reticulocyte hemoglobin content (CHr) has been validated in literature as the strongest independent predictor of iron deficiency and iron deficiency anemia, when compared to other laboratory markers (hemoglobin, ferritin, transferrin saturation, or mean corpuscular volume), both in children and in adults [1]. In pediatric patients, optimal CHr cut-off has been proven to be 27.5 pg for detecting iron deficiency (with a sensitivity of 83% and a specificity of 72%) [3] and 26 pg for detecting iron deficiency anemia (with a sensitivity of 83% and a specificity of 75%) [2]. In the totality of children described in our cohort (all displaying severe iron deficiency, defined by a transferrin saturation value of less than 10%), CHr levels were significantly lower than cut-off level of 26 pg ($p < 0.001$ for corresponding Wilcoxon test), and in 75% of children resulted even less than 20 pg.

TABLE 3: Descriptive characteristics of patients, divided into CERs = complete early responders (i.e., normal Hb value at day +30 for therapy onset), PERs = partial early responders (Hb value at day +30 at least 50% higher than the original one), and NERs = not early responders. p values come from Wilcoxon sum rank test.

(a)

	CERs ($n = 24$)		PERs + NERs ($n = 10$)		
	n	(%)	n	(%)	p value
Male	14	(63.64%)	8	(36.36%)	0.430
Female	10	(83.33%)	2	(16.67%)	
	Mean	(SD)	Mean	(SD)	p value
T0 Hb (g/dL)	7.00	(1.03)	6.46	(1.60)	0.134
T1 Hb (g/dL)	7.67	(1.02)	6.63	(1.68)	0.050
T2 Hb (g/dL)	11.33	(1.15)	8.70	(0.94)	<0.001
T0 ARC (n/mmc)	63820	(29399)	94280	(39813)	0.040
T1 ARC (n/mmc)	177077	(113504)	148200	(63023)	0.620
T2 ARC (n/mmc)	63300	(33954)	107560	(32749)	0.002
(T1 ARC − T0 ARC)/T0 ARC	2.92	(4.87)	0.58	(0.29)	0.023
T0 CHr (pg)	19.04*	(2.33)	16.73°	(1.44)	0.020
T1 CHr (pg)	22.95*	(2.38)	18.41°	(1.69)	0.001
T2 CHr (pg)	27.66*	(2.99)	20.73°	(3.38)	0.001
(T1 CHr−T0 CHr)/T0 CHr	0.21*	(0.14)	0.11°	(0.14)	0.042
	*$n = 19$		°$n = 9$		

(b)

	CERs + PERs ($n = 28$)		NERs ($n = 6$)		
	n	(%)	n	(%)	p value
Male	18	(81.82%)	4	(18.18%)	1.000
Female	10	(83.33%)	2	(16.67%)	
	Mean	(SD)	Mean	(SD)	p value
T0 Hb (g/dL)	6.78	(1.12)	7.13	(1.73)	0.790
T0 Hb (g/dL)	7.40	(1.20)	7.18	(1.90)	0.750
T0 Hb (g/dL)	11.00	(1.35)	8.47	(1.14)	0.001
T0 ARC (n/mmc)	71143	(35210)	80417	(36866)	0.580
T0 ARC (n/mmc)	178991	(105758)	120017	(61270)	0.120
T0 ARC (n/mmc)	70354	(36863)	104150	(39149)	0.040
(T1 ARC−T0 ARC)/T0 ARC	2.60	(4.56)	0.49	(0.23)	0.005
T0 CHr (pg)	18.56*	(2.49)	17.35°	(1.39)	0.300
T1 CHr (pg)	22.42*	(2.73)	18.07°	(0.91)	0.001
T2 CHr (pg)	27.09*	(3.30)	19.35°	(2.60)	<0.001
(T1 CHr−T0 CHr)/T0 CHr	0.22*	(0.14)	0.04°	(0.06)	0.006
	*$n = 22$		°$n = 6$		

The finding that CHr at T0 was significantly lower in patients who did not reach normal Hb levels at day +30 raises the intriguing possibility that CHr level at diagnosis might be a predictor of early response to oral iron. To our knowledge, no data about this issue are present in literature to date. Due to the limitations derived from the small sample size, our results need to be confirmed on larger cohorts of patients.

As reticulocyte indices allow a real-time evaluation of iron deficient erythropoiesis and of the effectiveness of iron replacement therapy [1], CHr has been validated in literature as an early predictor of response to parenteral iron therapy, in children receiving hemodialysis [10] and in adults [6].

Similar conclusion regarding response to exclusive oral iron therapy in a small cohort of children with severe iron deficiency anemia had been previously reported by our group [9]. Main outcome of our preliminary study [9] was to evaluate if oral iron supplementation should be proposed as first-line treatment in a small cohort of clinically asymptomatic patients with severe iron deficiency anemia. These patients, due to their Hb levels (median 6.3 g/dL, range

4.5–7), needed a tight follow-up; for that reason, the kinetic of response was assessed within 48 hours from the onset of iron administration (T1) and our data demonstrated the utility of ARC and CHr as accurate markers for the early detection of patients not responding to oral iron to be quickly switched to other therapies (parenteral iron supplementation or transfusion). These results prompted us to investigate the efficacy of reticulocyte parameters in monitoring the response to oral iron supplementation in a larger cohort of pediatric patients.

Despite the limitations derived from the retrospective nature of the study, analysis of reticulocyte parameters within one week from the beginning of therapy confirmed CHr to predict good early hematologic response to iron supplements after one week of therapy.

In particular, both CHr levels within 7 days from the beginning of therapy and the relative increase of CHr from T0 to T1 resulted significantly higher in patients who displayed normal hemoglobin levels or a hemoglobin concentration at least 50% higher than the original one at day +30.

4. Conclusions

Aim of the present study was to evaluate kinetic of response to oral iron in a cohort of pediatric patients with iron deficiency anemia and to investigate the usefulness of reticulocyte parameters CHr and ARC in monitoring early response to iron supplementation.

Despite the limitations derived from both the small number of patients and the retrospective nature of the study, according to data of literature, our data confirm that oral iron supplementation is an effective treatment for iron deficiency anemia, independently from base hemoglobin at diagnosis.

Moreover, our preliminary data suggest that reticulocyte parameters are early and accurate predictors of response to oral therapy and that pediatricians could take advantage of reticulocyte hemoglobin content both at diagnosis and during follow-up of iron deficiency anemia for assessing early erythropoietic response to iron replacement therapy.

A prospective multicentre study on a larger cohort of patients is ongoing in order to reinforce our conclusions.

Competing Interests

The authors have no competing interests to declare.

References

[1] E. Piva, C. Brugnara, F. Spolaore, and M. Plebani, "Clinical utility of reticulocyte parameters," *Clinics in Laboratory Medicine*, vol. 35, no. 1, pp. 133–163, 2015.

[2] C. Brugnara, D. Zurakowski, J. DiCanzio, T. Boyd, and O. Platt, "Reticulocyte hemoglobin content to diagnose iron deficiency in children," *The Journal of the American Medical Association*, vol. 281, no. 23, pp. 2225–2230, 1999.

[3] C. Ullrich, A. Wu, C. Armsby et al., "Screening healthy infants for iron deficiency using reticulocyte hemoglobin content," *The Journal of the American Medical Association*, vol. 294, no. 8, pp. 924–930, 2005.

[4] A. F. Bakr and G. Sarette, "Measurement of reticulocyte hemoglobin content to diagnose iron deficiency in Saudi children," *European Journal of Pediatrics*, vol. 165, no. 7, pp. 442–445, 2006.

[5] A. E. Mast, M. A. Blinder, and D. J. Dietzen, "Reticulocyte hemoglobin content," *American Journal of Hematology*, vol. 83, no. 4, pp. 307–310, 2008.

[6] C. Brugnara, M. R. Laufer, A. J. Friedman, K. Bridges, and O. Platt, "Reticulocyte hemoglobin content (CHr): early indicator of iron deficiency and response to therapy," *Blood*, vol. 83, no. 10, pp. 3100–3101, 1994.

[7] C. Borgna-Pignatti and M. Marsella, "Iron deficiency in infancy and childhood," *Pediatric Annals*, vol. 37, no. 5, pp. 329–337, 2008.

[8] X. Zeng and T. Wu, "Iron supplementation for iron deficiency anemia in children," *Cochrane Database of Systematic Reviews*, no. 2, Article ID CD006465, 2007.

[9] E. Parodi, M. T. Giraudo, M. Davitto et al., "Reticulocyte parameters: markers of early response to oral treatment in children with severe iron-deficiency anemia," *Journal of Pediatric Hematology/Oncology*, vol. 34, no. 6, pp. e249–e252, 2012.

[10] B. A. Warady, A. Kausz, G. Lerner et al., "Iron therapy in the pediatric hemodialysis population," *Pediatric Nephrology*, vol. 19, no. 6, pp. 655–661, 2004.

22

Evaluation of Iron Deficiency Anemia Frequency as a Risk Factor in Glaucoma

Penpe Gul Firat ⓘ,[1] Ersan Ersin Demirel,[2] Seyhan Dikci ⓘ,[3] Irfan Kuku,[4] and Oguzhan Genc[5]

[1]*Associate Professor, Inonu University School of Medicine, Department of Ophthalmology, Malatya, Turkey*
[2]*MD, Sarkısla State Hospital, Department of Ophthalmology, Sivas, Turkey*
[3]*Assistant Professor, Inonu University School of Medicine, Department of Ophthalmology, Malatya, Turkey*
[4]*Professor, Inonu University School of Medicine, Department of Hematology, Malatya, Turkey*
[5]*MD, Mujde Hospital, Department of Ophthalmology, Malatya, Turkey*

Correspondence should be addressed to Penpe Gul Firat; pfiratmd@gmail.com

Academic Editor: Duran Canatan

Purpose. Iron deficiency anemia is an important public health problem. Also it is considered to be a risk factor for many diseases. The study demonstrates the iron deficiency anemia frequency in glaucoma patients and compares with the normal subjects. We aimed to determine the iron deficiency anemia frequency in glaucoma patients. *Methods*. Prospective, controlled study in a single university hospital setting. A total of 130 normal subjects (Group 1) and 131 glaucoma patients (Group 2) were included. The erythrocytes parameters, hemoglobin, red blood cell, hematocrit, mean corpuscular volume, mean corpuscular hemoglobin concentration, mean corpuscular hemoglobin, and red blood cell distribution width, and iron status indicators, Fe (iron), total iron binding capacity, and ferritin of the cases, in normal subjects and glaucoma patients were compared. *Results*. There was no statistically significant difference for the erythrocyte parameters between the groups ($p \geq 0.05$). The number of the patients with iron deficiency anemia in both groups was similar. No statistically significant difference was found in the comparison of erythrocyte parameters and iron status indicators values according to the number of antiglaucomatous agents and visual field changes according to the presence of anemia in Group 2 ($p \geq 0.05$). A statistically significant difference was found only in MCH when the erythrocyte parameters and iron status indicators values of the cases in glaucoma patients were compared with the glaucoma duration ($p < 0.05$). *Conclusion*. The iron deficiency anemia frequency was like the normal population in glaucoma patients.

1. Introduction

Glaucoma is a chronic neuropathy that leads to progressive atrophy in the optic nerve head, degeneration in retinal ganglion cells, and visual field losses and causes visual loss due to optic atrophy when not treated. These changes usually exist together with intraocular pressure elevation (IOP) [1]. Increased IOP is not the only factor in glaucoma. Some publications in recent years have focused on the role of oxidative stress in the pathogenesis of glaucoma [2]. Oxidative stress can be defined as an imbalance between the high level of the intracellular concentrations of reactive oxygen species (ROS) in physiologic values while antioxidant level being insufficient. This imbalance has been shown to cause retinal ganglion cell death [3].

Anemia is clinically defined as a blood hemoglobin or hematocrit value under the valid reference range for the patient [4]. Iron deficiency is the most common form of anemia. It was demonstrated that oxidants were elevated, and the antioxidants were decreased in iron deficiency anemia (IDA) [5]. Besides iron is a vital element for myelin production [6]. Lack of iron is associated with hypomyelination which can affect all of the nervous systems, as well as the optic nerve, which is constituted mainly by myelinated fibers [7]. These findings highlight the importance of investigating the role of IDA on glaucoma. To date, the effects of IDA which can affect the oxidant– antioxidant system on glaucoma have not been studied.

The aim of this study was to determine the IDA frequency in glaucoma patients which is a neurodegenerative disease. We compared the IDA incidence in the normal population and the glaucoma patients to evaluate whether detecting and treating the anemia could slow down or stop the progress of the disorder.

2. Material and Method

A total of 131 glaucoma patients who were being followed up at our Glaucoma Unit and met the study inclusion criteria and 130 healthy individuals were included in the study. The healthy individuals were included in Group 1 and the patients with glaucoma in Group 2.

The study was conducted in accordance with the ethical standards stated in the Declaration of Helsinki and approved by our institutional ethics board. The patients were informed on the purpose of the study and the procedures to be performed in detail and consent was obtained.

Each subject underwent a full ophthalmic examination, including best-corrected visual acuity, IOP measurement with a Goldmann applanation tonometry, slit-lamp biomicroscopy, gonioscopy, stereoscopic fundus evaluation on the slit lamp using a 90-diopter lens, and visual field examination with Humphrey Field Analyzer (HFA) (Humphrey-Zeiss Systems, Dublin, CA, USA) Swedish Interactive Threshold Algorithm (SITA) 30-2 test. Each test was performed on the same machine with the same technician. The tests were repeated in the same week if an abnormality was found in the reliability indexes (fixation loss >20%, false positive response >25%, false negative response >25%). Both test strategies were investigated in terms of test duration and mean deviation (MD).

Inclusion criteria in normal subjects were IOP under 21 mmHg, normal optic disc, and visual field examination and the lack of any systemic disease or systemic drug use. Inclusion criteria in glaucoma patients were a minimum of one-year follow-up at our clinic, the presence of glaucomatous damage in the optic disc (glaucomatous cupping and/or glaucomatous optic nerve head changes), the use of at least one antiglaucomatous agent, and presence of glaucomatous visual field changes in a minimum of two computerized visual field examinations (30-2 SITA). History of laser treatment or trauma, presence of cornea or lens pathology, presence of uveitis, posterior segment pathology, neurodegenerative diseases of the central nervous system, and systemic diseases such as diabetes that can predispose to such disorders were accepted as exclusion criteria for both groups.

Erythrocyte parameters were studied with the Beckman Coulter LH 780, biochemical data, Fe and IBC with the Abbott Architect c16000, and Ferritin with the Siemens immulite 2000 device. IDA was defined as hemoglobin concentration <12.0 g/dL and serum ferritin concentration <15.0 μg/L [8].

Quantitative data were presented as mean ± standard deviation (SD) or median (min-max). Compliance with a normal distribution was determined with the Shapiro-Wilk test. The homogeneity of the variances was evaluated with the Levene test. One-way variance analysis and the Kruskal-Wallis test were used for statistical analyses and the t-test and Mann–Whitney U test were used for independent samples. When the one-way variance analysis result was important, multiple comparisons were made with the Tukey test. The anemia incidence of the subgroups in glaucoma was compared with Pearson Chi-Square test. A p value <0.05 was accepted as statistically significant. The study was powered to detect a hemoglobin concentration difference of 0.35 gr/dlt with a β error of 0.80 and an α error of 0.05 in a 2-tailed test.

3. Results

Patients who fulfilled the entry criteria were enrolled in this prospective, controlled study. There were 130 normal subjects (63 females, 67 males) in control group and 131 glaucoma patients (74 females, 57 males). The mean age of the normal subjects was 50,01 ± 13,6 years; the mean age of the glaucoma patients was 49,01 ± 10,7 years. There were no statistically significant differences in age (p=0.424) and gender (p=0.194) among the groups.

There were no statistically significant differences in the erythrocytes parameters and the iron status indicator values between the groups. (Table 1)

We detected 26 IDA patients in normal subjects and 24 patients with IDA in glaucoma group. No statistically significant difference was observed between the groups in terms of the number of patients with IDA (p=0.48, p>0.05, respectively).

The glaucoma group was consisting of primer open angle patients glaucoma (POAG) (n=57), pseudoexfoliation glaucoma (PEXG) patients (n=43), and normotensive glaucoma (NTG) patients (n=31). The number of patients with IDA was fourteen in POAG, five in PEXG, and seven in NTG patients. No statistically significant difference was found between the glaucoma subgroups regarding the IDA incidence (p=0.251, p>0.05).

No statistically significant difference was found regarding the number of antiglaucomatous agents used between the patients with and without IDA in glaucoma patients (p=0.68, p>0.05). Similarly, changes in the mean deviation (MD) in the right and left eye 30-2 computerized visual fields obtained at intervals of at least 6 months in these patients were not found to be statistically significant (p=0.44, p=0.21, p>0.05, respectively) (Table 2).

No statistically significant difference was found between the erythrocyte parameters and the iron status indicator values of the patients in glaucoma patients according to the number of antiglaucomatous agents used (Table 3).

There was no statistically significant difference between the erythrocytes parameters and the iron status indicator values according to the duration of glaucoma in glaucoma patients, but the difference in MCH values was statistically significant (p=0.03, p<0.05) (Table 4).

TABLE 1: Comparison of Fe, TIBC and ferritin values between Group 1 and Group 2.

Variables (mean±sd)	Group 1	Group 2	P*
Hb (g/dl)	13.73±1.8	13.48±1.7	0.21
Rbc (10^6/ml)	4.75±0.80	4.68±0.79	0.51
Htc (%)	40.94±5.29	40.41±4.93	0.40
MCV (fl)	87.20±7.87	87.62±7.19	0.62
MCHC (g/dl)	33.13±2.12	32.90±1.40	0.30
MCH (pg)	29.35±3.26	28.97±3.52	0.35
RDW (%)	14.29±1.81	13.81±2.28	0.06
Fe (μg/dl)	74.38±36.2	71.82±33.89	0.55
TIBC (μg/dl)	269.67±64.15	273.12±66.26	0.69
Ferritin (n/dl), [Median (Min-Max)]	70.60 (1-240)	70.07(2-294))	0.95
Plt 10^3/ml	241.22±80.82	268.39±72.00	**0.04***

Hb: hemoglobin; **Rbc: red blood cells**; **Htc:** hematocrit; **MCV: mean corpuscular volume**; **MCHC:** mean corpuscular hemoglobin concentration; **MCH: mean corpuscular hemoglobin**; **RDW:** red blood cell distribution width; **Fe:** iron; **TIBC:** Total iron binding capacity; **Plt:** platelet; **sd:** standard deviation; **Min:** minimum; **Max:** maximum.

TABLE 2: Comparison of the number of antiglaucomatous agents used and changes of visual fields patients in glaucoma patients according to presence of anemia.

	Patients With Anemia (Mean ± SD)	Patients Without Anemia (Mean ± SD)	P value
The number of antiglaucomatous agents used	2.36±0.7	2.85±1.3	0.68
MD Right eye	0.08±1.9	-0.55±2.6	0.44
MD Left eye	-2.21±4.3	-0.24±1.5	0.21

SD: standard deviation; **MD Right-Left:** changes in the mean deviation in the 2 separate visual fields with 6 monthly intervals.

4. Discussion

This study was undertaken to determine whether the IDA frequency is higher in glaucoma patients than the normal population. We could not find any statistically significant difference between the groups according to the IDA frequency. Although ocular findings of severe anemia have been defined more commonly in recent years, we could not find any study investigating the relationship between glaucoma and IDA. The severity of retinal findings is consistent with the severity of the anemia. Retinal ischemia findings of optic disc edema, retinal hemorrhages, and soft exudes can be seen in certain patients with anemia [9]. Venous congestion, retinal hemorrhages, and soft exudes can similarly also be seen in retinal vein occlusion and anterior ischemic optic neuropathy [10]. Although the pathophysiology is unknown, it is likely associated with retinal hypoxia [11].

Considering that IDA may accelerate the visual field loss in patients with glaucoma, we obtained two separate 30-2 visual field tests with an interval of six months in patients with and without iron deficiency anemia but the difference in mean deviations in visual field tests was not found to be statistically significant. We also showed that the need for antiglaucomatous agents also did not increase in glaucoma patients with IDA. A possible explanation can be the severity of anemia in our study. The range of hemoglobin level in anemia patients was 9-12 g/dl in normal group and 9.2-12 g/dl in glaucoma group. As shown in previous reports ocular side effects of anemia were seen in severe anemia cases. Retinal findings can be seen when the hemoglobin levels were less than 6 g/dl [12]. Our patients' anemia can be classified as

mild and moderate according to the WHO anemia classification [13]. Carraro et al. demonstrated the prevalence of retinopathy in patients with anemia or thrombocytopenia. They showed that retinopathy was closely associated with the severity of the anemia. But in their study acute blood loss was the main cause of the retinopathy and anemia not IDA [14].

We also demonstrated that the anemia frequencies in POAG, NTG, and PEXG are the same. Goldberg et al. studied the systemic factors including hemoglobin concentration and hematocrit levels in NTG and ocular hypertension patients. Similar to our study they found out that the hemoglobin and hematocrit levels were the same in NTG and ocular hypertension patients [15].

Iron is an essential element for many functions in the cell like oxygen transport, myelin synthesis, and oxidative phosphorylation. On the other hand if the iron is found in excess amount it can cause reactive oxygen species formation that can cause cellular degeneration and damage [16]. Disorders in iron metabolism have been shown to cause many neurodegenerative diseases such as Parkinson's disease, Alzheimer's disease, Huntington's disease, Hallervorden-Spatz disease, and Friedreich disease [17, 18]. Since glaucoma is also considered as a neurodegenerative disorder, IDA frequency in patients with glaucoma was compared with normal individuals and no statistically significant difference was found between the two groups in our study.

However, the neuronal affinity of iron and ferritin may increase in glaucoma patients. Considering that the serum iron and ferritin level may not be correlated with the brain iron and ferritin levels, we believe that detailed

TABLE 3: Comparisonthe hemogram, iron, TIBC, and ferritin valuesaccording to thenumber of antiglaucomatous agents used in Group 2.

The number of antiglaucomatous agents used The number of patients	1 (Mean± SD) n=28	2 (Mean ± SD) n=31	3 (Mean ± SD) n=36	4 (Mean ± SD) n=36	P value
Hb g/dl	13.48±1.50	12.85±1.90	13.45±2.04	14.11±1.54	0.14
Rbc 10^6/ml	4.87±0.55	4.46±0.45	5.00 ±1.73	4.83±0.46	0.28
Htc %	39.66±4.48	38.71±5.67	39.68±6.43	42.11±3.25	0.16
MCV fl	83.69±4.53	86.66±6.84	88.07±10.27	88.04±6.56	0.34
MCHC g/dl	33.25±2.09	32.77±1.00	32.56±1.76	32.87±1.32	0.65
MCH pg	28.40±2.15	28.85±2.40	29.52±3.87	27.48±6.02	0.69
RDW %	13.38±1.33	14.02 ±1.60	13.72±1.43	13.39±1.06	0.39
Fe μg/dl	69.69±31.24	74.42±32.25	75.44±42.62	84.00±41.39	0.71
TDBK μg/dl	293.07±65.82	284.95±80.11	261.22±66.25	253.81±52.5	0.25
Ferritin ng/ml Median (Min-Max)	69.90 (5-250)	67.46 (3-254)	67.58 (3-238)	70.88 (12-277)	0.93
Plt 10^3/ml	230.77±50.99	287.79±85.93	257.11±38.90	264.67±55.28	0,07

Hb: hemoglobin; Rbc: red blood cells; Htc: Hematocrit; MCV: mean corpuscular volume; MCHC: mean corpuscular hemoglobin concentration; MCH: mean corpuscular hemoglobin; RDW: red blood cell distribution width; Fe: iron; TIBC: total iron binding capacity; SD: standard deviation; Min: minimum; Max: maximum.

TABLE 4: Comparison of the hemogram, iron, TIBC, and ferritin values according to the duration of glaucoma in Group 2.

Duration of Glaucoma (mean±sd)	3 years	4 years	5 years	6 years and over	P value
Hb g/dl	12.71±2.03	13.36±1.73	13.45±1.68	14.09±1.70	0.13
Rbc 10^6/ml	4.72±1.24	4.63±0.62	4.98±1.11	4.67±0.64	0.64
Htc %	37.72±5.50	40.43±5.31	40.32±5.32	41.30±4.52	0.18
MCV fl	84.23±7.41	85.56±8.00	86.38±6.42	90.30±7.30	0.058
MCHC g/dl	32.54±1.45	32.58±1.53	32.95±1.83	33.10±1.28	0.59
MCH pg	28.35±2.89	26.48±6.83	28.47±2.34	30.27±2.6	0.03*
RDW %	14.29±1.90	13.69±1.40	13.56±1.18	13.27±0.86	0.14
Fe μg/dl	75.45±31.34	71.07±30.93	76.05±36.65	81.32±45.97	0.87
TDBK μg/dl	277.88±59.48	286.86±47.19	281.86±73.99	247.86±77.68	0.25
Ferritin n/dl. [Median (Min-Maks)]	21 (3-250)	26 (3-250)	58 (5-183)	71 (13-254)	0.14

Hb: hemoglobin; Rbc: red blood cells, Htc: hematocrit; MCV: mean corpuscular volume; MCHC: mean corpuscular hemoglobin concentration; MCH: mean corpuscular hemoglobin; RDW: red blood cell distribution width; Fe: iron; TIBC: total iron binding capacity; sd: Standart deviation; Min: minimum; Max: maximum.

neuropathology studies investigating brain iron and ferritin levels in glaucoma patients are required.

We therefore concluded that it was not necessary to change the frequency of follow-ups and number of antiglaucomatous agents in glaucoma patients who are found to have IDA.

The strengths of this study are that it is a prospective, controlled study. Also, to the best of our knowledge, this is the first study that demonstrates the IDA frequency in glaucoma. Limitation of our study is that the study includes mild and moderate anemia patients. Large sample sized studies with severe anemia patients are needed to better understand the effect of anemia on glaucoma.

Conflicts of Interest

The authors declare that they have no conflicts of interest.

References

[1] I. F. Gutteridge, "Normal tension glaucoma: diagnostic features and comparisons with primary open angle glaucoma," *Clinical and Experimental Optometry*, vol. 83, no. 3, pp. 161–172, 2000.

[2] A. Izzotti, A. Bagnis, and S. C. Saccà, "The role of oxidative stress in glaucoma," *Mutation Research—Reviews in Mutation Research*, vol. 612, no. 2, pp. 105–114, 2006.

[3] K. Kortuem, L. K. Geiger, and L. A. Levin, "Differential susceptibility of retinal ganglion cells to reactive oxygen species," *Investigative Ophthalmology & Visual Science*, vol. 41, no. 10, pp. 3176–3182, 2000.

[4] F. William and M. D. Kern, *Hemotology PDQ, 1*, İstanbul Medikal Yayıncılık, Baskı, İstanbul, Turkey, 2005.

[5] M. Aslan, M. Horoz, and H. Çelik, "Evaluation of oxidative status in iron deficiency anemia through total antioxidant capacity measured using an automated method," *Turkish Journal of Hematology*, vol. 28, no. 1, pp. 42–46, 2011.

[6] B. Todorich, J. M. Pasquini, C. I. Garcia, P. M. Paez, and J. R. Connor, "Oligodendrocytes and myelination: The role of iron," *Glia*, vol. 57, no. 5, pp. 467–478, 2009.

[7] A. S. Demaman, P. Melo, J. M. Homem, M. A. Tavares, and J.-J. Lachat, "Effectiveness of iron repletion in the diet for the optic nerve development of anaemic rats," *Eye*, vol. 24, no. 5, pp. 901–908, 2010.

[8] United Nations Children's Fund and United Nations University, *World Health Organizationiron Deficiency Anemia Assessment, Prevention, and Control: A Guide for Programme Managers*, WHO/NHD/01.3 World Health Organization, Geneva, Switzerland, 2001.

[9] S. Duke-Elder and J. H. Dobree, *Disease of Retina; System of Ophthalmology*, C.V. Mosby Co, 1967, Chapter IV.

[10] M. L. Aisen, B. R. Bacon, A. M. Goodman, and E. M. Chester, "Retinal abnormalities associated with anemia," *Arch Ophthalmol*, vol. 101, no. 7, pp. 1049–1052, 1983.

[11] B. Kacer, L.-O. Hattenbach, S. Hörle, I. Scharrer, P. Kroll, and F. Koch, "Central retinal vein occlusion and nonarteritic ischemic optic neuropathy in 2 patients with mild iron deficiency anemia," *Ophthalmologica*, vol. 215, no. 2, pp. 128–131, 2001.

[12] W. S. Foulds, *The Ocular Manifestations of Blood Diseases*, Trans Ophthalmol Soc UK, 1963.

[13] WHO, *Haemoglobin Concentrations for The Diagnosis of Anaemia and Assessment of Severity. Vitamin and Mineral Nutrition Information System*, World Health Organization, Geneva, 2011.

[14] M. C. Carraro, L. Rossetti, and G. C. Gerli, "Prevalence of retinopathy in patients with anemia or thrombocytopenia," *European Journal of Haematology*, vol. 67, no. 4, pp. 238–244, 2001.

[15] I. Goldberg, F. C. Hollows, M. A. Kass, and B. Becker, "Systemic factors in patients with low-tension glaucoma," *British Journal of Ophthalmology*, vol. 65, no. 1, pp. 56–62, 1981.

[16] P. Naomi, F. Visanjia Joanna et al., "Iron deficiency in parkinsonism: region-specific iron dysregulation in parkinson's disease and multiple system atrophy," *Journal of Parkinsons Disease*, vol. 3, pp. 523–537, 2013.

[17] L. M. Sayre, G. Perry, and M. A. Smith, "Redox metals and neurodegenerative disease," *Current Opinion in Chemical Biology*, vol. 3, no. 2, pp. 220–225, 1999.

[18] S. Shoham and M. B. Youdim, "Iron involvement in neural damage and microgliosis in models of neurodegenerative diseases," *Cellular and Molecular Biology*, vol. 46, no. 4, pp. 743–760, 2000.

23

Prevalence of Anemia and Iron Deficiency among Palestinian Pregnant Women and its Association with Pregnancy Outcome

Mahmoud A. Srour ⓘ,[1,2] **Samah S. Aqel,**[1] **Khaled M. Srour,**[3]
Khalid R. Younis,[1] **and Fekri Samarah ⓘ**[4]

[1]*Department of Medical Laboratory Sciences, Faculty of Health Professions, Al-Quds University, East Jerusalem, State of Palestine*
[2]*Department of Biology & Biochemistry, Birzeit University, Birzeit, State of Palestine*
[3]*Anatomy and Physiology Department, Faculty of Medicine, Al-Quds University, East Jerusalem, State of Palestine*
[4]*Department of Medical Laboratory Sciences, Arab-American University, Jenin, State of Palestine*

Correspondence should be addressed to Mahmoud A. Srour; msrour@birzeit.edu

Academic Editor: Ajit C. Gorakshakar

Background. Anemia is a public health problem especially among pregnant women. This study aimed to investigate the prevalence of anemia and iron deficiency among pregnant women and its association with pregnancy outcome in Hebron Governorate in southern Palestine. *Methods.* This is a cross-sectional study that included 300 pregnant women in their first trimester and 163 babies. Maternal anthropometric and socioeconomic and newborns' data were collected. Complete blood count for study subjects and maternal serum ferritin were measured. *Results.* The prevalence of iron deficiency anemia among pregnant women was 25.7% and 52% of them had depleted iron stores. When pregnant women were grouped into three hemoglobin (Hb) tertile groups, a significant difference was observed between maternal Hb and newborns' birth weight ($P= 0.009$), height ($P= 0.022$), head circumference ($P= 0.017$), and gestational age ($P= 0.012$). There was a significant association between maternal serum ferritin and frequency of low birth weight ($P= 0.001$) and frequency of preterm delivery ($P= 0.003$). No significant association was observed between maternal anthropometric measures or the socioeconomic status and pregnancy outcomes. *Conclusion.* Iron deficiency is a moderate public health problem among the study subjects. Maternal Hb and serum ferritin significantly affect pregnancy outcomes.

1. Introduction

Anemia is a widespread public health problem associated with an increased risk of morbidity and mortality, especially in pregnant women and young children. Anemia also negatively influences the social and economic development in countries with high prevalence of anemia [1, 2]. In general, it is assumed that 50% of the cases of anemia are due to iron deficiency [3, 4]. Iron deficiency anemia (IDA) is considered to be one of the top ten contributors to the global burden of disease [1, 2].

Iron deficiency is the most common nutritional deficiency worldwide, particularly among pregnant women. Because of the increased iron requirements during pregnancy, pregnant women are recognized as the group most vulnerable to iron deficiency anemia [2, 5]. In Eastern

Mediterranean region, the WHO estimates the prevalence of anemia to be 32.4% in nonpregnant and 44.2% in pregnant women [2]. Anemia during pregnancy is a significant concern. During pregnancy, the fetal demand for iron increases maternal daily iron requirements around 10-fold, increasing from 6 mg/day to 22 mg/day in first and third trimesters of pregnancy, respectively. This increased demand for iron is covered mostly from maternal iron stores, which makes pregnant women at higher risk of developing iron deficiency and IDA [6].

The consequences of IDA during pregnancy are often serious and long lasting for both the mother and fetus. Mothers with anemia often experience increased fatigue levels, reduced exercise performance, and reduced mental performance [7]. Furthermore, severe anemia (Hb < 90 g/L) is related to an increased risk of premature delivery with subsequent low birth weight, small for gestational-age babies, and spontaneous abortion [6–10]. Additionally, maternal IDA may contribute to low iron status and poor health of infants. Also, pregnant women with anemia are at a greater risk of perinatal mortality and morbidity [10, 11]. Fetal iron metabolism is completely dependent upon maternal iron delivery via the placenta and so the effects of anemia on the fetus are directly related to the extent of maternal iron deficiency with increased mortality linked to severe IDA [6].

The prevalence of IDA varies among countries but is a major public health problem in the developing world, reflecting differences in race, socioeconomic factors, nutritional habits, medical care, and the frequency of parasitic illnesses [7].

In Palestine, the Ministry of Health (MoH) has protocols for IDA management and prevention that involves free iron supplements for pregnant women. In 2016, the overall prevalence of anemia among pregnant women (Hb <110 g/L) who visited maternal and child healthcare (MCH) centers of MoH was 29.5% (18.7% in West Bank region and 40.3% in Gaza Strip) [12]. Earlier in 2009 Khader et al. [13] reported an overall prevalence of anemia of 38.6% among pregnant women attending/accessing the UNRWA (United Nations Relief and Works Agency) clinics in Palestine with a substantial difference between those living in West Bank (31.1%) and Gaza Strip (44.9%). In the latter report [13], anemia prevalence revealed a significant increase in Gaza strip in 2009 (44.9%) compared to an earlier survey (35.7%) conducted in 2004 by UNRWA. The former report [12] surveyed the general population in Palestine excluding refugees who were surveyed by UNRWA [13]. Although these data revealed a high prevalence of anemia among pregnant women in Palestine, the association of anemia among Palestinian pregnant women with pregnancy outcome was not investigated. Therefore, this study aimed to assess the prevalence of anemia and IDA among pregnant women in Hebron Governorate (south of Palestine) and to investigate the association between maternal anemia and pregnancy outcome.

2. Materials and Methods

2.1. Study Subjects and Design. The study included 11 maternal and child healthcare (MCHC) centers distributed all over Hebron Governorate, Palestine. All pregnant women in their first trimester and presenting for the first time during current pregnancy at one of the MCHC centers covered in this study were asked to participate in this study. All participants were presenting at the MCHC centers for general medical examination related to the current pregnancy in the period March to October 2015. Pregnant women included in this study were contacted immediately after delivery (6-9 months after time of enrollment of pregnant women) and asked to include their newborns in the study. Inclusion criteria included apparently healthy according to the physical examination and laboratory data obtained at their first (current) visit, being not on iron supplementation, no previous pregnancy complications, and free of pregravid chronic diseases. A total of 300 pregnant women and 163 newborns born to them were included in the study.

All study subjects were briefed about the study and gave a written informed consent for themselves and on behalf of their babies. The principles of Helsinki Declaration were applied.

The Hebron Governorate (study region) is located in the southern part of West Bank and has a population of 0.729 million from around 3 million in West Bank, Palestine [14].

2.2. Data Collection and Analysis of Blood Samples. Anthropometric and socioeconomic data from the subjects were collected using a structured questionnaire. All pregnant women at their first trimester who met the inclusion criteria were asked to donate a blood sample and provide all information required to fill up the first part of the questionnaire concerned with the mothers. Collection of blood samples from pregnant women took place during their first visit to collaborating centers for the purpose of medical examination concerning current pregnancy. Participants were contacted immediately after delivery and asked for a permission to collect a blood sample from their newborns and provide all information needed to fill the second part concerned with the newborns. Blood samples were collected from newborn babies on the 5th to 7th day following delivery when babies were presenting at the MCHC center for their first vaccination date.

Blood samples were used for testing of Complete Blood Count (CBC) using Medonic (version CA 620; Boule Medical, Sweden) or Drew (version 6.3 model 2902-0531; Drew Scientific group, USA) hematology analyzers immediately after sample collection. Hematology analyzers were calibrated using the appropriate calibrators. Reliability of tests was assessed by running appropriate controls every day. Anemia was determined by hemoglobin concentration level less than 110 g/L for pregnant women based on the recommendations of WHO [15]. The severity of anemia was assessed based on WHO recommendations as follows: severe for Hb < 70 g/L, moderate for Hb 70-99 g/L, and mild for Hb 100-109 g/L [15].

Serum from mothers was collected, stored at -18°C, and used later for analysis of serum ferritin. Serum ferritin was determined using ferritin reagent kits and the automated chemistry analyzer machine (Abbott, USA) per the instructions of the manufacturer. For calibration, six ferritin standards (corresponding to ferritin levels of 0, 10, 50, 250, 500, and 1000 ng/ml) were used per the instructions of manufacturer. The ferritin standard calibrators were traceable to the WHO standards. Additionally, the ferritin controls (low, medium, and high) were assayed in each run for verification of the accuracy and precision of the test.

2.3. Statistical Analysis. Descriptive statistics including (mean and standard deviation) were calculated for all variables using SPSS software (Version 23). Inferential statistics were used to reach conclusions and make generalizations about the characteristics of populations based on data collected from the study subjects. These statistical tests include independent sample t-test, one-way ANOVA, and Chi-Square tests. A P-value < 0.05 was considered statistically significant.

TABLE 1: General characteristics of the study subjects/pregnant women at first trimester.

General characteristics					
	n	Mean ± SD	95% CI	Minimum value	Maximum value
Age (years)	300	26.3 ± 5.9	25.6 – 26.9	15	45
BMI (kg/m^2)	300	24.8 ± 4.1	24.3 – 25.2	15.2	41.2
No. of children	300	2.1 ± 2.0	1.9 – 2.4	0	10
No. of abortions	300	0.66 ± 1.18	0.53 – 0.79	0	8
Educational level (years)	300	11.6 ± 3.2	11.3 – 12.0	0	16
Monthly income (NIS)*	264	1832 +-1154	1700 - 1963	700	7000
Biochemical status					
Hb (g/L)	300	118 ± 14	117 – 120	73	153
Hct (%)	300	34.1 ± 3.7	33.7 – 34.5	24.5	49.3
Serum ferritin (ng/mL)	300	20.2 ± 23.2	17.5 – 22.8	1.1	192.0

*NIS: New Israeli Sheqel, the currency used mostly in Palestine.

TABLE 2: General characteristics of the newborns (pregnancy outcome).

General characteristics					
	n	Mean ± SD	95% CI	Minimum value	Maximum value
Birth weight (gm)	163	3022 ± 585	2932 - 3113	1900	4350
Birth height (cm)	96	48.3 ± 2.7	47.8 – 48.9	43	55
Head circumference (cm)	96	34.6 ± 1.4	34.3 – 34.9	31	37
Gestational age (weeks)	122	38.5 ± 1.5	38.5 – 38.7	33	40
Biochemical status					
Hb (g/L)	79	162 ± 22	157 – 167	111	214

3. Results

The general characteristics of pregnant women are described in Table 1. The average serum ferritin and Hb levels were within the normal range. However, out of 300 pregnant women, 77 women (25.7%) had Hb levels below 110 g/L and thus were considered anemic based on the recommendation of WHO [15]. Of the anemic pregnant women, 51 (17%) had mild anemia, 26 (8.7%) had moderate anemia, and none of the women had severe anemia, based on recommendation of WHO for assessment of anemia severity [15]. Analysis of serum ferritin levels showed that 156 pregnant women (52%) had serum ferritin levels below 15 ng/mL which indicates depleted iron stores (iron deficiency) based on the recommendations of the WHO [16]. Seventy-seven of the pregnant women (25.7%) were found to meet the clinical criteria (Hb < 110 g/L and serum ferritin < 15 ng/mL). These results indicate that all cases of anemia observed among our study subjects were due to iron deficiency. For the newborns, their average weight, gestational age, and Hb level were within the normal reference range (Table 2).

In order to examine the association between maternal characteristics and pregnancy outcome on one side with the maternal Hb levels on the other side, the mothers were divided into three Hb tertile groups (Table 3). A statistically significant difference was observed among the Hb tertile groups when compared with maternal serum ferritin, where serum ferritin levels increased with increasing Hb levels (Table 3). For the pregnancy outcome (newborns) a statistically significant difference was observed among maternal

Hb tertile groups when compared with birth weight, birth height, and head circumference of newborns as well as with gestational age (Table 3). The results showed that birth weight, height, and head circumference of newborns as well as gestational age was increasing with increased maternal Hb levels.

As shown in Table 4, a statistically significant difference was observed between maternal serum ferritin levels when compared with maternal BMI kg/m^2. For the pregnancy outcome, a significant difference between maternal serum ferritin levels was observed when compared with birth height and head circumference of newborns as well as with gestational age, where birth height, head circumference, and gestational age were lower in mothers with iron deficiency (serum ferritin <15 ng/mL) compared to mothers with normal serum ferritin (serum ferritin ≥ 15 ng/mL) (Table 4). The latter findings confirm the significant differences among Hb tertile groups when compared with these parameters (Table 3). Additionally, a statistically significant difference was observed between maternal serum ferritin levels when compared with frequency of low birth weight and frequency of preterm delivery (Table 4).

The correlation between maternal iron status and anthropometric indices versus pregnancy outcome was assessed by Pearson's correlation (Table 5). A significant positive correlation was observed between maternal Hb levels and newborns' birth weight, birth height, head circumference and gestational age. Similarly, a significant positive correlation was observed between maternal Hematocrit (Hct) levels and newborns' birth weight, birth height, gestational

TABLE 3: **Maternal characteristics and pregnancy outcome by Hb tertile groups.** Statistical analysis was performed by one-way ANOVA, except for frequency of low birth weight and frequency of preterm delivery that were analyzed by Kruskal-Wallis test.

| | All | HbTertile groups | | | |
| | (Mean ± SD) | HbT1 | HbT2 | HbT3 | P-value |
		Hb< 110 g/L	Hb 110- 120 g/L	Hb> 120 g/L	
Maternal characteristics (n= 300)*					
Serum ferritin (ng/mL)	20.2 ± 23.2	14.8 ± 30.2	15.9 ± 10.6	25.0 ± 22.6	0.001
Age (years)	26.3 ± 5.9	27.1 ± 6.2	25.8 ± 6.3	26.1 ± 5.4	0.324
BMI (kg/m^2)	24.8 ± 4.1	24.3 ± 3.2	24.4 ± 4.5	25.1 ± 4.2	0.250
No. of children	2.1 ± 2.0	2.4 ± 2.1	2.2 ± 2.2	2.0 ± 1.9	0.268
No. of abortions	0.66 ± 1.2	0.73 ± 1.03	0.52 ± 0.94	0.69 ± 1.35	0.503
Educational level (years)	11.6 ± 3.2	11.9 ± 3.5	11.4 ± 3.0	11.6 ± 3.1	0.657
Monthly income (NIS)	1832 ± 1154	1888 ± 1262	1667 ± 913	1883 ± 1201	0.375
Pregnancy outcome					
Birth weight (gm)	3022 ± 585 (n= 163)[1]	2817 ± 568	3030 ± 577	3144 ± 571	0.009
Birth height (cm)	48.3 ± 2.7 (n= 96)[1]	47.3 ± 2.5	48.3 ± 2.5	49.1 ±2.8	0.022
Head circumference (cm)	34.6 ± 1.4 (n= 96)[1]	34.1 ± 1.5	34.5 ± 1.2	35.0 ± 1.3	0.017
Gestational age (weeks)	38.5 ± 1.5 (n= 122)[1]	37.8 ± 1.5	38.6 ± 1.4	38.8 ± 1.6	0.012
	Frequency (%)	HbT1	HbT2	HbT3	P-value
Frequency of low birth weight (< 2500 gm)	39 (23.9%)	16 (9.8%)	9 (5.5%)	14 (8.6%)	0.053
Frequency of preterm delivery (< 37 weeks)	16 (13.1%)	8 (6.6%)	4 (3.3%)	4 (3.3%)	0.53

*n= 300 for all maternal characteristics except for monthly income it was 264. [1]The indicated numbers of samples were assessed for each parameter.

age, and Hb levels. Also, a significant positive correlation was observed between maternal serum ferritin levels and newborns' birth height, gestational age, and Hb levels. No significant correlation was found between maternal age, BMI, number of children, number of abortions, educational level, and monthly income on one side and pregnancy outcome on the other side (Table 5).

4. Discussion

The prevalence of IDA among pregnant women from Hebron Governorate was 25.7% and 52% of them had depleted iron stores (iron deficiency). These data indicate that anemia among pregnant in Hebron region is a public health problem that can be classified as moderate [15]. The prevalence of anemia among pregnant women reported in this study was within the average rates reported for several Arab countries [17–21] concerning pregnant women in their first trimester. In Jordan, Al-Mehaisen et al. [19] reported an overall prevalence of anemia of 34.7% among pregnant women in rural areas, and the prevalence rate ranged from 18.9% among women in first trimester to 32.7% in second trimester to 42.5% in third trimester. In Kuwait, the prevalence of anemia among pregnant women was reported at 24.1% [20]. In the latter report [20] the prevalence of anemia varied with the stage of pregnancy, being lowest in first trimester (14.8%), highest in

second trimester (49.2%), and intermediate in third trimester (36%). In Saudi Arabia, the prevalence of anemia among pregnant women in their first trimester was reported at 29.6% [18] and 27.7% [21] in two different regions of Saudi Arabia. In our study, the percentage of pregnant women with depleted iron stores (52%) is higher than those with anemia (25.7%) in first trimester and this may indicate that the prevalence of anemia would become more common and more severe in second and third trimester.

Anemia or iron deficiency during pregnancy is associated with intrauterine growth retardation, premature birth, low birth weight, increased labor time, higher risk of infection, elevated maternal and prenatal mortality, muscle dysfunction, and low physical capacity [8, 9, 22–24]. In accordance with previous reports [9–11], our study revealed a significant difference among maternal Hb tertile groups when compared to newborns' birth weight, height, and head circumference as well as gestational age. The birth weight, height, and gestational age were lowest with maternal HbT1 (< 110 g/L) and highest with maternal HbT3 group (> 120 g/L). Although HbT1 (in our study included Hb values from 73 to 109 g/L) was not as low as Hb < 70 g/L, which is considered as severe anemia [15] the adverse effect of moderate/mild anemia on pregnancy outcome was clearly demonstrated. Additionally, there was a significant association between maternal low serum ferritin and frequency of low birth weight and frequency of preterm delivery.

Table 4: **Maternal characteristics and pregnancy outcomes by maternal serum ferritin levels.** Statistical analysis was performed by independent sample *t*-test, except for frequency of low birth weight and frequency of preterm delivery that were analyzed by Chi-square test.

	All (Mean ± SD)	Serum ferritin		P-value
		Normal (≥ 15 ng/mL)	Iron deficiency (< 15 ng/mL)	
Maternal characteristics (n= 300)*				
Age (years)	26.3 ± 5.9	26.0 ± 5.4	226.3 ± 6.3	0.436
BMI (kg/m²)	24.8 ± 4.1	25.3 ± 4.4	24.2 ± 3.7	0.017
No. of children	2.1 ± 2.0	2.0 ± 1.9	2.3 ± 3.1	0.158
No. of abortions	0.66 ± 1.2	0.59 ± 1.1	0.72 ± 1.2	0.328
Educational level (years)	11.6 ± 3.2	11.8 ± 2.8	11.5 ± 3.5	0.439
Monthly income (NIS)	1832 ± 1154	1835 ± 1096	1829 ± 1209	0.961
Pregnancy outcome				
Birth weight (gm)	3022 ± 585 (n= 163)[1]	3123 ± 538	2945 ± 610	0.053
Birth height (cm)	48.3 ± 2.7 (n= 96)[1]	49.1 ± 2.3	47.9 ± 2.8	0.026
Head circumference (cm)	34.6 ± 1.4 (n= 96)[1]	35.0 ± 1.1	34.4 ± 1.4	0.025
Gestational age (weeks)	38.5 ± 1.5 (n= 122)[1]	38.9 ± 1.5	38.1 ± 1.5	0.008
	Frequency	Normal (≥ 15 ng/mL)	Iron deficiency (< 15 ng/mL)	P-value
Frequency of low birth weight (< 2500 gm)	39 (23.9%)	9 (5.5%)	30 (18.4%)	0.001
Frequency of preterm delivery (< 37 weeks)	16 (13.1%)	2 (1.6%)	14 (11.5%)	0.003

*n= 300 for all maternal characteristics except for monthly income it was 264.
[1]The indicated numbers of samples were assessed for each parameter.

Table 5: Pearson's correlation coefficients between pregnancy outcome (newborns) and maternal iron status and anthropometric/socio-economic factors.

Maternal data↓	Newborn data				
	Birth weight	Birth height	Head circumference	Gestational age	Hb
Hb	**0.191**∗	**0.307**∗∗	**0.257**∗	**0.275**∗∗	0.197
Hct	**0.171**∗	**0.224**∗	0.178	**0.228**∗	**0.235**∗
Serum ferritin	0.008	**0.216**∗	0.174	**0.254**∗∗	**0.287**∗∗
Age	0.025	0.103	0.124	0.038	0.052
BMI	0.061	0.074	0.022	-0.016	0.008
No. of Children	0.126	0.107	0.130	0.147	-0.052
No. of abortions	0.046	0.054	0.088	-0.037	0.001
Educational level	-0.023	-0.138	-0.080	-0.062	0.170
Monthly income	0.095	-0.033	-0.020	0.167	0.106

∗ Correlation is significant at the 0.05 level (2-tailed). ∗∗ Correlation is significant at the 0.01 level (2-tailed).

The birth weight is affected by a complex and independent factors in addition to maternal Hb and serum ferritin. The anthropometry of the mother and her nutritional intake are thought to be among the most important [25, 26]. Among the anthropometry measures, prepregnancy BMI has received especial interest and was addressed by many studies. Despite this, the direct relationship between prepregnancy BMI and fetal growth is still not known [27]. Several reports have

shown that underweight women or those with low BMI are at high risk of having low birth babies and other adverse pregnancy outcome [27–30]. Also, high BMI (but still in the normal category) has a favorable effect on pregnancy outcome, a BMI in the overweight/obese/severely obese categories has been reported to increase the risk of adverse obstetric and neonatal outcomes such as maternal diabetes, preterm delivery, macrosomia, increasing risk of admission of baby to intensive care unit, and perinatal death [30–32]. In the present study no significant correlation was observed between maternal anthropometric measures (age and BMI) and pregnancy outcome. Also, no statistically significant difference was observed among maternal Hb tertile groups when compared with maternal age and BMI; the maternal Hb showed a slight increase with increasing BMI (Table 3). Our findings concerning BMI and pregnancy outcome are contradictory to previous reports [30–32] and may be due to the limited number of overweight/obese women among the study subjects.

Furthermore, several studies have investigated the effect of socioeconomic status of the mother on pregnancy outcome. Anemia has been linked to poverty [1, 24, 33], which in turn is considered as a consequence of many factors including low monthly income and low levels of education. Therefore, in this study we have examined the association of the mother's socioeconomic status (monthly income, level of education, and parity) with maternal Hb, maternal serum ferritin, and low birth weight and did not find a significant correlation. In consistence with our findings, a previous study that investigated a cohort of pregnant women from Nablus-Palestine did not find a significant association between monthly income, level of education, and size of family and prevalence of anemia among this group [34]. While Khader et al. [13] reported a significant association between parity and prevalence of anemia among Palestinian pregnant women living in Refugee camps in West Bank and Gaza but no significant association was found with regard to level of education. A recent report from rural areas of Jordan has found no significant association between socioeconomic status of mothers and prevalence of anemia among pregnant women [19]. In contrast to our findings, a study from Malaysia found that older age of the mother, parity of four or above, Indian origin, and per capita monthly income are significant risk factors for low birth weight [27]. Another study from Nigeria found that less educated pregnant women had significantly higher prevalence of anemia compared to educated women, and no significant association between parity and prevalence of anemia [35]. Thus, further studies are needed to study the effect of the socioeconomic status of mothers' on the pregnancy outcome using a larger sample size and preferably from different regions in Palestine. Additionally, the role of some factors in the contradictory results concerning anthropometric parameters among different studies from different geographic regions such as prevalence rate of anemia, ethnicity, and local environmental factors may be better tackled by meta-analysis studies.

A limitation in our study is that only one blood sample was collected from pregnant women and that was in their first trimester. However, anemia usually becomes more common and more severe as pregnancy progress. Thus, a second blood sample collected at the end of second trimester or beginning of third trimester could provide more information on the association between maternal anemia in second or third trimester and pregnancy outcome compared to first trimester.

5. Conclusion

Our study indicated that IDA is a moderate public health problem among pregnant women in Hebron Governorate and more than half of study subjects have depleted iron stores. Maternal Hb and serum ferritin were found to affect pregnancy outcome (birth weight, height, and gestational age). Newborns born to women with low Hb levels tended to have lower birth weight and height, head circumference, and lower gestational age. No significant association was observed between maternal anthropometric measures (age and BMI) or the socioeconomic status (level of education, monthly income, and parity) and pregnancy outcome. The high prevalence of anemia in our subjects was probably due to low iron intake and poor dietary habits rather than food insecurity or disease. Therefore, the etiological factors associated with maternal anemia during pregnancy in Palestine should deserve more attention.

Disclosure

The current address of Khaled M. Srour is University of Toledo Medical Center, Internal Medicine Department, Toledo, OH, USA. The current address of Samah S. Aqel is Al-Ramah clinic, Directorate of Primary Health Care of Hebron, Ministry of Health, Hebron, State of Palestine.

Conflicts of Interest

The authors declare that there are no conflicts of interest regarding the publication of this paper.

Acknowledgments

We would like to acknowledge the Ministry of Health and the Health Work Committees for giving us the permission to meet the study subjects at their maternal and child healthcare centers.

References

[1] E. McLean, I. Egli, M. Cogswell, B. de Benoist, and D. Wojdyla, "Worldwide prevalence of anemia in preschool aged children, pregnant women and non-pregnant women of reproductive age," in *The guide book: Nutritional Anemia. Basel*, J. Badham, M. B. Zimmermann, and K. Kraemer, Eds., pp. 11-12, Sight and Life Press, Basel, Switzerland, 2007.

[2] World Health Organization and Centers for Disease Control and Prevention, *The global prevalence of anaemia in 2011*, WHO, Geneva, Switzerland, 2015, http://www.who.int/nutrition/publications/micronutrients/global_prevalence_anaemia_2011/en/.

[3] S.-R. Pasricha and H. Drakesmith, "Iron Deficiency Anemia: Problems in Diagnosis and Prevention at the Population Level," *Hematology/Oncology Clinics of North America*, vol. 30, no. 2, pp. 309–325, 2016.

[4] T. O. Scholl, "Iron status during pregnancy: setting the stage for mother and infant," *American Journal of Clinical Nutrition*, vol. 81, no. 5, pp. 1218S–1222S, 2005.

[5] S. Killip, J. M. Bennett, and M. D. Chambers, "Iron deficiency anemia," *American Family Physician*, vol. 75, no. 5, pp. 671–678, 2007.

[6] T. O. Scholl, "Maternal iron status: Relation to fetal growth, length of gestation, and iron endowment of the neonate," *Nutrition Reviews*, vol. 69, no. 1, pp. S23–S29, 2011.

[7] C. Breymann, X.-M. Bian, L. R. Blanco-Capito, C. Chong, G. Mahmud, and R. Rehman, "Expert recommendations for the diagnosis and treatment of iron-deficiency anemia during pregnancy and the postpartum period in the Asia-Pacific region," *Journal of Perinatal Medicine*, vol. 39, no. 2, pp. 113–121, 2011.

[8] L. H. Allen, "Anemia and iron deficiency: effects on pregnancy outcome," *American Journal of Clinical Nutrition*, vol. 71, no. 5, pp. 1280S–1284S, 2000.

[9] A. G. Ronnenberg, R. J. Wood, X. Wang et al., "Preconception hemoglobin and ferritin concentrations are associated with pregnancy outcome in a prospective cohort of Chinese women," *Journal of Nutrition*, vol. 134, no. 10, pp. 2586–2591, 2004.

[10] H. S. Lee, M. S. Kim, M. H. Kim, Y. J. Kim, and W. Y. Kim, "Iron status and its association with pregnancy outcome in Korean pregnant women," *European Journal of Clinical Nutrition*, vol. 60, no. 9, pp. 1130–1135, 2006.

[11] J. Shao, J. Lou, R. Rao et al., "Maternal serum ferritin concentration is positively associated with newborn iron stores in women with low ferritin status in Late Pregnancy1-3," *Journal of Nutrition*, vol. 142, no. 11, pp. 2004–2009, 2012.

[12] State of Palestine, Ministry of Health, and Nutrition Department, "National nutritional surveillance system," Tech. Rep., 2016.

[13] A. Khader, H. Madi, F. Riccardo, and G. Sabatinelli, "Anaemia among pregnant Palestinian women in the Occupied Palestinian Territory," *Public Health Nutrition*, vol. 12, no. 12, pp. 2416–2420, 2009.

[14] "Palestinian Central Bureau of Statistics," 2016, http://www.pcbs.gov.ps/Portals/_Rainbow/Documents/gover_e.htm.

[15] World Health Organization, *Haemoglobin concentrations for the diagnosis of anaemia and assessment of severity. Vitamin and Mineral Nutrition Information System*, World Health Organization, Geneva, Switzerland, 2011, http://www.who.int/vmnis/indicators/haemoglobin/en/.

[16] World Health Organization and Centers for Disease Control and Prevention, *Worldwide prevalence of anaemia 1993-2005: WHO global database on anaemia*, B. de Benoist, E. McLean, E. Egli, and M. Cogeswell, Eds., WHO, 2018, http://www.who.int/vmnis/publications/en/.

[17] K. Bagchi, "Iron deficiency anaemia - An old enemy," *Eastern Mediterranean Health Journal*, vol. 10, no. 6, pp. 754–760, 2004.

[18] F. Habib, E. Habib Zein Alabdin, M. Alenazy, and R. Nooh, "Compliance to iron supplementation during pregnancy," *Journal of Obstetrics & Gynaecology*, vol. 29, no. 6, pp. 487–492, 2009.

[19] L. Al-Mehaisen, Y. Khader, O. Al-Kuran, F. Abu Issa, and Z. Amarin, "Maternal anemia in rural Jordan: Room for improvement," *Anemia*, vol. 2011, Article ID 381812, 7 pages, 2011.

[20] F. Ahmed and M. A. Al-Sumaie, "Risk factors associated with anemia and iron deficiency among Kuwaiti pregnant women," *International Journal of Food Sciences and Nutrition*, vol. 62, no. 6, pp. 585–592, 2011.

[21] P. Rasheed, M. R. Koura, B. K. Al-Dabal, and S. M. Makki, "Anemia in pregnancy: A study among attendees of primary health care centers," *Annals of Saudi Medicine*, vol. 28, no. 6, pp. 449–452, 2008.

[22] S. Rahmati, A. Delpishe, M. Azami, M. R. H. Ahmadi, and K. Sayehmiri, "Maternal anemia during pregnancy and infant low birth weight: A systematic review and meta-analysis," *International Journal of Reproductive BioMedicine*, vol. 15, no. 3, pp. 125–134, 2017.

[23] R. Suryanarayana, M. Chandrappa, A. Santhuram, S. Prathima, and S. Sheela, "Prospective study on prevalence of anemia of pregnant women and its outcome: A community based study," *Journal of Family Medicine and Primary Care*, vol. 6, no. 4, pp. 739–743, 2017.

[24] L. Lin, Y. Wei, W. Zhu et al., "Prevalence, risk factors and associated adverse pregnancy outcomes of anaemia in Chinese pregnant women: a multicentre retrospective study," *BMC Pregnancy and Childbirth*, vol. 18, no. 1, 2018.

[25] S. Muthayya, "Maternal nutrition & low birth weight—what is really important?" *Indian Journal of Medical Research*, vol. 130, no. 5, pp. 600–608, 2009.

[26] E. R. Smith, A. H. Shankar, L. S. Wu et al., "Modifiers of the effect of maternal multiple micronutrient supplementation on stillbirth, birth outcomes, and infant mortality: a meta-analysis of individual patient data from 17 randomised trials in low-income and middle-income countries," *The Lancet Global Health*, vol. 5, no. 11, pp. e1090–e1100, 2017.

[27] H. Yadav and N. Lee, "Maternal factors in predicting low birth weight babies," *Medical Journal of Malaysia*, vol. 68, no. 1, pp. 44–47, 2013.

[28] C. Anuranga, R. Wickramasinghe, R. P. Rannan-Eliya, S. M. Hossain, and A. T. Abeykoon, "Trends, inequalities and determinants of low birth weight in Sri Lanka.," *The Ceylon Medical Journal*, vol. 57, no. 2, pp. 61–69, 2012.

[29] S. Munim and H. Maheen, "Association of gestational weight gain and pre-pregnancy body mass index with adverse pregnancy outcome.," *Journal of the College of Physicians and Surgeons–Pakistan : JCPSP*, vol. 22, no. 11, pp. 694–698, 2012.

[30] Z. Yu, S. Han, J. Zhu, X. Sun, C. Ji, and X. Guo, "Pre-pregnancy body mass index in relation to infant birth weight and offspring overweight/obesity: a systematic review and meta-analysis," *PLoS ONE*, vol. 8, no. 4, Article ID e61627, 2013.

[31] E. Oteng-Ntim, J. Kopeika, P. Seed, S. Wandiembe, and P. Doyle, "Impact of Obesity on Pregnancy Outcome in Different Ethnic Groups: Calculating Population Attributable Fractions," *PLoS ONE*, vol. 8, no. 1, 2013.

[32] A. K. Phillips, S. C. Roy, R. Lundberg et al., "Neonatal iron status is impaired by maternal obesity and excessive weight gain during pregnancy," *Journal of Perinatology*, vol. 34, no. 7, pp. 513–518, 2014.

[33] S. E. Lee, S. A. Talegawkar, M. Merialdi, and L. E. Caulfield, "Dietary intakes of women during pregnancy in low- and middle-income countries," *Public Health Nutrition*, vol. 16, no. 8, pp. 1340–1353, 2013.

[34] A. W. M. Abu-Hasira, *Iron deficiency among pregnant women in Nablus district; prevalence, knowledge, attitude and practices. MSc*, An-Najah National University, Nablus, Palestine, 2007.

[35] G. N. Okwu and A. I. Ukoha, "Studies on the predisposing factors of iron deficiency anaemia among pregnant women in a Nigerian community," *Pakistan Journal of Nutrition*, vol. 7, no. 1, pp. 151–156, 2008.

24

Low Hemoglobin among Pregnant Women in Midwives Practice of Primary Health Care, Jatinangor, Indonesia: Iron Deficiency Anemia or β-Thalassemia Trait?

Ari Indra Susanti,[1] Edhyana Sahiratmadja,[2] Gatot Winarno,[3] Adhi Kristianto Sugianli,[4] Herman Susanto,[3] and Ramdan Panigoro[2]

[1] Program Study of Midwifery, Division of Maternal and Child Health, Department of Public Health, Faculty of Medicine, Universitas Padjadjaran, Bandung, Indonesia
[2] Department of Biochemistry and Molecular Biology, Faculty of Medicine, Universitas Padjadjaran, Bandung, Indonesia
[3] Department of Obstetrics and Gynecology, Faculty of Medicine, Universitas Padjadjaran and Dr. Hasan Sadikin General Hospital, Bandung, Indonesia
[4] Department of Clinical Pathology, Faculty of Medicine, Universitas Padjadjaran and Dr. Hasan Sadikin General Hospital, Bandung, Indonesia

Correspondence should be addressed to Edhyana Sahiratmadja; e.sahiratmadja@unpad.ac.id

Academic Editor: Duran Canatan

Low hemoglobin (Hb) or anemia is common among pregnant women in developing countries which may cause adverse pregnancy outcomes and maternal deaths. Our study aimed to assess Hb level measured by midwives in primary health care facility at rural area of Jatinangor, Indonesia, and to explore whether the anemia was due to iron deficiency (IDA) or β-thalassemia trait (β-TT). Pregnant women ($n = 105$) had finger prick test for Hb level during a regular antenatal care examination from October to November 2016. Hb level by finger prick test was compared with venous blood, measured by complete blood count (CBC). Indices including MCV and MCH and indices of Shine & Lal, Mentzer, Srivastava, Engels & Frase, Ehsani, and Sirdah were analyzed to differentiate anemia due to IDA and anemia due to suspect β-TT. HbA2 was measured to confirm β-TT. Anemic pregnant women were found in 86.7% by finger prick test compared to 21.9% ($n = 23$) by CBC. The prevalence of β-TT in our study was 5.7%. Hb measurement among pregnant women in low resource area is highly important; however, finger prick test in this study showed a high frequency of anemia which may lead to iron oversupplementation. A standard CBC is encouraged; MCV and MCH would help midwives to identify β-TT.

1. Introduction

Iron deficiency is the leading nutrient deficiency in the world, resulting in iron deficiency anemia (IDA) that affects infants, young children, and women of child-bearing age [1]. In pregnancy, lower hemoglobin occurs as a physiological phenomenon especially in the second trimester. Iron need is increased as a result of higher iron demand to accommodate the requirement of fetal placental unit [2]. Since anemia in pregnancy may lead to adverse pregnancy outcomes and maternal deaths [3], iron supplementation and proper nutrition are needed to fulfill the iron deficiency in pregnancy [4].

Iron deficiency is not the only etiology of anemia in the developing countries. Other coinfections, for example, helminthes, tuberculosis, and HIV, or other diseases such as diabetes mellitus may exist [5]. Interestingly, iron deficiency has a protective role for malarial infection, and iron supplementation in this malarial endemic area may thus increase the infection susceptibility [6]. Therefore, a good control of anemia in low- and middle-income countries needs to be considered [7]. Furthermore, low Hb can be caused by hemoglobinopathies, especially in area where thalassemia trait prevalence is high [8]. Individuals with thalassemia carrier may have enough iron due to erythropoiesis by hepcidin suppression, and excessive iron supplementation may subsequently increase the risk for various complications [9]. Whether the anemia in pregnancy in this area is due to iron deficiency or other causes needs to be further explored.

In areas with limited resources, anemia in pregnancy has been often examined by low cost test, which is an incredibly useful tool, that is, capillary finger-pricked test. On the other hand, in area where thalassemia prevalence is high, thalassemia trait is performed with inexpensive tool that has a good validity test, including Naked Eye Single Tube Red Cell Osmotic Fragility Test (NESTROFT) [10]. NESTROFT is, however, sometimes not possible to be done in the field because it needs some preparation. Other tools that can predict thalassemia trait are venous complete blood count (CBC) indices, which vary from indices using RBC, MCV, and MCH parameters, including Shine & Lal, Mentzer, Srivastava, Engels & Frase, Ehsani, and Sirdah index, to indices using RDW parameter including Green & King index [11]. In the case of pregnant women, HbA2 level is used to predict β-thalassemia trait (β-TT) [12]. The definitive differential diagnosis between β-TT and IDA can be based on the result of HbA2 electrophoresis, serum iron levels, and a ferritin calculation [13].

In Indonesia, the prevalence of anemia among pregnant women is declining over the time, but the number is still as high as more than 35% [14]. Since this country is located in the thalassemia belt, exploring thalassemia carrier in anemic pregnant women especially by midwives in limited source setting becomes an important issue. Midwives play a major role in antenatal care in the primary health care facility in rural area. Iron tablets are often prescribed without proper blood examination but by recognizing clinical symptoms [15]. This study aimed to explore the hemoglobin (Hb) level among pregnant women measured by midwives in the primary health care facility in rural area of West Java Province, Indonesia. The etiology of anemia in pregnancy was also assessed whether the anemia was due to iron deficiency or β-TT.

2. Materials and Methods

2.1. Pregnant Women Inclusion. The study was conducted using cross-sectional analytic comparative design. All pregnant women who visited the primary health care facility at Jatinangor, West Java, between October and November 2016 were invited to take part in this study after consent. In brief, while waiting in the waiting room for a regular antenatal care, the pregnant women and their husbands were given information about anemia including the possibility and the effect of anemia due to IDA and β-TT in the pregnancy. Known diseases such as diabetes mellitus and positive HIV were excluded.

2.2. Anemia Status Measurement and Hemoglobin Analyses. The anemia status (Hb level < 11 g/dL) [16] of pregnant women was determined from capillary blood from a finger-pricked test (EasyTouch® GCHb) by midwives who had a preeducated

TABLE 1: Characteristics and distribution of anemia among pregnant women ($n = 105$) in Jatinangor Puskesmas, West Java, Indonesia, using finger prick and CBC methods.

	Finger prick	CBC
Hb value (g/dL); mean (SD)	9.5 (1.4)	11.7 (1.1)
Anemia status; n (%)	91 (86.7%)	23 (21.9%)
Mild (Hb: 8–11 g/dL)	75	23
Moderate (Hb: 6.5–8 g/dL)	16	—

Note. CBC, complete blood count; Hb, hemoglobin; SD, standard deviation.

finger-pricked technique according to Indonesian Ministry of Health document (MOH, number 43, 2013). After signing the informed consent form, venous blood samples were drawn and stored at 2–8°C before being transported to Dr. Hasan Sadikin General Hospital, Bandung. The distance between the primary health care facility and the hospital was approx. 50 km and the time between the blood draw and measurement was about 4 hours. Automated hematology analyzer with impedance method for complete blood count (CBC) measurement (Sysmex XP-100, Japan) was used to measure 8 parameters including Hb, mean corpuscular volume (MCV), and red blood count (RBC). Various indices were calculated including index of Shine & Lal ($MCV^2 * MCH/100$), Mentzer (MCV/RBC), Srivastava (MCH/RBC), Engels & Frase ($MCV - RBC - (5 * Hb)$), Ehsani ($MCV - 10 * RBC$), and Sirdah ($MCV - RBC - 3 * Hb$), with cut-off of IDA and suspect β-TT as shown in Table 1. To confirm β-TT, hemoglobin capillary electrophoresis was performed to measure HbA2 levels (MG300, Sebia, France). Elevated HbA2 level ($\geq 3.5\%$) was designated as β-TT. Study protocol had been reviewed and ethical clearance was granted by Ethical Committee of Faculty of Medicine, Universitas Padjadjaran, number 453/UN6.C1.3.2/KEPK/PN/2016.

2.3. Statistical Analyses. Data was collected into paper-based form and inputted into predesigned Excel sheet (Microsoft Corp., USA). The data distribution of CBC result was tested for normality using Shapiro-Wilk test; when the test pointed out that p value was >0.05, the mean and standard deviation were calculated and when p value was <0.05, the median and min-max value were calculated.

Characteristics of the pregnant women were described and the frequencies of anemia using finger prick test and CBC were tabulated and compared; p value was considered significant when $p < 0.05$ (Student's t-test). Concordance of Hb level between finger prick test and CBC test and also between various indices and HbA2 analyses were calculated to determine Cohen's kappa value [17]. Analyses were performed on STATA 12.0 (Stata Corp., Texas, USA).

3. Results

3.1. Anemia Prevalence in Pregnancy. In total, there were 105 pregnant women included in this study with median age of 29 (range: 18–39) years. The finger prick test's result showed that 91 (86.7%) pregnant women had anemia, of whom 71.4% had mild anemia (Hb > 8 g/dL) and 15.2% had moderate anemia

Table 2: Anemia status among pregnant women ($n = 105$) in Jatinangor Puskesmas, West Java, Indonesia, stratified by gravidity and trimester of pregnancy.

	Anemia N = 23	Not anemia N = 82	p value
Gravidity			
Primigravida	7	23	
Multigravida (2-3)	12	47	
Grand multigravida (≥4)	4	12	0.997
Trimester			
(1) (<12 weeks)	—	10	
(2) (12–26 weeks)	7	35	0.021*
(3) (>26 weeks)	16	37	

Note. * p value was set as <0.05 (Spearman's correlation).

(Hb: 6.5–8 g/dL). Interestingly, while using CBC method, mild anemia was found in only 23 (21.9%) women (Table 1). There was, thus, a significant difference in frequency of anemia in pregnant women using finger prick test and CBC, that is, 86.7% and 21.9%, respectively, and this discordance result in both measurements had an agreement level (Cohen's kappa) of 0.056, which was very poor. Since the anemia prevalence using CBC was around the national prevalence of anemia published earlier [14], we used the CBC value for further analyses.

Anemia status in pregnant women was shown according to the gravida and pregnancy trimester (Table 2). There was a correlation between trimester and anemia status; that is, anemia was more prevalent in later stage of pregnancy ($p = 0.021$, Spearman's correlation), while there was no correlation between anemia status and the number of gravidas ($p = 0.997$).

3.2. Analyses of Complete Blood Count Indices. Further analyses of anemic pregnant women ($n = 23$) using CBC showed that single parameter of MCV <76 fL and MCH <24 pg and index of Shine & Lal could detect suspect β-TT for 5, 6, and 7 pregnant women, respectively, compared to other indices which could detect much lower number (Table 3). A total of 6 pregnant women had HbA2 result of >3.5, of whom 5 had β-TT and 1 was suspected as having probably HbE because the HbA2 result was very high. The HbA2 result indicated that the prevalence of β-TT in our study among pregnant women was at least 5.7%. Interestingly, when the CBC indices were compared with HbA2 analyses, discordance results were found with Cohen's kappa ranging from 0.20 to 0.25, which had a fair quality of agreement. Since the number of anemic pregnant women was low ($n = 23$), we did not calculate the sensitivity and specificity between both CBC indices and HbA2 analyses.

4. Discussions

During a regular antenatal care in the primary health care facility in a rural area in Jatinangor, Indonesia, Hb level is measured to control the well-being of both mother and baby.

Table 3: Concordant result of CBC indices to HbA2 electrophoresis among pregnant women ($n = 23$) in Jatinangor Puskesmas, West Java, Indonesia.

Indices	HbA2 < 3.5 (n 17)	HbA2 ≥ 3.5 (n 6)	Total	K
RBC count				
IDA < 5	17	5	22	0.228
Susp. β-TT > 5	—	1	1	
MCV*				
IDA >76	15	3	18	0.232
Susp. β-TT < 76	2	3	5	
MCH*				
IDA > 24	14	3	17	0.203
Susp. β-TT < 24	3	3	6	
Shine & Lal*				
IDA > 1530	13	3	16	0.251
Susp. β-TT < 1530	4	3	7	
Mentzer				
IDA > 13	17	5	22	0.228
Susp. β-TT < 13	—	1	1	
Srivastava				
IDA > 38	17	5	22	0.228
Susp. β-TT < 38	—	1	1	
Ehsani				
IDA > 15	17	5	22	0.228
Susp. β-TT < 15	—	1	1	
Sirdah				
IDA > 27	17	5	22	0.228
Susp. β-TT < 27	—	1	1	
Engels Fraser				
IDA < 0	17	6	23	n.d.
Susp. β-TT > 0	—	—	—	

Note. Susp. β-TT, suspect β-thalassemia trait; IDA, iron deficiency anemia; K, Cohen's kappa. * The indices with high suspect β-thalassemia trait cases. Formula to calculate indices as shown in the bracket: index of Shine & Lal (MCV^2 * MCH/100), Mentzer (MCV/RBC), Srivastava (MCH/RBC), Engels Frase (MCV – RBC – (5 * Hb)), Ehsani (MCV – 10 * RBC), Sirdah (MCV – RBC – 3 * Hb).

Our study showed that anemia in pregnancy status measured by midwives using inexpensive and easy to perform capillary finger prick test was very high, reaching almost 90% of pregnant women. Capillary finger prick test is a simple test to perform; nevertheless, this test requires proper technique. Therefore, the use of finger prick test by midwives in primary health care facility needs to be further reviewed.

When the Hb level is measured using CBC, result showed that anemia among pregnant women in our study only occurred in around 20%, in line with the national prevalence of anemia published earlier [14]. The discrepancy result shown using finger prick test and standard CBC seems too high and may lead to overprescription of iron supplementation. Iron is indeed needed more in second and third semesters as a result of increased fetal placental unit [18]. This conforms to our study, showing that anemia was more prevalent in third semester ($p = 0.021$). Iron deficiency anemia in later phase of pregnancy is associated with the birth weight of the neonates [19] and may play a role as a major killer in pregnant women [7]. Appropriate iron supplementation is needed in pregnancy and WHO has guidelines for iron supplementation in pregnant women and individuals where infection and hemoglobinopathies prevalence are high [1].

The first blood taken in life among healthy individual happens particularly in pregnant women. Study in the neighboring country Thailand showed that the main causes of anemia among pregnant women are IDA and thalassemia carriers [20]. In Indonesia, Thalassemia ranks 6th for catastrophic diseases; therefore, there is a rising interest to screen thalassemia carrier in the general population. Our study has shown β-TT prevalence as high as 5.7%, conforming to the national prevalence which is around 6 to 10%. Although the national guidelines for thalassemia trait screening exist [21], thalassemia trait screening in general population is not regularly conducted yet. Moreover, the knowledge about etiology of anemia among pregnant women other than iron deficiency such as hemoglobinopathies is not well known among students midwifery (Sahiratmadja et al., unpublished data), making the question on how to distinguish IDA and thalassemia trait a major concern, especially in the limited resource area. IDA can be diagnosed by simple and easy detection. Red blood cells are smeared in object glass and could be seen as small or microcytic cells with hypochromic color. More accurately, IDA can be diagnosed by calculating the CBC performed by a hematology analyzer. Furthermore, the β-TT pregnant women are often misdiagnosed as those suffering from iron deficiency anaemia; thus, they are given unnecessary iron medication. In this setting, a reliable screening test becomes a need of the hour for screening purposes.

In meta-analysis study to distinguish individuals with β-TT and IDA, Hoffmann et al. (2015) have noted that microscopic smear examinations and CBC are difficult to be performed in rural area since the source and personnel to examine the smear are scarce, and CBC analyzer is expensive and not portable [22]. For example, in rural area where equipment or expertise is scarce, One Tube Osmotic Fragility Test (OTOFT) is a simple test that can be done to examine carriers [23]. Interestingly, another study also showed that HbA2 is reliable to measure β-TT when IDA also coexists [24]. Ideally, HbA2 is more reliable as indicated to detect β-TT cases in pregnant women [12], but this measurement is costly. One obstacle in HbA2 measurement is that α-thalassemia could be coinherited with β-thalassemia, making HbA2 level have normal value, leading to difficulty in screening α-thalassemia using HbA2 level [25]. To confirm the definitive diagnosis, DNA analysis is needed.

Further study needs to be designed to calculate the cost-effectiveness screening in primary care [26], that is, the strategy of timing of screening of thalassemia carrier. Whether the screening is more beneficial during premarital screening [27, 28] or in young adults [29] needs further exploration. Moreover, knowledge of etiology of anemia among student midwives needs to be strengthened for thalassemia problem.

A simple standard CBC, that is, low MCV and low MCH, may be of important role to detect carriers and a good training program for the midwives leading the process is urgently required.

Limitation of this study was that iron status was not assessed, as this study was not designed for iron status study, particularly since this study was done in a limited setting area. Other limitation is that low number of anemic pregnant women in our study is considered low; however, the consistent results of the currently used method for Hb, that is, prick test, showed no doubt that the finger prick method has poor reliability.

5. Conclusion

Low hemoglobin level by finger prick test measured by midwives showed much higher prevalence of anemia, leading to iron oversupplementation. Since Indonesia is located in thalassemia belt area, a reliable measurement to distinguish anemia of iron deficiency or thalassemia carrier is highly needed. Simple single parameter of CBC such as MCV and MCH would help midwives to identify β-TT among pregnant women; therefore, wherever it is possible, a standard CBC to detect β-TT is encouraged.

Disclosure

Ari Indra Susanti and Edhyana Sahiratmadja are co-first authors.

Conflicts of Interest

The authors declare that there are no conflicts of interest.

Authors' Contributions

Ari Indra Susanti, Edhyana Sahiratmadja, Gatot Winarno, Adhi Kristianto Sugianli, Herman Susanto, and Ramdan Panigoro conceived the study and participated in the design and data analyses. Ari Indra Susanti and Edhyana Sahiratmadja were involved in data acquisition. All authors contributed towards drafting and agree to be accountable for all respects of the work. Edhyana Sahiratmadja, Adhi Kristianto Sugianli, Herman Susanto, and Ramdan Panigoro critically reviewed the manuscript. All the authors read and approved the manuscript.

Acknowledgments

The authors are grateful to all midwives from primary health care Puskesmas, Jatinangor, who participated in this study, especially Ms. Nia Kurniawati and Ms. Lilis Kurniati. Special thanks are due to Nessa Nuriftifa and Alvinsyah Pramono who helped in assisting the presentation of "Anemia in Pregnancy" to the pregnant women and are also due to Depi Setiadi for logistic preparation. Professor Ida Parwati from Dept. of Clinical Pathology, Dr. Hasan Sadikin General Hospital, Bandung, is also thanked for her fruitful and collaborative study. This study was financially supported by Academic Leadership Grant (ALG) for Thalassemia Study.

References

[1] World Health Organization (WHO), "Iron deficiency anaemia assessment, prevention, and control: a guide for programme managers," World Health Organization (WHO), Geneva, Switzerland, 2001. http://www.who.int/nutrition/publications/en/ida_assessment_prevention_control.pdf.

[2] N. A. Alwan and H. Hamamy, "Maternal iron status in pregnancy and long-term health outcomes in the offspring," *Journal of Pediatric Genetics*, vol. 4, no. 2, pp. 111–123, 2015.

[3] M. Khaskheli, S. Baloch, A. S. Baloch, S. Baloch, and F. K. Khaskheli, "Iron deficiency anaemia is still a major killer of pregnant women," *Pakistan Journal of Medical Sciences*, vol. 32, no. 3, pp. 630–634, 2016.

[4] R. J. Stoltzfus and M. L. Dreyfuss, "Guidelines for the Use of Iron Supplements to Prevent and Treat Iron Deficiency Anemia," http://www.who.int/nutrition/publications/micronutrients/guidelines_for_Iron_supplementation.pdf?ua=1.

[5] E. M. McClure, S. R. Meshnick, P. Mungai et al., "The association of parasitic infections in pregnancy and maternal and fetal anemia: a cohort study in coastal Kenya," *PLoS Neglected Tropical Diseases*, vol. 8, no. 2, Article ID e2724, 2014.

[6] L. Sangaré, A. M. van Eijk, F. O. Ter Kuile, J. Walson, and A. Stergachis, "The association between malaria and iron status or supplementation in pregnancy: a systematic review and meta-analysis," *PLoS One*, vol. 9, no. 2, article e87743, 2014.

[7] S.-R. Pasricha, H. Drakesmith, J. Black, D. Hipgrave, and B.-A. Biggs, "Control of iron deficiency anemia in low- and middle-income countries," *Blood*, vol. 121, no. 14, pp. 2607–2617, 2013.

[8] R. D. Merrill, A. A. Shamim, H. Ali et al., "High prevalence of anemia with lack of iron deficiency among women in rural Bangladesh: a role for thalassemia and iron in groundwater," *Asia Pacific Journal of Clinical Nutrition*, vol. 21, no. 3, pp. 416–424, 2012.

[9] E. Jones, S.-R. Pasricha, A. Allen et al., "Hepcidin is suppressed by erythropoiesis in hemoglobin e β-thalassemia and β-thalassemia trait," *Blood*, vol. 125, no. 5, pp. 873–880, 2015.

[10] S. Piplani, R. Manan, M. Lalit, M. Manjari, T. Bhasin, and J. Bawa, "NESTROFT—a valuable, cost effective screening test for beta thalassemia traitin north indian punjabi population," *Journal of Clinical and Diagnostic Research*, vol. 7, no. 12, pp. 2784–2787, 2013.

[11] A. Vehapoglu, G. Ozgurhan, A. D. Demir et al., "Hematological indices for differential diagnosis of beta thalassemia trait and iron deficiency anemia," *Anemia*, vol. 2014, Article ID 576738, 7 pages, 2014.

[12] Z. Ou, Q. Li, W. Liu, and X. Sun, "Elevated hemoglobin A2 as a marker for β-thalassemia trait in pregnant women," *Tohoku Journal of Experimental Medicine*, vol. 223, no. 3, pp. 223–226, 2011.

[13] E. Urrechaga, "Red blood cell microcytosis and hypochromia in the differential diagnosis of iron deficiency and β-thalassaemia trait," *International Journal of Laboratory Hematology*, vol. 31, no. 5, pp. 528–534, 2009.

[14] J. S. Barkley, K. L. Kendrick, K. Codling, S. Muslimatun, and H. Pachón, "Anaemia prevalence over time in Indonesia: estimates from the 1997, 2000, and 2008 Indonesia Family Life Surveys," *Asia Pacific Journal of Clinical Nutrition*, vol. 24, no. 3, pp. 452–455, 2015.

[15] P. Bergsjø, B. Evjen-Olsen, S. G. Hinderaker, N. Oleking'ori, and K.-I. Klepp, "Validity of non-invasive assessment of anaemia in pregnancy," *Tropical Medicine and International Health*, vol. 13, no. 2, pp. 272–277, 2008.

[16] World Health Organization (WHO), "Haemoglobin concentrations for the diagnosis of anaemia and assessment of severity. Vitamin and mineral nutrition information system (WHO/NMH/NHD/MNM/11.1)," World Health Organization (WHO), Geneva, Switzerland, 2011. http://apps.who.int/iris/bitstream/10665/66914/1/WHO_NHD_01.3.pdf?ua=1.

[17] R. Kwiecien, A. Kopp-Schneider, and M. Blettner, "Concordance analysis: part 16 of a series on evaluation of scientific publications," *Deutsches Arzteblatt*, vol. 108, no. 30, pp. 515–521, 2011.

[18] A. I. Adanikin, J. O. Awoleke, B. A. Olofinbiyi, P. O. Adanikin, and O. R. Ogundare, "Routine iron supplementation and anaemia by third trimester in a nigerian hospital," *Ethiopian Journal of Health Sciences*, vol. 25, no. 4, pp. 305–312, 2015.

[19] F. M. Tabrizi and S. Barjasteh, "Maternal hemoglobin levels during pregnancy and their association with birth weight of neonates," *Iranian Journal of Pediatric Hematology and Oncology*, vol. 5, no. 4, pp. 211–217, 2015.

[20] B. Sukrat and S. Sirichotiyakul, "The prevalence and causes of anemia during pregnancy in maharaj nakorn chiang mai hospital," *Journal of the Medical Association of Thailand*, vol. 89, supplement 4, pp. S142–S146, 2006.

[21] T. D. Atmakusumah, P. A. Wahidiyat, A. S. Sofro et al., "Health Technology Assessment Indonesia," Dirjen Bina Pelayanan Medik Kementrian Kesehatan Republik Indonesia, 2009. Accessed 12 January 2017. http://www.academia.edu/9564064/Health_Technology_Assessment_Indonesia.

[22] J. J. M. L. Hoffmann, E. Urrechaga, and U. Aguirre, "Discriminant indices for distinguishing thalassemia and iron deficiency in patients with microcytic anemia: a meta-analysis," *Clinical Chemistry and Laboratory Medicine*, vol. 53, no. 12, pp. 1883–1894, 2015.

[23] M. S. Yazdani and S. Ahmed, "An 'on the spot' test for targeted screening in index families of thalassaemia," *Journal of the Pakistan Medical Association*, vol. 60, no. 7, pp. 521–523, 2010.

[24] M. Verhovsek, C.-C. So, T. O'Shea et al., "Is HbA 2 level a reliable diagnostic measurement for β-thalassemia trait in people with iron deficiency?" *American Journal of Hematology*, vol. 87, no. 1, pp. 114–116, 2012.

[25] J. Li, X.-M. Xie, C. Liao, and D.-Z. Li, "Co-inheritance of α-thalassaemia and β-thalassaemia in a prenatal screening population in mainland China," *Journal of Medical Screening*, vol. 21, no. 4, pp. 167–171, 2014.

[26] S. Bryan, E. Dormandy, T. Roberts et al., "Screening for sickle cell and thalassaemia in primary care: a cost-effectiveness study," *British Journal of General Practice*, vol. 61, no. 591, pp. e620–e627, 2011.

[27] N. A. AlHamdan, Y. Y. AlMazrou, F. M. AlSwaidi, and A. J. Choudhry, "Premarital screening for thalassemia and sickle cell disease in Saudi Arabia," *Genetics in Medicine*, vol. 9, no. 6, pp. 372–377, 2007.

[28] H. Hashemizadeh and R. Noori, "Premarital screening of beta thalassemia minor in north-east of iran," *Iranian Journal of Pediatric Hematology and Oncology*, vol. 3, no. 1, pp. 210–215, 2013.

[29] A. Amato, M. P. Cappabianca, M. Lerone et al., "Carrier screening for inherited haemoglobin disorders among secondary school students and young adults in Latium, Italy," *Journal of Community Genetics*, vol. 5, no. 3, pp. 265–268, 2014.

25

Ferric Carboxymaltose as Treatment in Women with Iron-Deficiency Anemia

Melvin H. Seid,[1] Angelia D. Butcher,[2] and Ashwin Chatwani[3]

[1]*Unified Women's Clinical Research, 1100-C South Stratford Road, Suite 310, Winston-Salem, NC 27103, USA*
[2]*Luitpold Pharmaceuticals, Inc., 800 Adams Ave, Suite 100, Norrisville, PA 19403, USA*
[3]*Department of Obstetrics and Gynecology, Temple University School of Medicine, Philadelphia, PA 19140, USA*

Correspondence should be addressed to Melvin H. Seid; melvin.seid@unifiedhc.com

Academic Editor: Duran Canatan

Objective. To evaluate safety and efficacy of intravenous ferric carboxymaltose (FCM) versus standard medical care (SMC) for iron-deficiency anemia (IDA) in postpartum women and women with heavy menstrual bleeding. *Study Design.* This open-label, multicenter study randomized women with IDA (hemoglobin ≤ 11.0 g/dL) to single doses of FCM (15 mg/kg [maximum 1000 mg]) or SMC (this treatment was determined by the investigator and there may have been no treatment). Safety data (primary outcome) were collected for 30 days. *Results.* Of 2045 subjects enrolled (FCM: $n = 1023$; SMC: $n = 1022$), 996 received FCM and 1022 received SMC. At least 1 serious adverse event (AE) was reported by 0.6% and 2.2% of subjects in the FCM and SMC groups, respectively; none were considered treatment related. The difference in serious AEs was primarily due to higher rates of uterine leiomyoma, uterine hemorrhage, and menorrhagia in SMC subjects with heavy menstrual bleeding. Common AEs were generally predictable, with higher rates of infusion site reactions in FCM subjects and gastrointestinal AEs in SMC subjects. Mean hemoglobin increases were greater in the FCM group than the SMC group. *Conclusion.* FCM was well tolerated and effectively increased mean hemoglobin levels in postpartum women or women with heavy menstrual bleeding and IDA. This trial is registered with ClinicalTrials.gov, NCT00548860.

1. Introduction

Iron deficiency is the most common cause of anemia [1, 2]. Women who are of reproductive age are particularly at risk owing to blood loss or increased iron demand attributed to menstruation, pregnancy, and lactation [3, 4]. Iron-deficiency anemia (IDA) is associated with adverse effects on cognitive function, physical activity, immune response, and pregnancy outcome. The World Health Organization defines IDA as hemoglobin < 12.0 g/dL in women who are not pregnant and <11.0 g/dL in women who are pregnant [4, 5]. Postpartum anemia reportedly affects up to 27% of women, and approximately 20% of women suffer excessive menstrual blood loss [3, 6]. IDA associated with childbirth or heavy menstrual bleeding can be potentially reversed with iron repletion therapy [7]. Iron therapy for IDA has been shown to reduce morbidity by improving physical activity and reducing fatigue and cognitive deficits [3, 4, 7].

Iron therapy can be administered orally or parenterally [3, 4, 8]. Oral iron is the treatment of choice for the majority of patients with IDA because it is safe, effective, inexpensive, and readily available. However, the tolerability of oral iron therapy can be problematic, with up to 40% of patients reporting gastrointestinal adverse events (AEs) [3, 9]. In addition, sustained response to oral iron treatment may be complicated by ongoing losses from heavy menstrual bleeding that exceed the gastrointestinal absorption of iron [8]. Parenteral iron administration is preferred for patients who cannot tolerate or are unresponsive to oral iron treatment and for patients who are unable to absorb sufficient iron in the gastrointestinal tract or for whom blood transfusions should be avoided [4, 8]. Intravenous (IV) low-molecular-weight iron dextran has been associated with an incidence of anaphylaxis or anaphylactoid reactions as high as 1.7% [10, 11]. The high incidence of these serious AEs is believed to be caused by the formation of antibodies to the dextran moiety. Newer parenteral iron products (iron sucrose and iron gluconate) do not contain the dextran moiety, and the incidence of anaphylaxis with these products is markedly lower [11, 12]. However, the physical characteristics of iron gluconate and iron sucrose limit the dose and administration rate.

Ferric carboxymaltose (FCM) is a Type I polynuclear iron (III)-hydroxide carbohydrate complex that produces a slow and controlled delivery of the complexed iron to endogenous iron binding sites [13, 14]. In randomized trials in postpartum women with anemia and women with heavy menstrual bleeding, treatment with FCM significantly improved hemoglobin levels compared with oral iron treatment [15–17]. In previous trials in women with IDA in the postpartum period or women with heavy menstrual bleeding, the total dose of FCM was individualized to restore a calculated iron deficit at baseline, with total FCM doses up to 2500 mg administered weekly over several weeks. Since the total iron requirement was found to be ≤1600 mg for approximately 90% of postpartum women or women with heavy menstrual bleeding in these studies, the data suggest that 1 to 2 doses of FCM 15 mg/kg would likely treat most of these subjects. Therefore, the objective of the current large, randomized clinical trial was to evaluate the safety and efficacy of a more convenient, single 15 mg/kg dose (maximum 1000 mg) of FCM compared with standard medical care (SMC) for treatment of IDA in women with IDA in the postpartum period or women with heavy menstrual bleeding.

2. Material and Methods

2.1. Study Design. An open-label, randomized study was conducted at 130 sites and consisted of a screening visit and 2 study visits at day 0 and day 30. Each site received institutional review board approval before initiation of the study, and informed consent was obtained from each subject prior to participation. This study was conducted in compliance with Good Clinical Practice guidelines and the Declaration of Helsinki.

2.2. Subjects. Women with IDA in the postpartum period were eligible to participate if they had hemoglobin levels ≤ 11.0 g/dL obtained at least 18 hours after delivery. Women with heavy menstrual bleeding were eligible if they had hemoglobin levels ≤ 11.0 g/dL or point-of-care hemoglobin levels ≤ 11.5 g/dL. Heavy menstrual bleeding was defined as ≥1 of the following within the preceding 6 months: (a) inability to control flow with tampons alone, (b) use of >12 pads per period or 4 tampons per day unless subject was unusually fastidious, (c) passage of clots, or (d) period duration >7 days.

Exclusion criteria included recent (≤3 months) gastrointestinal bleeding or significant acute blood loss (other than at delivery); a history of anemia other than IDA due to pregnancy/delivery or heavy menstrual bleeding; current treatment with myelosuppressive therapy or asthma therapy; and recent administration (≤1 month) of blood transfusion, IV iron, erythropoietin, or investigational drug. Women who were pregnant or had a history of hypersensitivity to FCM or were planning surgery or had an active infection including hepatitis B or C, known human immunodeficiency virus

seropositivity, a history of malignancy, hemochromatosis, significant cardiovascular disease, elevated liver enzymes, alcohol abuse, or drug abuse were also excluded from study participation. Subjects were also excluded from participation on day 0 if they had point-of-care hemoglobin levels > 12.0 g/dL or a systolic blood pressure > 160 or <80 mm Hg or a diastolic blood pressure > 100 or <40 mm Hg prior to randomization.

2.3. Treatment. Subjects were randomized in a 1 : 1 ratio using a central interactive voice response system to receive either IV FCM or SMC (treatment in the SMC group was determined by the investigator for individual patients and there may have been no treatment). Randomization was stratified by etiology of IDA (postpartum or heavy menstrual bleeding); baseline hemoglobin levels ≤ 8.0, 8.1 to 9.5, or >9.5 g/dL; cardiac risk category (low or high); and past response to oral iron (poor or not poor). Subjects with 1 or no cardiac risk factors were designated as having low cardiac risk. Subjects with 2 or more cardiac risk factors, including smoking, high blood pressure, high blood cholesterol, diabetes, overweight or obesity, physical inactivity, and family history of heart disease (father/brother before age 55 years or mother/sister before age 65 years), were designated as having high cardiac risk.

Subjects in the FCM group received FCM 15 mg/kg (up to a maximum of 1000 mg) in a slow IV infusion over 15 minutes on day 0. Prepregnancy weight was used to determine the FCM dose for postpartum subjects. Sitting pulse and blood pressure were monitored before, immediately after, and at 30 and 60 minutes after administration of IV iron.

Subjects in the SMC group were treated for IDA as determined by the investigator from day 0 through day 30. Ferrous sulfate 325 mg tablets (65 mg of elemental iron) were provided to the subject as study medication if the investigator determined it to be the best method of treatment. All subjects randomized to receive SMC were considered to have started treatment, as no treatment was an option.

2.4. Study Assessments. Safety was assessed by measurement of vital signs and findings on physical examination in addition to hematology, chemistry, and iron indices determined from blood samples obtained at day 0 and day 30. Treatment-emergent AEs were recorded from administration of study drug for FCM-treated subjects and after randomization for SMC subjects through completion of the study (day 30) or 30 days after last dose of study drug, whichever was later. When subjects returned to the clinic on day 30, AEs were elicited by use of nonspecific questions. Subjects were encouraged to report AEs at their onset, and all AEs, whether elicited, reported spontaneously, or observed by the physician or study staff, were recorded with date of onset, relationship to study medication based on investigator opinion, action taken, and date of resolution if the AE resolved. Allergic reactions were classified according to the National Cancer Institute Common Terminology Criteria for Adverse Events version 3.0, including grading of all events to quantify severity. Follow-up telephone calls to collect AEs were made 30 days after the last dose of study drug to all FCM-treated subjects

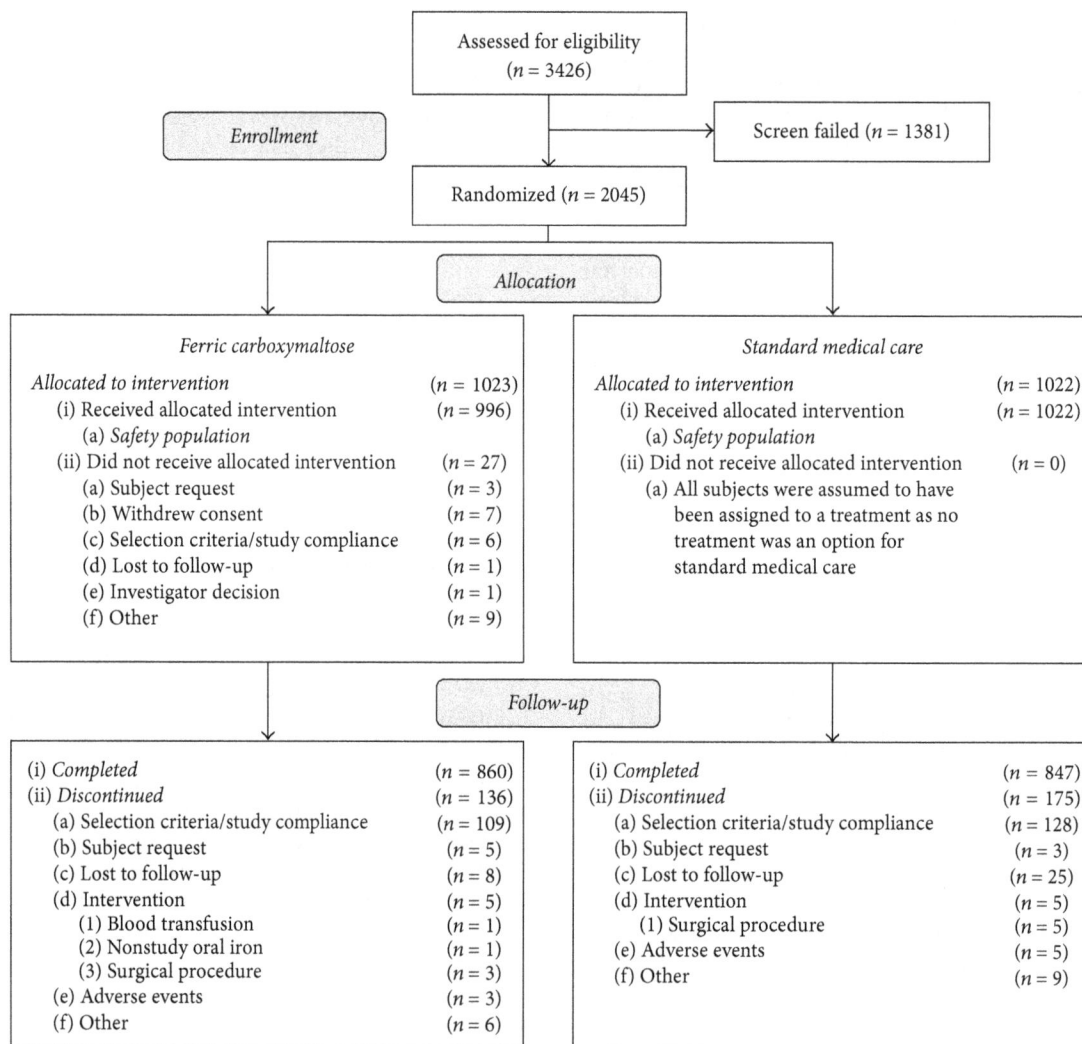

Figure 1

who terminated early and 30 days after last dose of study drug to all SMC subjects.

2.5. Study Endpoints and Analyses. The primary goal of this study was to assess safety. The safety population included all FCM-treated subjects who received a dose of FCM on day 0 and all randomized SMC subjects. A sample size of 750 subjects per group provided approximately 80% power to detect a statistically significant difference in the incidence of serious AEs, when the incidence was 5.25% for FCM and 2.5% for SMC. The primary endpoint was the incidence of serious AEs, including death, hospitalization, disability, congenital anomaly/birth defect, and life-threatening events. Other safety endpoints included incidence and severity of AEs and treatment-emergent abnormal clinical laboratory values. Quantitative endpoints were summarized descriptively using mean, standard deviation, median, and range, and investigators judged the clinical significance of laboratory abnormalities. Differences between treatment groups were assessed using Fisher's exact test. All tests were 2-tailed with 0.05 alpha level. Efficacy was assessed as the mean

change from baseline to highest postrandomization value for hemoglobin and ferritin levels, which were compared by cause of anemia across treatment groups and use of 1-way analysis of variance.

3. Results

3.1. Study Participants. A total of 2045 women were randomized to receive FCM ($n = 1023$) or SMC ($n = 1022$) (Figure 1). In the FCM group, 27 subjects discontinued the study before dosing and were excluded from the analysis. Reasons for discontinuation are summarized in Figure 1. No subjects randomized to receive SMC were excluded from the analysis. Thus, the safety population included 996 subjects in the FCM group and 1022 subjects in the SMC group. More than 80% of subjects in both treatment groups completed the study through day 30, including 860 (84.1%) in the FCM group and 847 (82.9%) in the SMC group. Reasons for discontinuation were similar between treatment groups (Figure 1). No notable differences were observed between the treatment groups for any demographic and baseline

TABLE 1: Demographic and baseline characteristics (safety population).

	FCM (n = 996)	SMC (n = 1022)
Demographic characteristics		
Mean (SD) age, years	31.2 (9.36)	31.4 (8.98)
Race, n (%)		
White	457 (45.9)	477 (46.7)
African American	391 (39.3)	387 (37.9)
Hispanic	122 (12.2)	135 (13.2)
Asian	5 (0.5)	8 (0.8)
Other	21 (2.1)	15 (1.5)
Mean (SD) height, cm[a]	163.4 (6.93)	163.1 (7.07)
Mean (SD) weight, kg[b]	82.0 (21.71)	82.8 (21.64)
Mean (SD) prepregnancy weight, kg[c]	72.4 (19.96)	73.3 (19.85)
Baseline characteristics		
Etiology of anemia, n (%)		
Postpartum	606 (60.8)	623 (61.0)
Heavy menstrual bleeding	390 (39.2)	399 (39.0)
Cardiac risk factor, n (%)[d]		
Low	709 (71.2)	723 (70.7)
High	287 (28.8)	299 (29.3)
Poor response to oral iron, n (%)[e]		
Yes	236 (43.1)	252 (44.4)
No	312 (56.9)	316 (55.6)
Mean (SD) hemoglobin, g/dL[f]	9.9 (1.32)	9.8 (1.29)

FCM = ferric carboxymaltose; SD = standard deviation; SMC = standard medical care.
[a] n = 996 for ferric carboxymaltose and n = 1019 for standard medical care.
[b] n = 992 for ferric carboxymaltose and n = 1013 for standard medical care.
[c] Prepregnancy weight for postpartum subjects only; n = 609 for ferric carboxymaltose and n = 625 for standard medical care.
[d] If a subject had ≤1 cardiac risk factor (specifically, smoking, high blood pressure, high blood cholesterol, diabetes, overweight or obese, physical inactivity, or family history of heart disease), the subject was categorized as low cardiac risk; if the subject had ≥2 risk factors, they were categorized as high cardiac risk.
[e] n = 548 for ferric carboxymaltose and n = 568 for standard medical care.
[f] n = 994 for ferric carboxymaltose and n = 1019 for standard medical care.

characteristic (Table 1). The cause of IDA was blood loss during delivery and/or antepartum IDA in approximately 60% of subjects and heavy menstrual bleeding in 40% of subjects. The majority of subjects did not receive prior iron treatment (FCM: 74.7%; SMC: 72.3%).

The mean dose of FCM during the study was 944 mg for all subjects, 926 mg for postpartum subjects, and 970 mg for subjects with heavy menstrual bleeding. Two subjects received an incorrect dose of FCM owing to the use of an incorrect body weight for weight-based dosing; in both cases, the incorrect dose was ≤1000 mg of FCM. Oral iron therapy (typically ferrous sulfate) was initially prescribed for 93% of subjects randomized to SMC; no treatment was received by 2.4% of SMC subjects. The SMC subjects who received oral ferrous sulfate as study medication had a mean compliance rate of 95.2%. Based on the number of pills taken versus the number of pills prescribed, similar prescribing and compliance rates in the SMC subjects were observed between the postpartum and heavy menstrual bleeding populations.

3.2. Safety. The incidence of serious AEs was statistically significantly higher among subjects in the SMC group (22/1022 [2.2%]) than among those in the FCM group (6/996 [0.6%]; $P = 0.004$). The investigators did not consider any serious AE in either treatment group to be related to study medication. In the FCM group, the incidence of serious AEs was similar for postpartum subjects and subjects with heavy menstrual bleeding (0.7% and 0.5%, resp.; $P > 0.9999$). In the SMC group, subjects with heavy menstrual bleeding had a higher incidence of serious AEs than postpartum subjects (4.3% and 0.8%, resp.; $P = 0.0003$). The increased incidence of serious AEs in the subjects with heavy menstrual bleeding receiving SMC was primarily due to higher rates of uterine leiomyoma, uterine hemorrhage, and menorrhagia.

Seven (0.7%) subjects in the FCM group and 22 (2.2%) subjects in the SMC group discontinued study drug early owing to the occurrence of AEs (Table 2). The proportion of subjects who discontinued study drug owing to AEs was similar between those with postpartum anemia and those with heavy menstrual bleeding in each treatment group.

TABLE 2: Adverse events leading to premature discontinuation of study drug by treatment group.

FCM ($n = 996$)		SMC ($n = 1022$)	
System organ class		*System organ class*	
Adverse event	n^a (%)	Adverse event	n^b (%)
General disorders and administration site conditions		*Gastrointestinal disorders*	
Injection site extravasation	5 (0.5)	Constipation	6 (0.6)
Injection site bruising	2 (0.2)	Nausea	6 (0.6)
Immune system disorders		Abdominal pain	5 (0.5)
Hypersensitivity	1 (0.1)	Vomiting	2 (0.2)
		Abdominal discomfort	1 (0.1)
		Small intestinal obstruction	1 (0.1)
		Abdominal hernia	1 (0.1)
		Abdominal adhesions	1 (0.1)
		Reproductive system and breast disorders	
		Uterine hemorrhage	2 (0.2)
		Menorrhagia	1 (0.1)
		Postpartum hemorrhage	1 (0.1)
		Vulvovaginal pruritus	1 (0.1)
		Drug exposure via breast milk	1 (0.1)

FCM = ferric carboxymaltose; SMC = standard medical care.
[a]One subject had multiple adverse events leading to premature discontinuation of study drug.
[b]Six subjects had multiple adverse events leading to premature discontinuation of study drug.

At least 1 AE was experienced by 27.3% (272/996) of subjects in the FCM group and 26.9% (275/1022) of subjects in the SMC group ($P = 0.841$). The incidence of injection site reactions (i.e., extravasation, pain, bruising, irritation, paresthesia, and coldness) was higher in the FCM group, and the incidence of gastrointestinal AEs (i.e., constipation, diarrhea, nausea, and vomiting) was higher in the SMC group (Table 3). Subjects in the FCM group had a significantly higher incidence of hypophosphatemia, dysgeusia, increased alanine aminotransferase, and immune system disorders (hypersensitivity, $n = 4$; latex allergy, $n = 1$) than subjects in the SMC group.

AEs are summarized separately in Table 4 for postpartum subjects and those with heavy menstrual bleeding within each treatment group. A larger percentage of subjects with heavy menstrual bleeding compared with postpartum subjects reported ≥1 AE in the FCM group (33.1 and 23.6%, resp.; $P = 0.0013$) and in the SMC group (31.3% and 24.1%, resp.; $P = 0.0115$). In both treatment groups, postpartum subjects and those with heavy menstrual bleeding had statistically significantly different rates of gastrointestinal events (FCM: $P = 0.0072$; SMC: $P = 0.0013$) and general disorders and administration site conditions (FCM: $P = 0.0285$; SMC: $P = 0.0002$).

Four subjects (0.4%) in the FCM group (2 postpartum and 2 heavy menstrual bleeding) and no subjects in the SMC group experienced hypersensitivity reactions during the study. All hypersensitivity events were Grade 1 in severity. Two subjects in the FCM group (1 postpartum and 1 heavy menstrual bleeding) were reported to have hypotension during the study; both AEs were Grade 1 in severity, and neither subject had a history of hypotension.

A significantly greater proportion of subjects in the FCM group than in the SMC group had a transient decrease in serum phosphorus (9.0% versus 0%; $P < 0.001$). The difference was more pronounced in subjects with heavy menstrual bleeding; 21.3% of subjects with heavy menstrual bleeding in the FCM group had a transient decrease in serum phosphorus compared with only 0.7% of subjects with postpartum anemia. These changes were not associated with clinical symptoms. No other treatment-emergent abnormal clinical chemistry values were observed.

3.3. Efficacy. Subjects treated with FCM and SMC experienced improvements in hemoglobin from baseline to the highest value during treatment, and subjects treated with FCM with either postpartum anemia or heavy menstrual bleeding experienced significantly greater mean increases in hemoglobin and ferritin levels from baseline to highest value compared with subjects treated with SMC (Figure 2 and Table 5). Mean hemoglobin levels at baseline were higher in postpartum subjects than in subjects with heavy menstrual bleeding (FCM: 10.2 versus 9.3 g/dL, $P < 0.001$; SMC: 10.1 versus 9.4 g/dL, $P < 0.001$). In the FCM group, the mean increase in hemoglobin from baseline to highest value was similar between subjects with postpartum anemia and those with heavy menstrual bleeding (2.35 versus 2.33 g/dL; $P = 0.808$). In the SMC group, the mean increase in hemoglobin was greater in postpartum subjects than in subjects with heavy menstrual bleeding (1.86 versus 1.47 g/dL; $P < 0.001$).

In both treatment groups, mean ferritin levels at baseline were higher in postpartum subjects than in subjects with heavy menstrual bleeding (FCM: 25.99 versus 8.89 ng/mL, $P < 0.001$; SMC: 26.55 versus 7.95 ng/mL, $P < 0.001$). In the FCM group, the mean increase in ferritin from baseline

TABLE 3: Treatment-emergent adverse events occurring in ≥2% of subjects either in treatment group or with a statistically significant[a] difference between the FCM and SCM treatment groups (safety population).

System organ class[b] Preferred term	FCM (n = 996) n (%)	SMC (n = 1022) n (%)
≥1 treatment-emergent AE	272 (27.3%)	275 (26.9)[c]
Gastrointestinal disorders	34 (3.4)	137 (13.4)
Constipation	9 (0.9)	79 (7.7)
Diarrhea	9 (0.9)	20 (2.0)[c]
Nausea	8 (0.8)	35 (3.4)
Vomiting	2 (0.2)	13 (1.3)
General disorders and administration site conditions	87 (8.7)	12 (1.2)
Injection site extravasation	24 (2.4)	0
Injection site pain	12 (1.2)	1 (0.1)
Injection site bruising	11 (1.1)	0
Injection site irritation	8 (0.8)	0
Injection site paresthesia	6 (0.6)	0
Injection site coldness	5 (0.5)	0
Immune system disorders	5 (0.5)	0
Investigations	25 (2.5)	11 (1.1)
ALT increased	18 (1.8)	6 (0.6)
Metabolism and nutrition disorders	8 (0.8)	1 (0.1)
Hypophosphatemia	6 (0.6)	0
Nervous system disorders	49 (4.9)	21 (2.1)
Headache	25 (2.5)	15 (1.5)[c]
Dysgeusia	7 (0.7)	0

AE = adverse event; ALT = alanine aminotransferase; FCM = ferric carboxymaltose; SMC = standard medical care.
[a] All comparisons between the FCM and SMC groups are statistically significant ($P \leq 0.05$) unless otherwise noted.
[b] Each subject is counted only once per system organ class.
[c] Not statistically significant from the FCM group.

to highest value was larger in subjects with postpartum anemia than in subjects with heavy menstrual bleeding (155.03 versus 92.69 ng/mL; $P < 0.001$). In the SMC group, a mean decrease was observed in the subjects with postpartum anemia compared with a mean increase observed in subjects with heavy menstrual bleeding (−2.32 versus 13.28 ng/mL; $P < 0.001$).

4. Discussion

Similar to 4 previous randomized, controlled trials of FCM [15–18], this large, open-label, randomized study supports that a single 15 mg/kg dose of IV FCM was safe and well tolerated for the treatment of subjects with IDA in the postpartum period and subjects with IDA caused by heavy menstrual bleeding. The current study evaluated the safety and efficacy of a more convenient, single 15 mg/kg dose (maximum 1000 mg) of FCM. Overall, the incidence of serious AEs was low in the present study. Differences in rates of common AEs between treatment groups were generally predictable, with a higher incidence of infusion site reactions (i.e., extravasation, pain, bruising, irritation, paresthesia, and coldness) in the FCM group and a higher

incidence of gastrointestinal AEs (i.e., constipation, diarrhea, nausea, and vomiting) in the SMC group. Subjects in the SMC group experienced more serious AEs than subjects in the FCM group; however, none of the reported serious AEs were considered related to study medication. Subjects with heavy menstrual bleeding who received SMC had an increased incidence of AEs primarily owing to higher rates of uterine leiomyoma, uterine hemorrhage, and menorrhagia in this subject subset. Comparison between the safety and efficacy of subjects with postpartum IDA and those with heavy menstrual bleeding was possible due to the fact that treatment randomization was stratified by etiology of anemia. Among postpartum women, the most common AEs were increased transaminase levels and injection site extravasation in the FCM group and constipation and nausea in the SMC group. Women with heavy menstrual bleeding experienced similar common adverse events, with headache, injection site extravasation, injection site pain, and dizziness in the FCM group and constipation, nausea, diarrhea, and vomiting in the SMC group.

Four subjects in the FCM group experienced Grade 1 hypersensitivity reactions, and no subject experienced

TABLE 4: Treatment-emergent adverse events occurring in ≥2% of subjects in either treatment group or with a statistically significant difference[a] between the FCM or SMC treatment groups by anemia etiology (safety population).

System organ class[b] Preferred term	FCM		SMC	
	Postpartum ($n = 606$) n (%)	HMB ($n = 390$) n (%)	Postpartum ($n = 623$) n (%)	HMB ($n = 399$) n (%)
≥1 treatment-emergent AE	*143 (23.6)*	*129 (33.1)*	*150 (24.1)[c]*	*125 (31.3)[c]*
Gastrointestinal disorders	13 (2.1)	21 (5.4)	66 (10.6)	71 (17.8)
Constipation	5 (0.8)	4 (1.0)	37 (5.9)	42 (10.5)
Diarrhea	3 (0.5)	6 (1.5)	8 (1.3)	12 (3.0)[c]
Nausea	1 (0.2)	7 (1.8)	15 (2.4)	20 (5.0)
Vomiting	1 (0.2)	1 (0.3)	5 (0.8)	8 (2.0)
General disorders and administration site conditions	43 (7.1)	44 (11.3)	1 (0.2)	11 (2.8)
Injection site extravasation	12 (2.0)	12 (3.1)	0	0
Injection site pain	4 (0.7)	8 (2.1)	0	1 (0.3)
Injection site bruising	5 (0.8)	6 (1.5)	0	0
Injection site irritation	5 (0.8)	3 (0.8)	0	0
Injection site paresthesia	1 (0.2)	5 (1.3)	0	0
Injection site coldness	3 (0.5)	2 (0.5)	0	0
Immune system disorders	3 (0.5)	2 (0.5)	0	0
Investigations	20 (3.3)	5 (1.3)	10 (1.6)[c]	1 (0.3)
ALT increased	17 (2.8)	1 (0.3)	6 (1.0)	0
AST increased	14 (2.3)	0	8 (1.3)[c]	0
Metabolism and nutrition disorders	1 (0.2)	7 (1.8)	1 (0.2)	0
Hypophosphatemia	0	6 (1.5)	0	0
Nervous system disorders	21 (3.5)	28 (7.2)	12 (1.9)[c]	9 (2.3)
Dizziness	0	9 (2.3)	0	3 (0.8)[c]
Headache	12 (2.0)	13 (3.3)	9 (1.4)[c]	6 (1.5)[c]
Dysgeusia	4 (0.7)	3 (0.8)	0	0

AE = adverse event; ALT = alanine aminotransferase; AST = aspartate aminotransferase; FCM = ferric carboxymaltose; HMB = heavy menstrual bleeding; SMC = standard medical care.
[a] All comparisons between the FCM and SMC groups are statistically significant ($P \leq 0.05$) unless otherwise noted.
[b] Each subject is counted only once per system organ class.
[c] Not statistically significant from the FCM group.

TABLE 5: Mean hemoglobin and ferritin levels at baseline and at the highest level after randomization (safety population).

	FCM		SMC	
	Postpartum ($n = 606$)	HMB ($n = 390$)	Postpartum ($n = 623$)	HMB ($n = 399$)
Hemoglobin, mean (SD), g/dL				
Baseline	10.20 (1.161)	9.34 (1.387)	10.11 (1.191)	9.40 (1.310)
Highest postrandomization result	12.53 (0.899)	11.68 (1.090)	11.97 (1.153)[a]	10.89 (1.246)[a]
Mean ferritin (SD), ng/mL				
Baseline	25.99 (22.730)	8.89 (15.529)	26.55 (24.973)	7.95 (15.072)
Highest postrandomization result	180.97 (96.798)	101.62 (89.312)	24.23 (16.743)[a]	20.94 (53.122)[a]

FCM = ferric carboxymaltose; HMB = heavy menstrual bleeding; SD = standard deviation; SMC = standard medical care.
[a] $P < 0.001$ for between-group comparison.

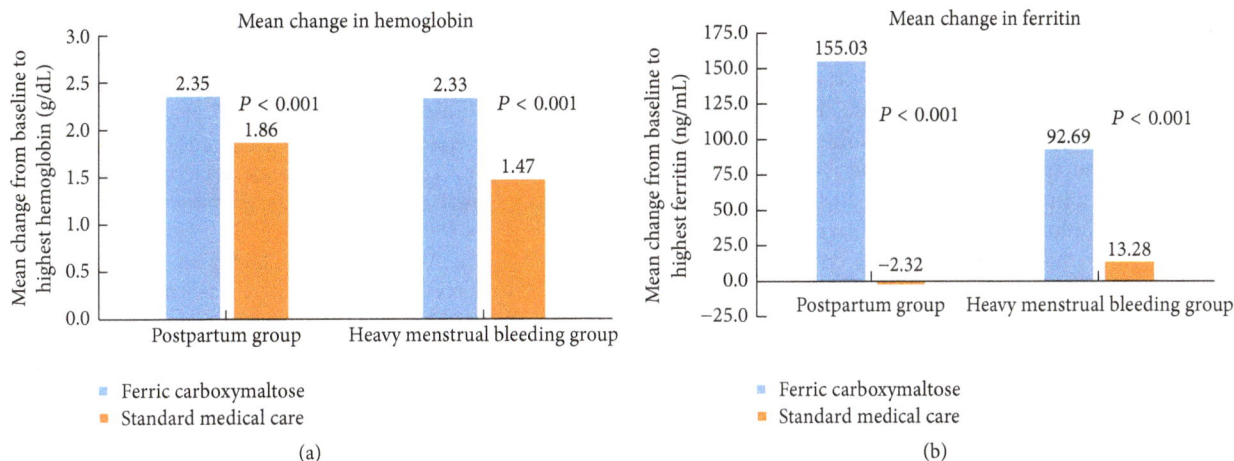

Figure 2

anaphylaxis or an anaphylactoid reaction. Based on previous studies conducted on low-molecular-weight iron dextran the rate of anaphylaxis or anaphylactoid reactions was reported to be 1.7% [10, 11]. While the present study is not an iron dextran investigation, if we use this rate of anaphylaxis or anaphylactoid reactions as a guide, the probability of observing ≥1 reaction among 1023 subjects was >99.9%.

Barish and colleagues published findings of a single dose ($n = 735$) and multidose ($n = 703$) safety trial of FCM versus SMC (including approved oral or IV iron preparations) for the treatment of IDA associated with a variety of medical conditions including gastrointestinal disorders, chronic kidney disease, heavy menstrual bleeding, and postpartum-related anemia [19]. The maximum single dose of FCM was 750 mg compared with 1000 mg used in the current study. FCM was well tolerated, and there were no clinically important differences in safety outcomes between the 2 groups. Supporting the results of the current study, the incidence of AEs was similar between the FCM and SMC treatment groups in the Barish et al. study, with more gastrointestinal AEs reported in the SMC group.

We observed a higher incidence of hypophosphatemia in the FCM group compared with the SMC group. The majority of hypophosphatemia events occurred in women with heavy menstrual bleeding who received FCM. Transient decreases in serum phosphorus have been reported in other studies of FCM [15–17, 20]. In a study evaluating the efficacy of FCM for women with heavy menstrual bleeding, 70% of subjects receiving FCM experienced a transient decrease in serum phosphorus [16]. The authors hypothesized that the transient decrease is due to an observed increase in the full length (uncleaved) form of fibroblast growth factor 23, an osteocyte-derived hormone that regulates phosphate and vitamin D homeostasis [20, 21]. The effects of FCM on serum phosphorus are transient and appear to be unassociated with other clinically significant events.

Similar to the previously reported trials, efficacy outcomes in the current trial demonstrated that FCM was superior to SMC in improving hemoglobin and correcting IDA [15–17]. Treatment differences were smaller than those

reported for previously published trials in postpartum subjects and subjects with heavy menstrual bleeding [16, 17]. This is likely explained by the higher baseline hemoglobin values for postpartum subjects in this trial, as specified by the inclusion criteria. Furthermore, the total dose of FCM was generally higher in the prior studies, as the FCM dose was individualized by using the Ganzoni method to calculate the total amount of iron needed for repletion, which was typically administered in up to 3 infusions [15–17]. In this study, all subjects randomized to receive FCM were given a single dose of 15 mg/kg, not to exceed 1000 mg. FCM was also superior in replenishing tissue stores of iron as measured by ferritin levels compared with SMC. The results of this trial are consistent with others demonstrating that oral iron does not restore tissue iron stores in this population [15–18]. The mean decrease in ferritin for women with heavy menstrual bleeding in the SMC group is consistent with an inability of oral iron to replenish tissue stores of iron. The finding suggests that oral intake of iron may be insufficient for many women with heavy menstrual bleeding to replace the rapid loss of iron from menstruation.

The safety and efficacy of FCM compared with currently available IV iron could not be assessed in this trial because more than 90% of subjects in the SMC group received oral iron. In a noninferiority study in 2584 subjects, FCM was found to be noninferior to IV iron sucrose in subjects with non-dialysis-dependent chronic kidney disease [22]. In another study of subjects with a broad range of IDA etiologies, 503 subjects were randomly assigned to receive FCM versus standard of care IV iron [22]. FCM was superior to the IV iron standard of care in increasing hemoglobin levels. FCM was given as 2 injections of 750 mg separated by 1 week in both of these trials.

In conclusion, this study demonstrated that a single dose of FCM up to 1000 mg, given by IV infusion, is safe and effective in the treatment of IDA in postpartum women and women with heavy menstrual bleeding. FCM improves hemoglobin levels and replenishes iron stores more effectively than oral iron.

Conflicts of Interest

Melvin H. Seid has received clinical trial support from Luitpold Pharmaceuticals, Inc., AMAG Pharmaceuticals, Actavis (now Allergan), and Pharmacosmos. Melvin H. Seid has served on the speaker's bureau for American Regent, a subsidiary of Luitpold Pharmaceuticals, Inc. Angelia D. Butcher is an employee of Luitpold Pharmaceuticals, Inc. Ashwin Chatwani has received clinical trial support from Luitpold Pharmaceuticals, Inc.

Acknowledgments

This study was supported by research grants from Luitpold Pharmaceuticals, Inc., which was responsible for the study design and analysis and interpretation of the data. Luitpold Pharmaceuticals provided full access to the study data to the authors and this remains ongoing. Editorial support was provided by WebbWrites, LLC, Durham, NC, and Peloton Advantage, LLC, Parsippany, NJ, and was funded by Luitpold Pharmaceuticals, Inc.

References

[1] C. Brugnara, "Iron deficiency and erythropoiesis: new diagnostic approaches," *Clinical Chemistry*, vol. 49, no. 10, pp. 1573–1578, 2003.

[2] N. J. Kassebaum, R. Jasrasaria, M. Naghavi et al., "A systematic analysis of global anemia burden from 1990 to 2010," *Blood*, vol. 123, no. 5, pp. 615–624, 2014.

[3] A. J. Friedman, Z. Chen, P. Ford et al., "Iron deficiency anemia in women across the life span," *Journal of Women's Health*, vol. 21, no. 12, pp. 1282–1289, 2012.

[4] K. Jimenez, S. Kulnigg-Dabsch, and C. Gasche, "Management of iron deficiency anemia," *Gastroenterology and Hepatology*, vol. 11, no. 4, pp. 241–250, 2015.

[5] World Health Organization, *Assessing the Iron Status of Populations*, WHO, Geneva, Switzerland, 2007.

[6] L. M. Bodnar, K. S. Scanlon, D. S. Freedman, A. M. Siega-Riz, and M. E. Cogswell, "High prevalence of postpartum anemia among low-income women in the United States," *American Journal of Obstetrics and Gynecology*, vol. 185, no. 2, pp. 438–443, 2001.

[7] V. Markova, A. Norgaard, K. J. Jorgensen, and J. Langhoff-Roos, "Treatment for women with postpartum iron deficiency anaemia," *Cochrane Database of Systemic Reviews*, vol. 8, Article ID CD010861, 2015.

[8] M. Auerbach and J. W. Adamson, "How we diagnose and treat iron deficiency anemia," *American Journal of Hematology*, vol. 91, no. 1, pp. 31–38, 2016.

[9] Z. Tolkien, L. Stecher, A. P. Mander, D. I. A. Pereira, and J. J. Powell, "Ferrous sulfate supplementation causes significant gastrointestinal side-effects in adults: a systematic review and meta-analysis," *PLoS ONE*, vol. 10, no. 2, Article ID e0117383, 2015.

[10] S. Fishbane, V.-D. Ungureanu, J. K. Maesaka, C. J. Kaupke, V. Lim, and J. Wish, "The safety of intravenous iron dextran in hemodialysis patients," *American Journal of Kidney Diseases*, vol. 28, no. 4, pp. 529–534, 1996.

[11] S. Fishbane, "Safety in iron management," *American Journal of Kidney Diseases*, vol. 41, supplement 5, pp. S18–S26, 2003.

[12] G. M. Chertow, P. D. Mason, O. Vaage-Nilsen, and J. Ahlmén, "Update on adverse drug events associated with parenteral iron," *Nephrology Dialysis Transplantation*, vol. 21, no. 2, pp. 378–382, 2006.

[13] K. A. Lyseng-Williamson and G. M. Keating, "Ferric carboxymaltose: a review of its use in iron-deficiency anaemia," *Drugs*, vol. 69, no. 6, pp. 739–756, 2009.

[14] J. E. Toblli and M. Angerosa, "Optimizing iron delivery in the management of anemia: patient considerations and the role of ferric carboxymaltose," *Drug Design, Development and Therapy*, vol. 8, pp. 2475–2491, 2014.

[15] D. B. Van Wyck, M. G. Martens, M. H. Seid, J. B. Baker, and A. Mangione, "Intravenous ferric carboxymaltose compared with oral iron in the treatment of postpartum anemia: a randomized controlled trial," *Obstetrics and Gynecology*, vol. 110, no. 2, part 1, pp. 267–278, 2007.

[16] D. B. Van Wyck, A. Mangione, J. Morrison, P. E. Hadley, J. A. Jehle, and L. T. Goodnough, "Large-dose intravenous ferric carboxymaltose injection for iron deficiency anemia in heavy uterine bleeding: a randomized, controlled trial," *Transfusion*, vol. 49, no. 12, pp. 2719–2728, 2009.

[17] M. H. Seid, R. J. Derman, J. B. Baker, W. Banach, C. Goldberg, and R. Rogers, "Ferric carboxymaltose injection in the treatment of postpartum iron deficiency anemia: a randomized controlled clinical trial," *American Journal of Obstetrics and Gynecology*, vol. 199, no. 4, pp. 435.e1–435.e7, 2008.

[18] C. Breymann, F. Gliga, C. Bejenariu, and N. Strizhova, "Comparative efficacy and safety of intravenous ferric carboxymaltose in the treatment of postpartum iron deficiency anemia," *International Journal of Gynecology and Obstetrics*, vol. 101, no. 1, pp. 67–73, 2008.

[19] C. F. Barish, T. Koch, A. Butcher, D. Morris, and D. B. Bregman, "Safety and efficacy of intravenous ferric carboxymaltose (750 mg) in the treatment of iron deficiency anemia: two randomized, controlled trials," *Anemia*, vol. 2012, Article ID 172104, 9 pages, 2012.

[20] M. Wolf, T. A. Koch, and D. B. Bregman, "Effects of iron deficiency anemia and its treatment on fibroblast growth factor 23 and phosphate homeostasis in women," *Journal of Bone and Mineral Research*, vol. 28, no. 8, pp. 1793–1803, 2013.

[21] H. Jüppner, M. Wolf, and I. B. Salusky, "FGF-23: more than a regulator of renal phosphate handling?" *Journal of Bone and Mineral Research*, vol. 25, no. 10, pp. 2091–2097, 2010.

[22] J. E. Onken, D. B. Bregman, R. A. Harrington et al., "A multicenter, randomized, active-controlled study to investigate the efficacy and safety of intravenous ferric carboxymaltose in patients with iron deficiency anemia," *Transfusion*, vol. 54, no. 2, pp. 306–315, 2014.

26

Prevalence of Iron Deficiency Anemia among University Students in Hodeida Province, Yemen

Abdullah Ahmed Al-alimi ⓘ, **Salem Bashanfer** ⓘ, **and Mohammed Abdo Morish**

Department of Medical Laboratory, Faculty of Medicine and Health Sciences, Hodeida University, Al Hudaydah, Yemen

Correspondence should be addressed to Salem Bashanfer; salembashanfer@yahoo.com

Academic Editor: Duran Canatan

Background. Iron deficiency anemia (IDA) is one of the most common types of nutritional anemia in the worldwide and considered a major public health problem in developing countries especially in Yemen. Therefore, this cross-sectional study was conducted to determine the prevalence and risk factors of IDA among apparently healthy Yemeni students at Hodeida University. *Method.* Five hundred blood samples (326 males and 174 females) were collected randomly from medical students at Hodeida University. Participants were subjected to different tests including complete blood counts (CBC), serum ferritin (SF), serum iron (SI), and total iron binding capacity (TIBC). Moreover, a questionnaire was designed to collect demographics, food and drink habits, and socioeconomic status. *Result.* The overall prevalence of IDA was 30.4% ($n = 152$), of whom 54.00% were females ($n = 82$) and 46.0% were males ($n = 70$). Students aged 20–22 years were found more anemic with prevalence 59.2% than students aged 17–19 years (25.0%) and 23–25 years (15.8%). Statistical analysis showed regularly having breakfast had significant ($p < 0.001$) role in preventing development of IDA compared with irregularly having breakfast. Infrequent consumption of vegetables/fruits; meat, fish, chicken; tea drinking; low household income; smoking and khat *(Catha edulis)* chewing showed a significant role ($p < 0.001$) in provoking of IDA, whereas consumption of coffee and cola showed insignificant influence ($p = 0.585$; $p = 0.513$) on IDA. *Conclusion.* This study revealed that the majority of university students, especially females, have IDA that might become worse by malnutrition, lifestyle habits, and lack of awareness. Our results suggest that IDA can be prevented by providing proper knowledge on the healthful diet, improved lifestyle, and harmful effect of IDA to the students.

1. Introduction

Anemia is a major public health problem in the worldwide with prevalence of 43% in developing countries and 9% in developed nations [1]. It is widespread in individuals at any stage of life, although pregnant-reproductive women and young children are most susceptible, which may increase the risk of impaired cognitive and physical development and increased mortality and morbidity rate [2].

Despite its multifactorial etiology, anemia might be nutritional (iron, folic acid, and vitamin B12), inherited (thalassemia and sickle cell), environmental pollutants (lead), infectious (malaria), socioeconomic (low maternal level of education and low household income), demographic factors (age and gender), autoimmune (hemolytic anemia), malabsorption (achlorhydria), and chronic (cancer); iron

deficiency anemia IDA is the most common cause of anemia [3]. According to WHO report in 2001, around two billion individuals in the worldwide have been estimated to suffer from anemia with 50% of all anemia was documented to IDA [4].

Until today, IDA is still the most prevalent and common type of micronutrient deficiency in the developing countries [5], which results from long-term negative iron imbalance. Usually, deficiency of iron develops gradually and does not have clinically apparent symptoms until anemia becomes severe [6].

The etiology of IDA during puberty might be due to increased iron demand/loss or decreased iron intake, chronic blood loss, iron malabsorption (celiac disease), pregnancy, or parasitic infection (helminthiasis), which may lead to decreased intellectual and work performance and learning difficulties [6, 7]. Poor activity, mental, and educational performances among children that have strong relations with IDA may also continue into adulthood and cause low work efficiency which has effects on the economic productivity [3].

In the Middle East region, the reported prevalence of IDA in rural and urban people varies from 17 to 70% among preschool children; 12.6–50% among school children; 14–42% among adolescents; and 11% to more than 54% among pregnant women [3, 8, 9].

Yemen is one of the poorest countries in the Middle East. It has a very high population growth, severe urban-rural imbalances, food and water scarcity, female illiteracy, widespread poverty, and economic stagnation. According to UN agencies, about half of Yemen's population of about 26.8 million lives below the poverty line [10].

Previous studies have shown that the prevalence of IDA in Yemen varies between 73.5% and 81% among children and pregnant women, respectively [3, 11]. Most of the previous studies on anemia in Yemen were conducted on school children and pregnant women and their predictive factors. Yet there is no information about the prevalence and risks factors of IDA among Yemeni adolescents in educated communities at the university stage. Consequently, the current study aims to determine the prevalence and risk factors of IDA among apparently healthy Yemeni medical students at Hodeidah University, Yemen.

2. Methodology

2.1. Study Design. This a cross-sectional study designed to determine the prevalence among university students by analyzing blood samples to measure serum iron (SI), serum ferritin (SF), total iron binding capacity (TIBC), and complete blood pictures (CBC). Moreover, a questionnaire survey was conducted to participants to evaluate their health condition and lifestyle and social habits. The survey was conducted by Faculty of Medicine and Health Sciences, University of Hodeidah, between March and June 2017.

2.2. Study Subjects. The present study included 500 medical students randomly selected between the ages of 17 and 25 years and excluded female students with heavy and clotted menstrual cycle. The protocol of this study was approved by Faculty of Medicine and Health Sciences, University of Hodeida, Yemen. Questionnaires were administered randomly to each student to survey dietary drink habits, socioeconomic status, demographic information, and medical history (blood disorder). Participants were informed about the objectives of the study and experiments protocol.

2.3. Data and Samples Collections. The questionnaire was designed to collect demographic and socioeconomic information of the participants which includes household income (low < 50,000 YER; fair 50,000–200,000 YER; and good > 200,000 YER) and regular or irregular breakfast intake with tea or juice. The types of foods taken (fruits, vegetables, meat, fish, and chicken) were classified into the following: no, infrequently (<2 servings/week), and frequently (>2

servings/week); tea consumption: no, within or after meal, and frequently (>4 times/day); coffee and cola consumption (yes or no/week) after meal; fitness, khat (*Catha edulis*) chewing, and smoking habit defined as yes or no. Moreover, participants medical history included blood disorders or any type of anemia were classified as yes or no.

Five ml of venous blood was collected from each student and divided into two tubes and 2 ml was drawn into K3EDTA tubes to measure hematological parameters, whereas 3 ml was drawn into a plain tube with no anticoagulant to measure serum iron (SI), serum ferritin (SF), and total iron binding capacity (TIBC); biochemical tests were performed to samples with low Hb and MCV based on WHO guidelines [12] to confirm the diagnosis of IDA.

2.4. Hematological and Biochemical Parameters. Hemoglobin (Hb), red blood cell count (RBC), hematocrit (Hct), mean corpuscular volume (MCV), mean corpuscular hemoglobin (MCH), mean corpuscular hemoglobin concentration (MCHC), white blood cell count (WBC), red cell width distribution (RWD), and platelets were determined and measured using hematology analyzer Sysmex KX-21N.

Students with Hb levels lower than cut-off values were considered to be anemic if Hb < 13.0 g/dl, MCV < 76 fl, and RWD > 14.5% for male and Hb < 12.0 g/dl, MCV < 76 fl, and RWD > 14.5% for female.

SF (Omega Diagnostics), SI (QCA), and TIBC (QCA) were measured according to manufactured kit manual.

Students who had SF < 15 μg/L, Hb < 13 g/dl, SI < 10 μmol/L, and TIBC ≥ 68 μmol/L were defined as IDA.

2.5. Statistical Analysis. Statistical analysis of the data was achieved using Statistical Package for Social Sciences (SPSS) version 18. All quantitative variables were examined for normality by Shapiro-Wilks test before analysis. Continuous variables were presented as mean and standard deviations. We used independent sample t-test and one-way analysis of variance (ANOVA) to compare the mean and median proportions between IDA and nonanemic students for parameters such as SI, SF, TIBC, hemoglobin, and MCV. Differences between proportions were considered statistically significant if 95% CI did not overlap. In categorical variables, percentages and frequency counts were presented using cross-tabulation test. Pearson's chi-square test was used to investigate the association between the dependent variables (IDA) and the independent variables were grouped as socioeconomic information, dietary, drinks, and chewing khat habits of students.

3. Results

3.1. Prevalence of Anemia among Students. A total number of 500 blood samples were screened for anemia. Cross-tabulation was performed to describe the association between IDA and age, gender, foods and drink habits, household income, and social habits.

Table 1 shows the overall prevalence of IDA by age and gender; 30.4% students were found anemic, of whom 47.1%

TABLE 1: Levels of Hb, MCV, SF, SI, and TIBC parameters and prevalence of iron deficiency anemia among Yemeni University students according to age and gender.

Parameters	Nonanemic students				IDA students				p value
	Male	%	Female	%	Male	%	Female	%	
Gender	256	78.5	92	54.0	70	21.5	82	46.0	<0.001
Age by years									
17–19	12	4.7	24	26.1	10	14.3	28	34.1	
20–22	189	73.8	54	58.7	45	64.3	45	54.9	<0.001
23–25	55	21.5	14	15.2	15	21.4	09	11.0	
Hb (g/dL) Mean ± SD	14.41 ± 0.84		13.10 ± 0.60		12.00 ± 0.80		10.82 ± 0.63		<0.001
MCV (fL) Mean ± SD	87.80 ± 6.20		88.44 ± 4.00		72.40 ± 4.45		72.30 ± 3.45		<0.001
SF (ng/ml) Median IQR	41.00 (33.63, 48.90)		34.50 (33.05, 37.30)		5.35 (3.65, 8.00)		5.8 (4.41, 7.93)		<0.001
SI (μmol/L) Median IQR	31.95 (29.10, 33.03)		28.2 (25.03, 29.70)		11.20 (9.00, 12.00)		9.3 (8.10, 10.74)		<0.001
TIBC (μmol/L) Median IQR	59.65 (47.65, 70.20)		74.6 (52.70, 76.30)		108.1 (96.75, 113.95)		111.0 (102.1, 115.84)		<0.001

IDA = iron deficiency anemia; Hb = hemoglobin; MCV = mean corpuscular volume; SI = serum iron; SF = serum ferritin; SD = standard deviation; IQR = interquartile rang.

were female ($n = 82$) and 21.5% were male ($n = 70$). Also the higher prevalence of IDA (59.2%) was found among students aged 20–22 years compared to students aged 17–19 (25.0%) and 23–25 (15.8%) years which revealed that the prevalence of IDA was decreasing with increase of students' age. Similarly, in the case of nonanemic students, the older age group was found to be 69.8% in 20–22 years followed by other two age groups (17–19 years: 10.4%; 23–25 years: 19.8%). Moreover, the mean of hemoglobin level for IDA male and female students was found to be 12.00 g/dl (SD ± 0.80) and 10.82 g/dL (SD ± 0.63) with low statistically significant ($p < 0.001$) compared to nonanemic male (14.41 g/dl; SD ± 0.84) and nonanemic female students (13.10 g/dl; SD ± 0.60). Similarly, the median of SF, SI, and TIBC for IDA male and female students had low significantly level compared to nonanemic male and female students groups ($p < 0.001$).

Figure 1 illustrates that, out of 326 male students, 73.0% had hemoglobin levels in the range of 13–15 g/dL, 21.8% in the range of 10–12 g/dL, 0.9% in the range of 7–9 g/dL, and 4.3% in the range of 16–18 g/dL. However, 68.4% of female students had hemoglobin range 10–12 g/dL, 26.4% in the range of 13–15 g/dL, and 5.2% in the range of 7–9 g/dL. Also, it was found that no female students were found with hemoglobin range 16–18 g/dL.

3.2. Risk Factors Enhance the Prevalence of IDA Students.

Table 2 shows the association between IDA and different parameters: regular and irregular breakfast intake; dietary habits which include food (frequency intake of fruits, vegetables, meat, and fish); coffee and cocoa consumption directly after meal per week (yes or no); tea consumption (no and within and after meals, >4 caps/day); socioeconomic factors (family income, fitness, khat chewing, and smoking).

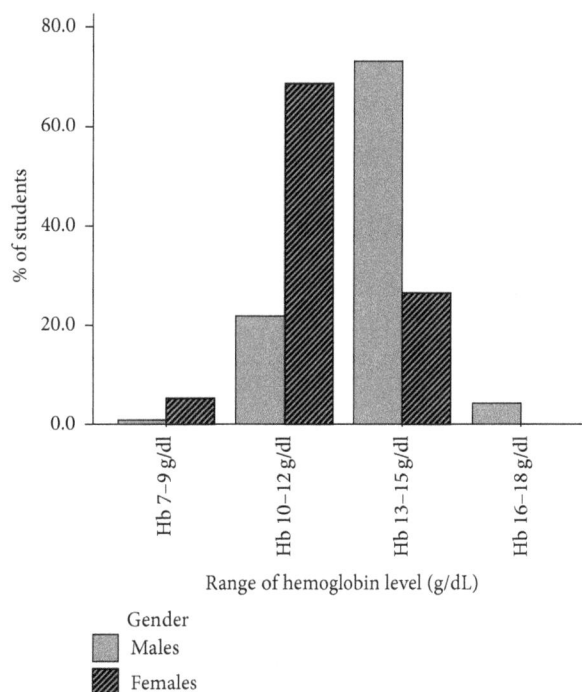

FIGURE 1: Percentage of hemoglobin concentrations for male and female students.

Depending on the analysis in the present study, an important relationship between IDA and breakfast, drinks, weekly intake of meat, vegetables, and fruits in students at university stage was demonstrated. It was found that students who had a regular breakfast intake (76.7%) or frequently consume fruits and vegetables (46.6%) and red meat (32.5%) per week

TABLE 2: Distribution of anemic (IDA) and nonanemic students according to risk factors (social habits).

Variables	Answers	Nonanemic students (n = 348)		IDA students (n = 152)		Chi-square value	p value
		Total	%	Total	%		
breakfast intake	Regular	267	76.7	62	40.8	60.705	<0.001
	Irregular (nonregular)	81	23.3	90	59.2		
Vegetables and Fruits/week	No	58	16.7	47	30.9	37.235	<0.001
	Infrequently (<2 times/week)	128	36.8	77	50.7		
	Frequently (>3 times/week)	162	46.6	28	18.4		
Eating red meat, fish, chicken/week	No	77	22.1	69	45.4	29.131	<0.001
	Infrequently (<2 times/week)	158	45.4	55	36.2		
	Frequently (>2 times/week)	113	32.5	28	18.4		
Drinking cocoa after meal/week	Yes	81	23.3	32	21.1	0.299	0.585
	No	267	76.7	120	78.9		
Drinking coffee after meal/week	Yes	139	39.9	56	36.8	0.427	0.513
	No	209	60.1	96	63.2		
Drinking tea/day	No	102	29.3	08	5.30	73.993	<0.001
	within every meal	104	29.9	27	17.8		
	after every meal	102	29.3	60	39.5		
	Yes >4 caps	40	11.5	57	37.5		
Family income	Very good (>200,000 YER)	180	51.7	29	19.1	74.779	<0.001
	Good (50,000–200,000 YER)	141	40.5	71	46.7		
	Low (<50,000 YER)	27	7.8	52	34.2		
Diet (fitness)	Yes	29	8.3	12	7.9	0.027	0.869
	No	319	91.7	140	92.1		
Showing khat (Catha edulis)	Yes	164	47.1	38	25.0	21.510	<0.001
	No	184	52.9	114	75.0		
Smoking	Yes	76	21.8	4	2.6	29.040	<0.001
	No	272	78.2	148	97.4		
Being aware of anemia	Yes	138	39.7	39	25.7	9.064	0.003
	No	210	60.3	113	74.3		

had a better iron status (nonanemic) than students who had irregular breakfast intake or insufficient portions of fruits and meat. Indeed, the prevalence of IDA was more significant among students who had irregular breakfast intake (59.2%); no (30.9%) or infrequent vegetables/fruits intake (50.7%); no (45.4%) or infrequent meat intake (36.2%) than nonanemic group who had irregular breakfast (23.3%), no (16.7%) or infrequent fruits intake (36.8%), and no (22.1%) or infrequent meat intake (45.4%). The present study further showed that students of families with low household monthly income < YER 50,000 (1 USD = 450 YER) had significant ($p < 0.001$) related factor which contributed to higher prevalence of IDA (34.2%) compared to their nonanemic counterparts (7.8%).

Moreover, the prevalence of IDA was significant among students who had regular tea daily intake > 4 caps/day (37.5%) and direct intake after meal (39.5%) compared to nonanemic group, 11.5% and 29.3%, respectively. Astonishingly, there was no statistically significant difference between IDA and non-IDA students with respect to drinking coffee or cola and fitness. Additionally, there were statistically significant differences among nonanemic (47.1%) (21.8%) compared to IDA students (25.0%) (2.6%), with respect to khat chewing and smoking. Regarding awareness and unawareness of anemia among the university students, among IDA students, it was found that high significantly proportion [74.3% (113/152); $p = 0.003$] of students were unaware and 25.7% (39/152) were aware about anemia whereas 60.3% (210/326) and 39.7% (138/326) of nonanemic students were unaware and aware about anemia, respectively.

4. Discussion

Iron deficiency anemia is the most nutritional anemia in developed countries and become a significant health burden in the world. Many studies have demonstrated the association of IDA with impaired cognitive performance and impaired work productivity in adults [13, 14]. Previous studies have been shown the prevalence of iron deficiency anemia (34.2%) among Yemeni children aged ≤ 15 years in rural areas [3]. The current study is considered the first study to demonstrate the prevalence and risk factors of IDA among medical university students in Hodeida province, Yemen. Our findings showed the prevalence of IDA among medical university students (30.4%), of whom (54.00%) were female (n = 82) and (46.00%) were male (n = 70), which agrees with previous WHO's report that estimated the prevalence of anemia among females at reproductive age was more than 50% [15].

Possible causes of the high prevalence rate of IDA among females population may include inadequate intake of dietary iron, poor bioavailability, a concurrent inadequate intake of dietary micronutrients, lack of awareness of iron deficiency, and nutritional status. Initially females are more prone to be anemic than males particularly at reproductive age because of menstruation and due to socioeconomic customs; they get a diet of lower quality compared to males [16, 17]. Moreover, the higher prevalence of anemia among females in our population could be contributed to the traditional cultural practices in some families in which they tend to give more priority and more rights to the males than females especially in food sharing.

A previous study on Bengali University students revealed that 55.3% of students were IDA, of whom 63.3% were female and 36.7% were male, with high significant difference (p < 0.001) [6]. Another study reported in India showed that the prevalence of IDA among medical students was found to be 32.0%, of whom 44.0% were females and 20.0% males [18]. In addition, the prevalence of IDA among university students was found to be 23.9% in Saudi Arabia, 29.0% in United Arab of Emirates, and 3.8% of IDA in Iran [19–21], while the prevalence of IDA in this study was found to be 30.4%.

The high prevalence of IDA among adolescents may due to increase necessity of iron for rapid growth, menarche, and low intake of iron-rich food. Moreover, inappropriate dietary choices and frequently consumption of tea, coffee and cola with meals are associated risk factors for anemia [22].

The highest prevalence of IDA among our population could be linked to poverty which resulted in insufficient nutrition and inadequate health care as well as educated states [3]. Besides sex and age, this study investigated some possible risk factors significantly associated with IDA among the participants students as follows: the low-income families, no or infrequent intake of breakfast, red meat, fish, chicken, vegetables, and fruits, and some lifestyle habits (drinking tea, chewing khat, and smoking), and unawareness about anemia and its causes.

In our current study, regular breakfast intake revealed statistically significant (p < 0.001) difference among IDA (40.8%) than nonanemic students (76.7%). Similarly, students who consume irregular breakfast intake were demonstrated to have a higher IDA (59.2%) than nonanemic group (23.3%). Healthy breakfast food that contains heme and non-heme iron such as fat, meat, proteins, bread, fiber, grains, pulses, legumes, fruits, vegetables, minerals, and vitamins especially vitamin C is necessary to provide energy and enhanced iron absorption [23]. Earlier study on Bengali students revealed that, among anemic students, 41.0% regularly and 59.0% irregularly had breakfast intake compared to 68.7% regular and 31.3% irregular breakfast intake of nonanemic students [6]. Missing breakfast meals among university students might be due to low household income, waking up late, not being hungry in the morning, dislike of served food, or cutting calories to lose weight as in females.

The frequent (46.6%), infrequent (36.8%), or no (16.7%) consumption of vegetables and fruits; frequent (32.5%), infrequent (45.4%), or no (22.1%) consumption of red meat, fish, or chicken of nonanemic students compared to the frequent (18.4%), infrequent (50.7%), or no (30.9%) consumption of vegetables and fruits; frequent (18.4%), infrequent (36.2%), or no (45.4%) consumption of red meat, fish, or chicken of IDA students was statistically significant different (p < 0.001). Previous studies on Bengali students and Saudi women have demonstrated that low consumption of meat, vegetables, or fruits is associated with IDA [6, 24].

On the one hand, the current study revealed statistically significant difference (p < 0.001) between nonanemic and IDA students based on tea consumption, which agrees with previous studies reporting that the intake of tea was significantly higher among anemic subjects [25, 26], while disagreeing with another study where no association was found between the anemic and nonanemic subjects with respect to tea consumption [27]. On the other hand, the current study revealed that there were no statistically significant differences found with regard to coffee or cola consumption, while a previous study reported coffee consumption as a factor in iron deficiency anemia among pregnant women [28]. Moreover, another study reported that cola consumption significantly increased the risk of anemia, but no association was found with respect to coffee consumption [29].

The harmful effect of tea, coffee, and cocoa on anemia may be justified as they contain polyphenols (tannins) that inhibit absorption of iron from intestine [25]. Additionally, our students are not aware of foods and drinks that contain high amount of inhibitors which have an influence on iron absorption. These inhibitors are found in phytates (bread, wheat bran, breakfast cereals, oats, and rice); tannins or polyphenols (tea, coffee, cocoa, and certain vegetables); calcium (milk and cheese); and phosphate [30].

Several studies had been conducted about the association of chewing khat and higher prevalence of anemia, which could be explained by the loss of appetite [31]. Besides, khat contains a substantial amount of tannin, which reduces the bioavailability of non-heme iron from the diet that is mainly based on foods of plant sources in the population [32, 33].

Currently chewing khat has become an epidemic over East Africa especially in Ethiopia, Somalia, and South Arabia from the old to young, male and female, urban and rural settings as well as in our country. Furthermore, chewing khat has become a common practice among high school, college, and university students [34]. The association of IDA with chewing khat that causes the loss of appetite and reduces iron absorption is well documented [31]; the authors reported that the subject who chewed khat every day had a 29% higher risk of anemia than those who did so occasionally or never [31]. By contrast, findings of the present study showed that the prevalence of IDA (25.0%) was significantly lower among students who were chewing khat every day compared to nonanemic students (47.1%). Our study suggests that chewing khat every day leads to the insufficient intestinal absorption of bioavailable iron and then smoking could increase hemoglobin levels among nonanemic students who are chewing khat and smoking. In general, this study is in agreement with studies reporting that chewing khat may lead to loss of appetite which may cause a general malnutrition resulting in IDA. Also, the habit of chewing khat reinforces the appearance and the development of other habits like cigarette smoking and consuming plenty of liquids (cola, black tea, coffee, and cold water).

Smoking habit has been found to be associated with a higher prevalence of IDA in many studies [35]. Although cigarettes smoking causes increase of hemoglobin and hematocrit levels which could be related to the effect of exposure to carbon monoxide which reduces oxygen tension and causes hypoxia in the body [36]. Hypoxia consequently increases production of erythrocytes from blood forming organs and elevates levels of hemoglobin and hematocrit, while serum ferritin may be low [37]. However, the effect of smoking on other iron indices is not clear [36]. In this study, it was found that 21.8% of nonanemic students were cigarette smokers compared to 2.6% of IDA, with statistically significant association ($p < 0.001$). This could be explained by the chewing khat coexisting with smoking among our population.

Findings of the present study further showed that students of families with household monthly income < YER 50,000 (1 USD = 450 YER) had significant ($p < 0.001$) related factor which contributed to higher prevalence of IDA (34.2%) compared to their nonanemic couterparts (7.8%). Recently, Yemen is classified among the lower middle income countries with >50% of the population lives below the poverty line and had a very low purchasing power [10]. Low family's income and poverty had been documented in many studies as important factors provoking the prevalence of IDA and resulting in low overall food intakes and poor diets with low micronutrient content [38]. In Iran, 30–50% of women and children, especially those in low-income families, are suffering from iron deficiency [39–41].

5. Conclusion

IDA is highly prevalent and considered as serious health problems among university students, in Hodeidah province, Yemen. Our findings showed that more than half of the female students were found to be IDA than males. Most of cases IDA were occurring due to the lack of healthy iron-rich foods in daily food, drinking tea, irregular intake of breakfast, low household monthly income, and chewing khat, all of those were identified as the significant risk factors increasing the prevalence of IDA among university students. To prevent the prevalence of IDA among students, a proper health education to increase knowledge about anemia and its causative factors, benefits of taking iron-rich food, and avoiding unhealthy food and drink intake is needed.

Conflicts of Interest

The authors declare that they have no conflicts of interest.

References

[1] F. Habibzadeh, "Anemia in the Middle East," *Lancet*, vol. 379, no. 1, 2012.

[2] M.-N. Khaskheli, S. Baloch, A. S. Baloch, S. Baloch, and F. K. Khaskheli, "Iron deficiency anaemia is still a major killer of pregnant women," *Pakistan Journal of Medical Sciences*, vol. 32, no. 3, pp. 630–634, 2016.

[3] E. M. Al-Zabedi, "Prevalence and Risk Factors of Iron Deficiency Anemia among Children in Yemen," *American Journal of Health Research*, vol. 2, no. 5, p. 319, 2014.

[4] *WHO/UNICEF/UNUIron deficiency anemia: assessment, prevention, and control*, World Health Organization, Geneva, 2001.

[5] M. Hashizume, O. Kunii, S. Sasaki et al., "Anemia and iron deficiency among schoolchildren in the Aral Sea Region, Kazakhstan," *Journal of Tropical Pediatrics*, vol. 49, no. 3, pp. 172–177, 2003.

[6] K. B. Shill, P. Karmakar, M. G. Kibria et al., "Prevalence of iron-deficiency anaemia among university students in Noakhali Region, Bangladesh," *Journal of Health, Population and Nutrition*, vol. 32, no. 1, pp. 103–110, 2014.

[7] F. A. Oski, "Iron deficiency in infancy and childhood," *The New England Journal of Medicine*, vol. 329, no. 3, pp. 190–193, 1993.

[8] K. Bagchi, "Iron deficiency anemia-an old enemy," *Eastern Mediterranean Health Journal*, vol. 10, pp. 754–760, 2004.

[9] A. O. Musaiger, "Iron deficiency anaemia among children and pregnant women in the arab gulf countries: The need for action," *Nutrition and Health*, vol. 16, no. 3, pp. 161–171, 2002.

[10] *World Development Indicators 2010*, The World Bank, Washington, DC, USA, 2014.

[11] A. S. Bin Braik and A. A. Bahaj, "Prevalence of and risk factors of anemia among pregnant women Mukalla - Hadhramout – Yemen," *Tikrit Journal of Pharmaceutical Sciences*, vol. 2, no. 1, 2006.

[12] WHO, *Hemoglobin concentrations for the diagnosis of anemia and assessment of severity. Vitamin and mineral nutrition information system*, World Health Organization, Geneva, Switzerland, 2011.

[13] R. J. Stoltzfus, "Iron deficiency: Global prevalence and consequences," *Food and Nutrition Bulletin*, vol. 24, no. 4, pp. S99–S103, 2003.

[14] S. More, V. B. Shivkumar, N. Gangane, and S. Shende, "Effects of iron deficiency on cognitive function in school going adolescent females in rural area of central India," *Anemia*, vol. 2013, Article ID 819136, 5 pages, 2013.

[15] WHO, *The prevalence of anemia in women: A tabulation of available information*, WHO/MCH/MSM/92.2 World Health Organization, 1992.

[16] P. Thankachan, S. Muthayya, T. Walczyk, A. V. Kurpad, and R. F. Hurrell, "An analysis of the etiology of anemia and iron deficiency in young women of low socioeconomic status in Bangalore, India," *Food and Nutrition Bulletin*, vol. 28, no. 3, pp. 328–336, 2007.

[17] N. Hwalla, A. Al Dhaheri, H. Radwan et al., "The Prevalence of Micronutrient Deficiencies and Inadequacies in the Middle East and Approaches to Interventions," *Nutrients*, vol. 9, no. 12, p. 229, 2017.

[18] R. Bano, N. Ahmad, BC. Sharma, and A. Agarwal, "Nutritional anemia in the medical students," in *Indian Medical Gazette*, vol. 1, pp. 16–18, 2012.

[19] F. Al-Sayes, S. Qusti, M. Gari, and M. Babaker, "Serum Transferrin Receptor Assay in Iron-Deficiency Anemia and Anemia of Chronic Diseases," *Journal of King Abdulaziz University-Medical Sciences*, vol. 18, no. 3, pp. 3–16, 2011.

[20] A. H. Sultan, "Anemia among female college students attending the University of Sharjah, UAE: prevalence and classification," *Journal of the Egyptian Public Health Association*, vol. 82, no. 3-4, pp. 261–271, 2007.

[21] S. Shams, H. Asheri, A. Kianmehr et al., "The prevalence of iron deficiency anaemia in female medical students in Tehran," *Singapore Medical Journal*, vol. 51, no. 2, pp. 116–119, 2010.

[22] A. A. Mohamed, A. A. A. Ali, N. I. Ali, E. H. Abusalama, M. I. Elbashir, and I. Adam, "Zinc, parity, infection, and severe anemia among pregnant women in Kassla, Eastern Sudan," *Biological Trace Element Research*, vol. 140, no. 3, pp. 284–290, 2011.

[23] C. G. Neumann, N. O. Bwibo, S. P. Murphy et al., "Animal Source Foods Improve Dietary Quality, Micronutrient Status, Growth and Cognitive Function in Kenyan School Children: Background, Study Design and Baseline Findings," *Journal of Nutrition*, vol. 133, no. 11, 2003.

[24] J. M. Al-Quaiz, "Iron deficiency anemia: a study of risk factors," *Saudi Medical Journal*, vol. 22, no. 6, pp. 490–496, 2001.

[25] S. Belgnaoui and B. Belahsen, "Anemia and Iron deficiency Anemia During Pregnancy in an Agricultural Region of Morocco : Effects of Dietary Intake and Iron Supplementation," *RJBS*, vol. 2, pp. 118–126, 2007.

[26] M. Nelson and J. Poulter, "Impact of tea drinking on iron status in the UK: A review," *Journal of Human Nutrition and Dietetics*, vol. 17, no. 1, pp. 43–54, 2004.

[27] A. M. Abdelhafez and S. S. El-Soadaa, "Prevalence and risk factors of anemia among a sample of pregnant females attending primary health care centers in Makkah, Saudi Arabia," *Pakistan Journal of Nutrition*, vol. 11, no. 12, pp. 1113–1120, 2012.

[28] L. M. Muñoz, B. Lönnerdal, C. L. Keen, and K. G. Dewey, "Coffee consumption as a factor in iron deficiency anemia among pregnant women and their infants in Costa Rica," *American Journal of Clinical Nutrition*, vol. 48, no. 3, pp. 645–651, 1988.

[29] A. Gad, J. Al-Quaiz, T. Khoja et al., "Anemia among primary school children (5-12 years) in Riyadh Region, Saudi Arabia: a community-based study," *Canadian Journal of Clinical Nutrition*, vol. 1, no. 1, pp. 27–34, 2013.

[30] M. Tseng, H. Chakraborty, D. T. Robinson, M. Mendez, and L. Kohlmeier, "Adjustment of iron intake for dietary enhancers and inhibitors in population studies: Bioavailable iron in rural

and urban residing Russian women and children," *Journal of Nutrition*, vol. 127, no. 8, pp. 1456–1468, 1997.

[31] H. Kedir, Y. Berhane, and A. Worku, "Khat chewing and restrictive dietary behaviors are associated with anemia among pregnant women in high prevalence rural communities in Eastern Ethiopia," *PLoS ONE*, vol. 8, no. 11, Article ID e78601, 2013.

[32] A. Al-Motarreb, M. Al-Habori, and K. J. Broadley, "Khat chewing, cardiovascular diseases and other internal medical problems: the current situation and directions for future research," *Journal of Ethnopharmacology*, vol. 132, no. 3, pp. 540–548, 2010.

[33] N. Wabe and M. Mohammed, "What science says about khat (Catha edulis Forsk)? Overview of chemistry, toxicology and pharmacology," *Journal of Experimental and Integrative Medicine*, vol. 2, no. 1, p. 29, 2012.

[34] A. Gashawa, "Tewodros Getachewb, (2014), The Chemistry of Khat and Adverse Effect of Khat Chewing," *American Scientific Research Journal for Engineering, Technology, and Sciences (ASRJETS)*, vol. 9, no. 1, pp. 35–46, 2014.

[35] C. Plante, *Carole Blanchet and Huguette Turgeon O'Brien 2004. iron Deficiency and anemia among Women in nunavik*, Institut national de santé publique du Québec Nunavik Regional Board of Health and Social Services, 2004.

[36] M. E. Cogswell, P. Weisberg, and C. Spong, "Cigarette smoking, alcohol use and adverse pregnancy outcomes: implications for micronutrient supplementation," *Journal of Nutrition*, vol. 133, no. 5, pp. 1722S–1731S, 2003.

[37] E. J. Van Liere and J. C. Stickney, "Effect of hypoxia on the blood," in *Hypoxia*, pp. 31–60, The University of Chicago Press, 1963.

[38] B. Thompson, "Food-based approaches for combating iron deficiency," in *Sight And Life, Basel*, Switzerland Michael B. Zimmermann Swiss Federal Institute of Technology, Zurich, Switzerland, 2007.

[39] M. R. Kadivar, H. Yarmohammadi, A. R. Mirahmadizadeh, M. Vakili, and M. Karimi, "Prevalence of iron deficiency anemia in 6 months to 5 years old children in Fars, Southern Iran," *Medical Science Monitor*, vol. 9, no. 2, pp. CR100–CR104, 2003.

[40] M. Karimi, R. Kadivar, and H. Yarmohammadi, "Assessment of the prevalence of iron deficiency anemia, by serum ferritin, in pregnant women of Southern Iran," *Medical Science Monitor*, vol. 8, no. 7, pp. CR488–CR492, 2002.

[41] M. Karimi, M. Mirzaei, and A. Dehghani, "Prevalence of anemia, iron deficiency and iron deficiency anemia in 6-60 month old children in Yazd's rural area," *International Pediatrics*, vol. 19, no. 3, pp. 180–184, 2004.

Permissions

List of Contributors

Iftikhar Hussain and Jessica Bhoyroo
Vital Prospects Clinical Research Institute, PC, Tulsa, OK 74136, USA

Angelia Butcher, Todd A. Koch and Andy He
Luitpold Pharmaceuticals, Inc., Norristown, PA 19403, USA

David B. Bregman
Department of Pathology, Albert Einstein College of Medicine, Bronx, NY 10461, USA
Luitpold Pharmaceuticals, Inc., Norristown, PA 19403, USA

Jose E. Dutra-de-Oliveira and J. Sergio Marchini
Department of Internal Medicine, Ribeirão Preto School of Medicine, University of São Paulo, Av Bandeirantes 3900, 14049-900 Ribeirao Preto, SP, Brazil

Joel Lamounier
Department of Pediatrics, Medical School Belo Horizonte, Av Professor Alfredo Balena 190, 30130-100 Belo Horizonte, MG, Brazil

Carlos A. N. Almeida
Department of Pediatrics, Ribeirão Preto School of Medicine, University of São Paulo, Av Costábile Romano 2201, 14096-900 Ribeirao Preto, SP, Brazil

Abu Syed Mohammed Mujib, Abu Sayeed Mohammad Mahmud and Milton Halder
Industrial Microbiology Research Division, Bangladesh Council of Scientific and Industrial Research, Chittagong 4220, Bangladesh

Chowdhury Mohammad Monirul Hasan
Department of Biochemistry and Molecular Biology, University of Chittagong, Chittagong 4331, Bangladesh

Mauricio López-Sierra, Susana Calderón and Lilian Pilleux
Hematology Unit, Institute of Medicine, Faculty of Medicine, Universidad Austral de Chile, Bueras 1003 CP 5090000 Valdivia, Chile

Jorge Gómez
Institute of Public Health, Faculty of Medicine, Universidad Austral de Chile, Valdivia, Chile

Todd A. Koch
Luitpold Pharmaceuticals, Inc., Norristown, PA 19403, USA

Jennifer Myers
St. John's University, Jamaica, NY 11439, USA

Lawrence Tim Goodnough
Department of Pathology and Medicine (Hematology), Stanford, CA 94305, USA

Sheetal Patel and Ayesha Khalid
Department of Internal Medicine, New York Methodist Hospital, 506 Sixth Street, Brooklyn, NY 11215, USA

Seyed Monemian
Division of Hematology-Oncology, Department of Internal Medicine, New York Methodist Hospital, 506 Sixth Street, Brooklyn, NY 11215, USA

Harvey Dosik
Division of Hematology, Department of Internal Medicine, New YorkMethodist Hospital, 506 Sixth Street, Brooklyn, NY 11215, USA
Weill Cornell Medical College of Cornell University, 1300 York Avenue, New York, NY 10065, USA

Sarika More
Department of Pathology, Sri Lakshmi Narayana Institute of Medical Sciences, Osudu, Kudapakkam Post, Villanur Communie, Pondicherry 605502, India

V. B. Shivkumar and Nitin Gangane
Department of Pathology, Mahatma Gandhi Institute of Medical Sciences, Sevagram, Maharashtra, India

Sumeet Shende
Department of Forensic Medicine, Sri Lakshmi Narayana Institute of Medical Sciences, Pondicherry 605502, India

Maria Georgieva Angelova and Atanaska Naumova Bozhinova
Department of Chemistry and Biochemistry & Physics and Biophysics, University of Medicine-Pleven, 1 Kliment Ohridski Street, 5800 Pleven, Bulgaria

Vania Nedkova Nedkova-Kolarova and Tsvetelina Valentinova Petkova-Marinova
Department of Pediatrics, University of Medicine-Pleven, 1 Kliment Ohridski Street, 5800 Pleven, Bulgaria

Maksym Vladimirovich Pogorielov
Department of Hygiene and Ecology, Sumy State University, Medical Institute, 31 Sanatornaya Street, Sumy 40007, Ukraine

Andrii Nikolaevich Loboda
Department of Pediatrics with Medical Genetics, Sumy State University, Medical Institute, 31 Sanatornaya Street, Sumy 40007, Ukraine

Eugenia Prus and Eitan Fibach
Department of Hematology, Hadassah-Hebrew University Medical Center, Ein-Kerem, Jerusalem 91120, Israel

Fatih Akin, Ece Selma Solak, Cengizhan Kilicaslan and Saltuk Bugra Boke
Department of Pediatrics, Konya Training and Research Hospital, Meram, 42090 Konya, Turkey

Sukru Arslan
Department of Pediatric Nephrology, Konya Training and Research Hospital, 42090 Konya, Turkey

Charles F. Barish
Wake Gastroenterology and Wake Research Associates, Raleigh, NC 27612, USA

Todd Koch and Angelia Butcher
Luitpold Pharmaceuticals, Inc., Norristown, PA 19403, USA

David Morris
Webb Writes, LLC, Durham, NC 27705, USA

David B. Bregman
Department of Pathology, Albert Einstein College of Medicine, NY 10461, USA
Luitpold Pharmaceuticals, Inc., Norristown, PA 19403, USA

Ashok Bhardwaj, Dinesh Kumar, Sunil Kumar Raina, Pardeep Bansal and Vishav Chander
Department of Community Medicine, Dr. Rajendra Prasad Government Medical College, Kangra, Himachal Pradesh 176001, India

Satya Bhushan
Department of Biochemistry, Dr. Rajendra Prasad Government Medical College, Kangra, Himachal Pradesh 176001, India

Eloísa Urrechaga
Hematology Laboratory, Hospital Galdakao—Usansolo, Galdakao, 48960 Vizcaya, Spain

Luís Borque and Jesús F. Escanero
Department of Pharmacology and Physiology, Faculty of Medicine, University of Zaragoza, Zaragoza, Spain

Julia G. Shaw
Public Health Program, Division of Biology and Medicine, Brown University, Providence, RI 02912, USA

Lifespan Hospital Center for International Health Research, 55 Claverick Street, Suite 100, Providence, RI 02903, USA

Jennifer F. Friedman
Warren Alpert School of Medicine, Brown University, Providence, RI 02912, USA
Lifespan Hospital Center for International Health Research, 55 Claverick Street, Suite 100, Providence, RI 02903, USA

Betelihem Terefe
Department of Hematology and Immunohematology, University of Gondar, Gondar, Ethiopia

Asaye Birhanu and Aster Tsegaye
School of Medical Laboratory Science, Addis Ababa University, Addis Ababa, Ethiopia

Paulos Nigussie
Ethiopian Health and Nutrition Research Institute (EHNRI), Addis Ababa, Ethiopia

María Nieves García-Casal, Rafael Puche, Irene Leets, Zoila Carvajal and Carlos Ibarra
Laboratorio de Fisiopatología, Centro de Medicina Experimental, Instituto Venezolano de Investigaciones Científicas (IVIC), Caracas 1020-A, Venezuela

Maritza Landaeta-Jiménez and Elijú Patiño
Fundación Bengoa para la Salud y Nutrición, 8va Transversal con 7ma Avenida, Quinta Pacairigua, Altamira, Caracas 1050, Venezuela

Asa V. Thorisdottir and Inga Thorsdottir
Unit for Nutrition Research, Landspitali-The National University Hospital of Iceland, Eir´ıksgata 29, 101 Reykjavik, Iceland
Faculty of Food Science and Nutrition, University of Iceland, 101 Reykjavik, Iceland

Gestur I. Palsson
Children's Hospital, Landspitali-The National University Hospital of Iceland, 101 Reykjavik, Iceland

Mirza Sultan Ahmad, Hadia Farooq, Sumaira Noor Maham, Zonaira Qayyum, Abdul Waheed and Waqar Nasir
Fazle Omar Hospital Rabwah, Chenab Nagar, Pakistan

António Robalo Nunes
Hospital de Dia de Imuno-Hemoterapia, Hospital Pulido Valente, Centro Hospitalar Lisboa Norte (CHLN), Alameda das Linhas de Torres 117, 1769-001 Lisboa, Portugal

Ana Palricas Costa, Sara Lemos Rocha and Ana Garcia de Oliveira
Hospital de Dia de Imuno-Hemoterapia, Hospital de Santa Maria, CHLN, Avenida Prof. Egas Moniz, 1649-035 Lisboa, Portugal

Huguette Turgeon O'Brien
School of Nutrition, Laval University, 2425 rue de l'Agriculture, Qu'ebec City, QC, Canada G1V 0A6

Rosanne Blanchet
Interdisciplinary School of Health Sciences, University of Ottawa, 35 University Private THN140, Ottawa, ON, Canada K1N 6N5

Doris Gagné
Nutrition DG, 1187 rue du Saint-Brieux, Qu'ebec City, QC, Canada G1Y 2B9

Julie Lauzière
Department of Family Medicine and Emergency Medicine, University of Sherbrooke, 150 place Charles-Le Moyne, Longueuil, QC, Canada J4K 0A8

Carole Vézina
Inuulitsivik Health and Social Services Centre, Puvirnituq, QC, Canada J0M 1P0

Emilia Parodi
Pediatric and Neonatology Unit, Ordine Mauriziano Hospital, Largo Turati 62, 10128 Turin, Italy

Maria Teresa Giraudo
Department of Mathematics "G. Peano", University of Turin, Via Carlo Alberto 10, 10123 Turin, Italy

Fulvio Ricceri
Unit of Epidemiology, Regional Health Service ASL TO3, Via Sabaudia 164, Grugliasco, 10095 Turin, Italy

Ugo Ramenghi and Maria Luigia Aurucci
HematologyUnit, Department of Sciences of Public Health and Pediatrics, University of Turin, Piazza Polonia 94, 10126 Turin, Italy

Raffaela Mazzone
Hematology and Coagulation Laboratory, Città della Scienza e della Salute Hospital, Piazza Polonia 94, 10126 Turin, Italy

Penpe Gul Firat
Associate Professor, Inonu University School of Medicine, Department of Ophthalmology, Malatya, Turkey

Ersan Ersin Demirel
MD, Sarkısla State Hospital, Department of Ophthalmology, Sivas, Turkey

Seyhan Dikci
Assistant Professor, Inonu University School of Medicine, Department of Ophthalmology, Malatya, Turkey

Irfan Kuku
Professor, Inonu University School of Medicine, Department of Hematology, Malatya, Turkey

Oguzhan Genc
MD, Mujde Hospital, Department of Ophthalmology, Malatya, Turkey

Samah S. Aqel and Khalid R. Younis
Department of Medical Laboratory Sciences, Faculty of Health Professions, Al-Quds University, East Jerusalem, State of Palestine

Mahmoud A. Srour
Department of Biology & Biochemistry, Birzeit University, Birzeit, State of Palestine
Department of Medical Laboratory Sciences, Faculty of Health Professions, Al-Quds University, East Jerusalem, State of Palestine

Khaled M. Srour
Anatomy and Physiology Department, Faculty of Medicine, Al-Quds University, East Jerusalem, State of Palestine

Fekri Samarah
Department of Medical Laboratory Sciences, Arab-American University, Jenin, State of Palestine

Ari Indra Susanti
Program Study of Midwifery, Division of Maternal and Child Health, Department of Public Health, Faculty of Medicine, Universitas Padjadjaran, Bandung, Indonesia

Edhyana Sahiratmadja and Ramdan Panigoro
Department of Biochemistry and Molecular Biology, Faculty of Medicine, Universitas Padjadjaran, Bandung, Indonesia

Gatot Winarno and Herman Susanto
Department of Obstetrics and Gynecology, Faculty of Medicine, Universitas Padjadjaran and Dr. Hasan Sadikin General Hospital, Bandung, Indonesia

Adhi Kristianto Sugianli
Department of Clinical Pathology, Faculty of Medicine, Universitas Padjadjaran and Dr. Hasan Sadikin General Hospital, Bandung, Indonesia

Melvin H. Seid
UnifiedWomen's Clinical Research, 1100-C South Stratford Road, Suite 310, Winston-Salem, NC 27103, USA

Angelia D. Butcher
Luitpold Pharmaceuticals, Inc., 800 Adams Ave, Suite 100, Norrisville, PA 19403, USA

Ashwin Chatwani
Department of Obstetrics and Gynecology, Temple University School of Medicine, Philadelphia, PA 19140, USA

Abdullah Ahmed Al-alimi, Salem Bashanfer and Mohammed Abdo Morish
Department of Medical Laboratory, Faculty of Medicine and Health Sciences, Hodeida University, Al Hudaydah, Yemen

Index

www.ingramcontent.com/pod-product-compliance
Lightning Source LLC
Chambersburg PA
CBHW050454200326
41458CB00014B/5179